Preoperative Events

Their Effects on Behavior
Following Brain Damage

COMPARATIVE COGNITION
AND NEUROSCIENCE

Thomas G. Bever, David S. Olton,
and Herbert L. Roitblat, Senior Editors

Preoperative Events

Their Effects on Behavior Following Brain Damage

Edited by

Jay Schulkin
University of Pennsylvania

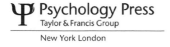
Psychology Press
Taylor & Francis Group

New York London

First Published by
Lawrence Erlbaum Associates, Inc., Publishers
10 Industrial Avenue
Mahwah, New Jersey 07430

Transferred to Digital Printing 2009 by Psychology Press
270 Madison Ave, New York NY 10016
27 Church Road, Hove, East Sussex, BN3 2FA

Design by Jodi Forlizzi, Inks Inc.

Library of Congress Cataloging-in-Publication Data

Preoperative events : their effects on behavior following brain damage
  / edited by Jay Schulkin.
       p.   cm.
    Includes bibliographies and index.
    ISBN 0-8058-0021-2. — ISBN 0-8058-0535-4 (pbk.)
    1. Brain damage—Surgery—Complications and sequelae—Prevention.
  2. Brain damage—Animal models.   3. Habituation (Neuropsychology)
  4. Preoperative care—Physiological aspects.   I. Schulkin, Jay.
    [DNLM: 1. Behavior—physiology.   2. Brain—surgery.   3. Brain
  Injuries—complications.   4. Brain Injuries—rehabilitation.
  5. Postoperative Complications—prevention & control.
  6. Preoperative Care.   WL 354 P927]
  RD594.P65   1989
  617'.481—dc19
  DNLM/DLC   89-1622
  for Library of Congress   CIP

Publisher's Note
The publisher has gone to great lengths to ensure the quality of this reprint
but points out that some imperfections in the original may be apparent.

Contents

List of Contributors

DAVID J. ALBERT, Department of Psychology, University of British Columbia.

J. JAY BRAUN, Department of Psychology, Arizona State University.

RICHARD G. BURRIGHT, Department of Psychology, State University of New York at Binghampton.

G. LINCOLN CHEW, Department of Psychology, Lethbridge University.

PETER J. DONOVICK, Department of Psychology, State University of New York at Binghampton.

PAUL FEDIO, Clinical Neuropsychology Section, Medical Neurology Branch, National Institute for Neurological Disorders and Stroke, National Institutes of Health.

JORDAN GRAFMAN, Cognitive Neuroscience Unit, Medical Neurology Branch, National Institute of Neurological Disorders and Stroke, National Institutes of Health.

CARLOS V. GRIJALVA, Department of Psychology, Brain Research Institute, University of California, Los Angeles.

ERNEST D. KEMBLE, Division of Social Sciences, University of Minnesota, Morris.

BRYAN KOLB, Department of Psychology, University of Lethbridge, Canada.

E. E. KRIECKHAUS, Department of Psychology, University of Massachusetts, Amherst.

FRANCOIS LALONDE, Cognitive Neuroscience Unit, Medical Neurology Branch, National Institute for Neurological Disorders and Stroke, National Institutes of Health.

FRANCO LEPORE, Groupe de Recherche en Neuropsychologie Experimentale, Université de Montréal.

ERNEST LINDHOLM, Department of Psychology, Arizona State University.

IRENE LITVAN, Experimental Therapeutics Branch, National Institute for Neurological Disorders and Stroke, National Institutes of Health.

ALICJA L. MARKOWSKA, Department of Neuropsychology, Nencki Institute of Experimental Biology, Warsaw, Poland.

DAVID S. OLTON, Department of Psychology, Johns Hopkins University.

J. BRUCE OVERMIER, Department of Psychology, University of Minnesota, Minneapolis.

BARBARA ROLAND, Department of Psychology, University of California, Los Angeles.

TIMOTHY SCHALLERT, Department of Psychology, University of Texas, Austin.

JAY SCHULKIN, Department of Anatomy and Institute of Neurological Sciences, University of Pennsylvania.

DEVENDRA SINGH, Department of Psychology, University of Texas, Austin.

ELIOT STELLAR, Department of Anatomy and Institute of Neurological Sciences, University of Pennsylvania.

MIKE L. WALSH, Department of Kinesiology, Simon Fraser University.

JEANNETTE P. WARD, Department of Psychology, Memphis State University.

Preface

This book is filled with essays on the subject of Behavioral Neuroscience: specifically the role of preoperative experiences on the behavioral consequences that result from brain damage. The field of recovery from brain damage has focused to a large extent on the postoperative rehabilitation and competence of the brain-damaged subject, and to a much less extent on the sometimes crucial role of preoperative experience. This book is the first to assemble exclusively a set of essays on the relationship of preoperative experience and postoperative performance. I hope the readers will benefit by our labors.

My own research in this field has its roots in the laboratory of my teacher, George Wolf. This was where I had my first scientific idea. The idea was simple. Since it had been discovered that rats exposed to the taste of salt preoperatively were protected against impairments in the behavioral regulation of salt hunger following damage to the central gustatory system, I thought that the hunger for salt preoperatively might protect the lateral hypothalamic-damaged animal against similar behavioral deficits. And we found just that.

I would like to thank my friends and colleagues for their help. In particular I would like to thank my colleagues at the University of Pennsylvania: Alan Epstein, Steve Fluharty, Paul Rozin, John Sabini, and Eliot Stellar. I also thank my friends and my parents for their encouragement.

The book is dedicated to my first two students: Ron Paulus and Andy Hartzell.

Jay Schulkin

Introduction

The neuroscientific literature contains the observation that one subject will show impairments following brain damage, whereas another will not (e.g., Finger & Stein, 1982; Hebb, 1949). For example, one subject (in this case a rat) is unable to regulate body sodium behaviorally following damage to the hypothalamus, whereas another subject retains this ability (Schulkin & Fluharty, 1985). Why? One part of the answer is that the subject's history plays an important role in determining whether it will be impaired by a brain lesion; another important factor of course is the location of the lesion, but for present purposes we are interested in those cases where the lesion is substantially the same but the postoperative effects are different.

Those subjects who fail to show the expected behavioral impairments following brain trauma are said to be "protected." By protection, I mean specifically that as a result of preoperative experience behavioral competence is retained (spared) following brain damage. This phenomenon is of general importance in understanding the differential effects of similar brain damage on behavior. It may also have clinical relevance in suggesting preoperative manipulations that may reduce deficits that result from neurosurgery.

Several striking facts regarding the effects of brain damage on behavior are evident in the divergent and confusing neuroscience literature. In one paradigm, animals retain what they acquired preoperatively, but are unable to acquire new relevant behaviors postoperatively (e.g., Schwartz & Teitelbaum, 1974). In another case, they lose what they acquired preoperatively, but they can acquire it again (e.g., Lashley, 1921). In a third case, they can neither retain the preoperative event, nor learn about new events (Morgan, 1951).

The research presented in this volume covers these three possibilities. But it is the first possibility that represents what is essentially meant by protection. What evidence there is of protective effects is dispersed throughout a diffuse array of research, and only on rare occasions has it been studied directly. Some of these rare occasions are assembled in this book.

A number of regularities should be enumerated. At the outset, note that where one does find protective effects they tend to be limited to the preoperative context. Behavioral responses in new contexts are often not protected (e.g., Held, Gordon, & Gentile, 1985; Marcotte & Ward, 1980). Another fact that stands out is that the more difficult the task, the less likely the animal will be protected (e.g., Mishkin, 1954). In addition, overtraining, rather than simply preoperative training, is at times required to produce protection (e.g., Orbach & Fantz, 1958). The results in several contexts also suggest that an impoverishment of preoperative experiences may contribute significantly to some of the lesion-induced behavioral impairments (e.g., Donovick, Burright, & Bengelloun, 1979; Hughes, 1965). Finally, the more complete the brain damage to a critical brain region the less likely one will see any protective effects (Geschwind, 1965, 1974; Powley & Keesey, 1970; Schallert, 1982; chap. 8).

Thus consider the following empirical generalizations that should orient the reader in reading the chapters that follow:

1. Protective effects following lesions tend to be highly specific for the task learned or experienced preoperatively and these protective effects depend on the parts of the brain that are damaged (chaps. 2, 7, and 11).

2. Preoperative overtraining, and not just preoperative training, is sometimes required for protection (chap. 11), although in some cases it can actually decrease or have no effect on postoperative performance (chaps. 12 and 13).

3. The degree of preoperative experience correlates with the range of protective effects. Therefore, an impoverishment of preoperative experiences may contribute significantly to the extent of the deficits (chaps. 1, 4, and 6; though also read, Dalrymple–Alford & Kelche, 1985).

4. The more difficult the task, the less likely it is that the animal will be protected.

5. The more complete the brain damage, and the greater the dependence on the brain region in executing the behavior, the less is the likelihood of any protection (chaps. 2, 8, 9, and 10).

6. Interoperative experiences can facilitate protection in animals with serial stage lesions (chap. 12).

7. This general line of research may have clinical relevance. The research suggests that specific preoperative training procedures might be used to lessen the severity of behavioral deficits following neurosurgery, and that

predamage experiences are relevant factors in the diagnosis of brain-damaged patients (chaps. 6, 14).

The book is conceptually divided into two sections. The first seven chapters have to do with regulatory or appetitive behavior. The next seven chapters have more to do with the learning of tasks. The range of inquiry is from fish to humans, from cortex to hypothalamus, from escape behavior to space perception. In some contexts there are protective effects from the preoperative experiences; in other cases there are not. And not all the authors are in agreement. This book is an invitation to think further on these issues and what they may be telling us about brain function.

Jay Schulkin

REFERENCES

Dalrymple–Alford, J. C., & Kelche, C. R. (1985). Behavioural effects of preoperative and postoperative differential housing in rats with brain lesions: A review. In Will, P. E., Schmit, P., & Dalrymple–Alford, J. C. (Eds.), *Brain plasticity, learning and memory.* New York: Plenum Press.

Donovick, P. J., Burright, R. G., & Bengelloun, W. A. (1979). The septal region and behavior: An example of the importance of genetic and experimental factors in determining effects of brain damage. *Neuroscience and Biobehavioral Reviews, 3,* 83–96.

Finger, S., & Stein, D. J. (1982). Environmental and experiential determinants of recovery of function. In *Brain damage and recovery,* New York: Academic Press.

Geschwind, N. (1965). Disconnexion syndromes in animals and man. In *Selected papers on language and the brain,* 1975. Boston: D. Reidel.

Geschwind, N. (1974). Late changes in the nervous system: An overview. In Stein, D. J., Rosen, J. F., & Butters, N. (Eds.), *Plasticity and recovery of function in the central nervous system.* New York: Academic Press.

Hebb, D. O. (1949). *The organization of behavior.* New York: Wiley.

Held, J. M., Gordon, J., & Gentile, A. M. (1985). Environmental influences on locomotor recovery following cortical lesions in rats. *Behavioral Neuroscience, 99,* 678–690.

Hughes, K. R. (1965). Dorsal and ventral hippocampus lesions and maze learning: Influence of preoperative environment. *Canadian Journal of Psychology, 19,* 325–332.

Lashley, K. S. (1921). Studies of cerebral function in learning. 11. The effects of long continued practice upon cerebral localization. *Journal of Comparative Psychology, 1,* 453–468.

Marcotte, R. R., & Ward, J. P. (1980). Preoperative overtraining protects against form learning deficits after lateral occipital lesions in Galago senagalensis. *Journal of Comparative and Physiological Psychology, 94,* 305–312.

Mishkin, M. (1954). Visual discrimination performance following partial ablations of the temporal lobe, 11. Ventral surface vs. hippocampus. *Journal of Comparative and Physiological Psychology, 47,* 187–193.

Morgan, C. T. (1951). The psychology of learning. In Stevens (Ed.), *Handbook of experimental psychology.* New York: Wiley, pp. 758–788.

Orbach, J., & Fantz, R. L. (1958). Differential effects of temporal neo-cortical resections on overtrained and non-overtrained visual habits in monkeys. *Journal of Comparative and Physiological Psychology, 51,* 126–129.

Powley, T. L., & Keesey, R. E. (1970). Relationship of body weight to the lateral hypothalamic feeding syndrome. *Journal of Comparative and Physiological Psychology, 70,* 25–36.

Schallert, T. (1982). Adipsia produced by lateral hypothalamic lesions: Facilitation of recovery by preoperative restriction of water intake. *Journal of Comparative and Physiological Psychology, 96,* 604–614.

Schulkin, J., & Fluharty, S. J. (1985). Further studies on salt appetite following lateral hypothalamic lesions: Effects of preoperative alimentary experiences. *Behavioral Neuroscience, 99,* 929–935.

Schwartz, M., & Teitelbaum, P. (1974). Disassociation between learning and remembering in rats with lesions in the lateral hypothalamus. *Journal of Comparative and Physiological Psychology, 87,* 384–398.

1

Preoperative Intermittent Feeding or Drinking Regimens Enhance Postlesion Sensorimotor Function

Timothy Schallert
Department of Psychology
University of Texas, Austin

A study of recovery of function can proceed more successfully with a thorough understanding of the preinjury condition of the organism being examined. In diagnostic neurology and neuropsychology, detailed patient histories can be of tremendous value. Though normative data are available, it is obvious that the effects of brain damage and prognosis can be determined more reliably with an accurate record of an individual's behavior prior to the damage. Although little is known about the variables that affect the level of posttraumatic function in people, potentially at least, past experience may be quite influential and, under certain circumstances, beneficial.

In animal models of brain damage, manipulation of preoperative experience can enhance postoperative outcome or the rate of recovery of ingestive and sensorimotor functions. Many of these effects have been reviewed in the present volume and elsewhere (Donovick, Burright, & Swidler, 1973; Finger & Stein, 1982; Gentile, Beheshita, & Held, 1987; Greenough, Fass, & DeVoogd, 1976; Grijalva & Lindholm, 1980; Hughes, 1965; Schallert, 1982; Schallert & Whishaw, 1978). A particularly thorough, cogent, and still-relevant overview of earlier experiments and ideas was written by Greenough et al. (1976).

Among the most dramatic and consistent transoperative effects involves the manipulation of ingestive behavior prior to brain damage. Preoperative regimens of restricted daily feeding reduce or prevent the period of deficient eating behavior that otherwise occurs following small lateral hypothalamic (LH) lesions (Grijalva & Lindholm, 1980; Grijalva, Lindholm, Schallert, & Bicknell, 1976; Powley & Keesey, 1970; Schallert & Whishaw, 1978; Fig. 1.1) or orbital frontal cortex damage (Glick & Greenstein, 1972; Kolb, Whishaw, & Schallert, 1977). The most established view of these data has been that the brain damage

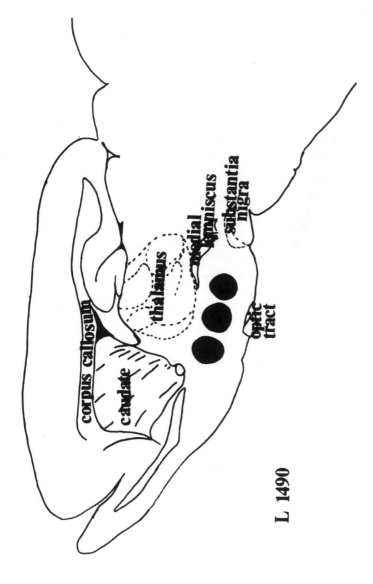

L 1490

FIG. 1.1. Parasaggital representation of three different lateral hypothalamic areas damaged in Schallert and Whishaw (1978). Lesions that included the more posterior area yielded a passive type of aphagia and sensory neglect. Lesions that included the more anterior area yielded an active type of aphagia and rejection reactions to many forms of sensory stimulation. Intermediate lesions yielded a mixed group of symptoms. A preoperative regimen of restricted daily feeding attenuated both types of impairment postoperatively. Brain section is 1.49 mm lateral to midline. Drawing adapted from König & Klippel, 1970.

lowers the set point for weight regulation and that the preoperative reduction of food intake simply brings the body weight nearer to the level chronically maintained by the animal after surgery (Keesey et al., 1976; Powley & Keesey, 1970; see Grijalva, Lindholm, & Roland, chap. 3 in this volume, for a more thorough discussion of the set point hypothesis). Consistent with this hypothesis, preoperative fattening prolongs the period of aphagia and enhances food-rejection behaviors (Kolb et al., 1977; Schallert & Whishaw, 1978, Fig. 1.2).

The set point explanation has been useful, but may not by itself sufficiently account for these effects (Grijalva et al., 1976; Kolb et al., 1977; Schallert, 1982; Schallert & Whishaw, 1978; Grijalva, this volume). For example, as we will discuss in a later section, preoperative weight manipulations do not affect food intake specifically. A variety of postoperative outcomes are influenced, including sensorimotor, thermoregulatory, and autonomic functions. In addition, a preoperative regimen of restricted daily watering reduces or prevents the period of adipsia that follows LH lesions. The *method* of water restriction was critical. Total water deprivation was not effective. Indeed, the animals did not have to be in a state of hydrational deficit at the time of surgery. Like the restricted feeding regimens, the drinking regimens also can greatly attenuate or

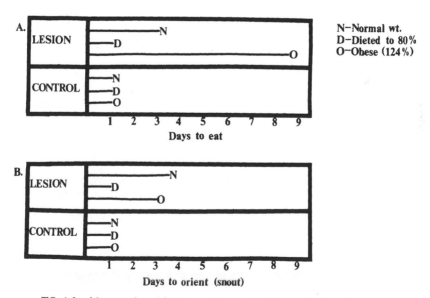

FIG. 1.2. Mean number of days to eat (A), or to orient to perioral stimulation with a von Frey hair (B), after bilateral lateral hypothalamic lesions or sham operations in rats subjected preoperatively to one of three conditions: D = dieted to 80% of normal via a 17-day restricted daily feeding regimen; O = obese, 124% of normal weight via a 17-day cafeteria-style "junk-food" diet; N = *ad libitum* feeding of standard lab chow. After Schallert and Whishaw, 1978.

abolish certain types of sensorimotor abnormalities (Schallert, 1982; Schallert & Whishaw, 1978; see also Fig. 1.2). Thus the set point type of explanation appears to be too limited (White, 1986).

VIEWS OF PREOPERATIVE
EFFECTS

Although the effects are well established, the means by which the preoperative manipulations work remain a puzzle. Insights about possible mechanisms might come from studying both pre- and postoperative factors that can influence recovery and maintenance of function. The present chapter, reflecting this approach, considers three ways to view some of these preoperative effects and introduces data that bear on these views.

1. *Interaction with recovery processes.* The preoperative events may truly interact with adaptations specifically involved in recovery. That is, postoperative mechanisms may be sensitized by the preoperative experience, or new ones may be created that linger long enough into the postoperative period to speed up or expand capacity for plasticity. Included would be mechanisms that facilitate restoration not only of local function but also of tissue remote from the damage that has become deactivated as a consequence of its interconnections with the damaged tissue.

2. *Improvement of baseline behavior.* There may be changes observable in the preoperative period that simply carry over to the postoperative period to improve behavior equally in operated and unoperated populations. In other words, baseline behavior may be altered, perhaps via conditioning mechanisms, or performance may become flexible in general and thereby more resistant to disruption.

3. *Tameness and testing familiarization.* Conditions may be introduced by the preoperative experience that permit the behavioral expression of recovery processes in the brain-damaged animal that otherwise are masked by the testing situation; specifically, via promotion of tameness or extension of the range of environmental familiarity conducive to successful behavior.

These viewpoints, which were developed in part through the influence of earlier papers on the topic (e.g., Finger & Stein, 1982: Greenough et al., 1976), should be treated as suggested frameworks for organizing some of the behavioral research. They are not meant to incorporate all preoperative effects nor explain any one effect completely, and one does not exclude another. Neurochemical and neuroanatomical effects of food or water restriction (e.g., Barney, Homeister, Muiderman, Laman, & Crumbaugh, 1988: Carlson, Glick, Hinds, & Baird, 1988; Krieger et al., 1980; Lonati-Galligani, 1988; Masoro, 1988; Mori,

Ishihara, & Iriuchijima, 1988; Perlmutter, Tweedle, & Hatton, 1985; Schulkin, 1988) are not discussed because there is not sufficient data relating to recovery to warrant their inclusion. Given the present state of the data, the three selected viewpoints should be regarded as preliminary.

View 1

It seems possible that there is a lingering effect of the preoperative intake regimens that facilitates recovery by an *interaction with postoperative mechanisms* in a manner analogous to postoperative manipulations known to enhance sensorimotor recovery, such as amphetamine (Davis, Cristostomo, Duncan, Propst, & Feeney, 1987; Feeney & Baron, 1987; Feeney et al., 1982; Feeney & Sutton, 1987; Hovda & Feeney, 1984; Macht, 1950), environmental enrichment (Dalrymple-Alford & Kelche, 1985; Donovick, Burright, & Swidler, 1973; Einon, Morgan, & Will, 1980; Finger & Stein, 1982; Gentile et al., 1987; Greenough et al., 1976; Held, Gordon, & Gentile, 1985; Kelche, Dalrymple-Alford, & Will, 1988; Rose, Davey, Love, & Dell, 1987; Rosenzweig & Bennett, 1976; Schwartz, 1964; Whishaw, Zaborowski, & Kolb, 1984; Will, Rosenzweig, & Bennett, 1976), exercise (Gentile et al., 1987), electrical stimulation (Harrell, Raubeson, & Balagwa, 1974), exposure to continuous darkness (Crowne, Richardson, & Ward, 1983), stress (Robinson & Whishaw, 1974; Wolgin & Teitelbaum, 1978), or neuroconvulsive agents (Feeney, Bailey, Boyeson, Hovda, & Sutton, 1987; Hernandez & Schallert, 1988). These postoperative manipulations may activate neurons closely connected with the damaged tissue that have become temporarily inhibited as a result of denervation (Feeney & Baron, 1987; Schallert, Hernandez, & Barth, 1986) or by affecting anatomical, transmitter release, or receptor coupling mechanisms involved in recovery from the deficit (Feldon & Weiner, 1988; Finger & Stein, 1982; Gentile et al., 1987; Marshall, 1984, 1985; Rosenzweig, 1984; Simansky, Bourbonais, & Smith, 1984). The data from Feeney and his colleagues (1982) are particularly interesting in this regard. They found that amphetamine facilitates recovery from a beam walking deficit caused by unilateral frontal cortex lesions. Norepinephrine is believed to be involved critically because the facilitative effect of amphetamine is reversed by noradrenergic blocking agents (Boyeson & Feeney, 1984).

Crowne et al. (1983) reported that placing rats in the dark postoperatively abolishes the orienting deficit typically found following unilateral medial cortex lesions, while Harrell and Balagura (1974) found that a preoperative period of darkness attenuates motor deficits caused by bilateral hypothalamic lesions. It is possible that catecholamines are involved in these effects as well because darkness activates an animal, yielding locomotion reminiscent of that produced by low doses of amphetamine. Other types of preoperative treatments, such as chronic drug administration or cortical damage, also are thought by some investigators to work by altering norepinephrine or dopamine function (Balagura &

Harrell, 1974; Balagura, Harrell, & Ralph, 1973; Glick & Greenstein, 1972a,b; Glick, Greenstein, & Zimmerberg, 1972; Hynes, Anderson, Gianutsos, & Lal, 1975; Kolb et al., 1977; Krieger, Crowley, O'Donohue, & Jacobowitz, 1980; Misantone, Schallert, & Lombardi, 1980). However, Whishaw, Sutherland, Kolb, and Becker (1986) reported that although noradrenaline appears to be critical for recovery in hemidecorticate rats housed singly in standard cages after surgery, noradrenaline depletion does not attenuate the enhanced recovery produced by an enriched environment.

The potential effect of a convulsant agent on recovery was also explored. A regimen of a subconvulsant dose of pentylenetetrazol versus vehicle was administered beginning at 18 hrs after a unilateral lesion of the somatosensory cortex, which in an undrugged condition yields a somatosensory asymmetry that lasts for several weeks or more (Barth & Schallert, 1987; Hernandez & Schallert, 1987). The pentylenetetrazol-treated rats recovered from this lesion significantly more rapidly than the vehicle-treated animals (Hernandez & Schallert, 1987). As with diazepam, the asymmetry, but not the absolute latencies to remove the stimuli, was affected by the drug at the time of daily testing. Thus, the drug did not work by altering the motor function required to carry out the task, but instead appeared to interact with processes related to the lesion. Pentylenetetrazol is believed to act in part by inhibiting GABAergic receptor activity, which would cause disinhibition. Thus, pentylenetetrazol, amphetamine, and the short-term lingering effects of intermittent schedules of reinforcement may share the characteristic of enhanced cerebral activation (see also Post, 1980), which could affect recovery by reversing functional depression in brain regions remote from the site of the damage (von Monakow, 1969).

Recent work suggests that the postoperative duration of preoperatively triggered changes need not last beyond a few days to be effective. There is evidence that during a short period after brain damage the mechanisms of recovery are particularly vulnerable to manipulation. In a model of brain damage, rats received unilateral anterior medial cortex (AMC) lesions (Fig. 1.3), which yielded a precisely quantifiable sensory asymmetry that reliably recovered within about 8 days. Adhesive patches were placed on the radial part of each forelimb. The lesioned animals removed the patch from the ipsilateral limb first, followed immediately by the contralateral patch. The magnitude of the asymmetry was estimated by decreasing the size of the ipsilateral stimulus relative to the size of the contralateral stimulus until the bias (order of responding to the ipsi versus contra patch) was neutralized. The contralateral/ipsilateral ratio decreased with recovery. One group of rats was exposed postoperatively to twice-daily injections of diazepam. A diazepam regimen beginning at 12 hrs after surgery and continuing for 3 postoperative weeks completely disrupted recovery from the lesion-induced sensory asymmetry for an indefinite period (Schallert et al., 1986; see also Watson & Kennard, 1945). Sedation or ataxia could be ruled out because the efficiency and speed (as opposed to the symmetry) of behavior were not

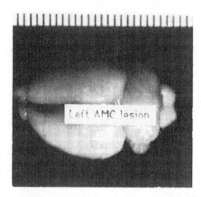

FIG. 1.3. Typical lesion of the anterior medial cortex (AMC), left hemisphere. Top border depicts scale in mm.

impaired. If the initial injection of diazepam was administered *after* recovery occurs, only a very transient asymmetry appeared, even if the exposure was chronic and the dose was raised (Schallert et al., 1986). It seems especially noteworthy that there may be a special stage of events after brain damage in which the recovery process is vulnerable to profound, perhaps permanent, disruption. The onset and length of this sensitive period were explored in a series of further experiments in which the time of initial postoperative injection of the drug regimen was systematically varied (Hernandez, Kiefel, Barth, Grant, & Schallert, 1988). The diazepam regimen was begun 12, 24, 48, 72, 96, or 120 hrs after brain damage.

There are several things to note about the results that might relate to the role of preoperative manipulations. First, it was necessary to administer diazepam prior to 96 hrs (approximately) to observe significant disruption of recovery in most rats. The action of preoperative manipulations that affect recovery would need to last long enough in the postoperative period to cover the duration of this 96-hr period (at least with AMC lesions). Second, recovery was impaired in 100% of the rats in the 12- and 24-hr groups and, for the other groups, only in those animals that had not yet shown any degree of recovery at the time of the diazepam regimen onset. Thus, the period of vulnerability appeared to vary according to the severity of the deficit, and likewise, the onset of recovery appeared to represent the initial time point at which recovery was not completely blocked by diazepam (Hernandez et al., 1988).

If it is assumed that preoperative manipulations interact specifically with mechanisms of recovery active during this period of vulnerability, and that the preoperative effect lingers only for a brief period after brain damage, then it would be predicted that preoperative manipulations should be effective in attenuating the effects only of relatively nonsevere lesions that yield a sufficiently early onset of recovery. As indicated in Schallert (1982), this appears to be the case. The behavioral effects of larger lesions are enduring and resistant to preoperative intake manipulations. Moreover, deficits that do not begin to recover until much later (e.g., more than 4 weeks) after surgery, such as motor deficits or inappropriate orienting to complex spatial-sensory information observed after posterolateral hypothalamic lesions, are not attenuated by preoperative intake regimens (Schallert, 1982; Schallert & Whishaw, 1984).

View 2

The evidence for the second hypothesis (*baseline improvement*) is more compelling. All animals subjected to intake restrictions become generally more reactive to sensory stimulation both pre- and postoperatively, particularly to cues associated with food (in the case of periodic restricted feeding) or water (in the case of periodic restricted watering). This is true for sham-operated rats as well (Schallert, 1982; Schallert & Whishaw, 1978). Sherrington (1900) noted that many reflexes are more easily elicited when an animal is hungry than when it is not, even if the reflex does not require for its operation a level of the nervous system above the spinal cord or caudal brain stem. Rats exposed to an intermittent schedule of access to water persistently orient to the drinking spout and follow the spout as it is pulled from the home cage. If the lesion is not too large (Fig. 1.5), this enhanced positive reactivity to water is followed by vigorous drinking behavior (Fig. 1.4). Undeprived control animals ignore the water spout, even if it is placed in front of the snout. Rats exposed to an intermittent schedule of food deprivation rear up for the food and will excitedly grab the food out of the experimenter's hand. Unlike undeprived rats, these animals hoard food when sated. Conditioning appears to play a role. Thus, even though they may be sated, with food pellets scattered on the floor, if the experimenter rattles the food hopper and opens the cage (as was done during the food restriction regimen), both sham-operated and lesioned rats in the restricted feeding groups rear up for the food and engage in vigorous eating behavior (see also Hsiao,

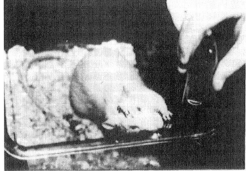

FIG. 1.4. Vigorous drinking response on the first day after bilateral lateral hypothalamic lesions. Recovery from adipsia and sensorimotor orienting impairment was facilitated by a preoperative restricted-watering regimen (Schallert, 1982).

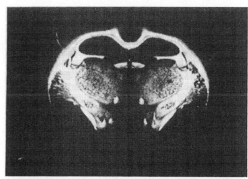

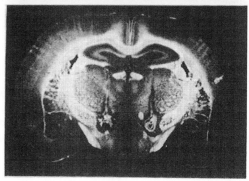

FIG. 1.5. (a) Coronal section through the rostrocaudal midpoint of damage to the lateral hypothalamic area. A preoperative restricted-watering regimen prevented the expected transient adipsia and orienting impairment that typically follows this type of lesion. (b) Relatively dorsally placed lesions in a rat adipsic for only 24 hr (water-restricted prelesion). (From Schallert, 1982.)

Wang, & Schallert, 1979; Schallert, Pendergrass, & Farrar, 1982; Weingarten, 1985).

Access to food or water must be intermittent to obtain the "reactivity" changes. Rats that are totally fasted or who are subjected to complete water deprivation do not exhibit the marked behavioral characteristics, neither pre- nor postoperatively. Consistent with the baseline-improvement hypothesis, recovery is not facilitated (Schallert, 1982).

It is worth emphasizing that restricted feeding or drinking regimens attenuate deficits in orienting to sensory stimulation, an effect that might not be anticipated. Animals without brain damage orient "playfully" and almost explosively to sensory stimulation when access to food or water is partly restricted preoperatively, though reactivity is especially intense to food or to water (Bolles, 1965, 1968; Ghent, 1951, 1957; Holeckova & Fabry, 1959; McFarland, 1970; Morgan, 1974; Osborne, 1977; Neuringer, 1969; Schallert, 1977, 1982; Schallert et al., 1982; Schallert & Whishaw, 1978; Stellar & Morgan, 1943; Young, 1949). Thus, it seems reasonable to suggest that the preoperative intermittent intake procedures can affect postoperative outcome simply by improving baseline reactivity in operated and unoperated populations (see also Ahern, Landin, & Wolf, 1978; Baker, 1955; Benjamin, 1959; Greenough et al., 1976; King & Gaston, 1973; Ruger & Schulkin, 1980; Singh, 1973, 1974; Will & Kelche, 1979).

A number of studies have found that preoperative exposure to otherwise-novel flavors (particularly attractive foods that in unoperated rats are more readily ingested than the familiar dry laboratory chow) facilitates recovery from the failure to eat these foods caused by diencephalic lesions or cortical damage (e.g., DiCara, 1970; Kolb et al., 1977; Schallert & Whishaw, 1978; Schulkin, 1988; Singh, chap. 4 in this volume). It is particularly clear in animals that were given samples of highly palatable foods while being subjected to a preoperative restricted feeding regimen, which appeared to exacerbate reactivity (Schallert & Whishaw, 1978). These data reinforce the view that improvement of behavior via conditioning mechanisms may be involved in a number of established trans-operative effects.

View 3

The third hypothesis (*tameness and testing familiarization*) developed from the results of a variety of experiments that stressed the importance of the testing situation and environment in the evaluation of recovery and maintenance of function. Long after apparently complete recovery from sensorimotor or in-gestive deficits caused by unilateral or bilateral lesions, the deficits can be reinstated if the environment is altered even slightly.

A good example of this lesion/environment interaction was observed in rats recovered from unilateral hemidecortication that were normally tested in the home (wire-mesh hanging) cage. If the cage was opened partway or the lighting altered, marked unilateral orienting (patch removal) asymmetries reappeared (Schallert & Whishaw, 1984). The magnitude and qualitative features of the reinstated asymmetry were identical to that observed in the most recently re-corded stage of recovery (sensorimotor recovery from the cortical damage occurs in an orderly sequence of definable events; Schallert & Whishaw, 1984, 1985). The deficits were not due to generalized severe distraction that might interfere with all behavior nonspecifically, because the *asymmetry* (involving active re-sponding to adhesive patches on both sides of the body), which had been neutralized via the recovery process, returned. The change in environment appeared to bring out specifically the otherwise-unseen dysfunction that was present in an earlier postoperative period.

Preoperative manipulations of food or water intake may facilitate postopera-tive orienting by familiarizing the animal with the experimenter and the testing situation (see also Greenough et al., 1976). In the given example, the testing situation involved an interaction between the animal and the experimenter who presented the sensory stimulation. If the cage is opened slightly, the food-nonrestricted animal is distracted (or stressed; Snyder, Stricker, & Zigmond, 1985) just enough to interfere with mechanisms that maintain the fragile state of so-called recovery without disrupting behavioral responding per se. Small doses of sedative-hypnotic drugs (Faugier–Grimaud, Frenois, & Stein, 1978; Schallert, 1987; Schallert et al., 1986) or the aging process (Schallert, 1983, 1987) also precipitate "recovered" deficits. An unfamiliar environment might interfere with complex neural processing in much the same way as aging or sedative-hypnotic drugs. Preoperative deprivation procedures may be among the fastest and most efficient means of taming an animal and reducing the stress of experimenter–rat encounters. Animals exposed to these intermittent regimens become very easy to handle and indeed appear to seek out actively interactions with the experimenter. Blind ratings consistently yield higher scores on "friendliness" and lower scores on "agitation" in the restricted-intake animals relative to handled-only controls.

A particularly striking example of how the environment can interact with brain damage was evident in rats apparently recovered from the transient aphagia, adipsia, and sensorimotor impairment caused by bilateral orbital frontal cortical lesions. Kolb et al. (1977) found that when these rats were tested in an environment that was much larger than the home cage or in one that was not enclosed completely by the familiar four walls and ceiling, they would not eat, drink, or orient to sensory stimulation.

Schallert and Whishaw (1978, and unpublished data) found that hypothalamus-damaged animals raised preoperatively in cages with a grid floor showed less impaired feeding and movement initiation when tested on a grid surface than when tested on a surface containing wood shavings, and that animals raised in cages with wood shavings showed less impaired feeding and movement initiation when tested on a surface containing wood shavings than when tested on a grid surface. Golani, Wolgin, and Teitelbaum (1979) and Schallert and Teitelbaum (1978) noted that the chronic akinesia or "warmup phenomenon" observed in rats tested in the open field after large hypothalamic lesions or intraventricular 6-OHDA were not present or were greatly ameliorated when the animals were examined in the home cage. Schallert, Petrie, and Whishaw (in press) found that neonatally dopamine-depleted rats, which display minor deficits in initiating behaviors when tested as adults, are much more severely impaired by unfamiliar or mildly distracting environmental stimuli than are sham-operated animals. Feeser and Raskin (1987) reported a similar result using a spontaneous alternation test. Whishaw, Nonneman, and Kolb (1981), having confirmed several previous reports that decorticate rats exhibit an abnormal grooming pattern, found that grooming behavior was perfectly normal as long as the animals were tested in their home cage.

Another experiment relevant to the third hypothesis was conducted by De-Vietti, Pellis, Pellis, and Teitelbaum (1985). They examined the behavior of rats drugged with anticholinergic atropine sulfate. They found that atropine caused thigmotaxis and stereotyped behaviors, as reported previously by Schallert, DeRyck, and Teitelbaum (1980), but also that these behaviors did not occur in animals that were frequently exposed to the various testing environments prior to being drugged. Schallert et al. (1980) had examined the behavior of saline-control animals when they were first exposed to the testing environments, and concluded that the atropine-induced stereotyped behaviors appeared to be similar to these *initial* undrugged reactions, as though atropine simply prolonged them. Predrug exposure to the testing environment might well have altered stereotyped reactions to an unfamiliar environment and thereby prevented the effects of atropine (see also Whishaw & Tomie, 1987; Lindner & Schallert, 1988).

In a recent study, we found that a preoperative regimen of restricted daily feeding, comparable to that described in Schallert and Whishaw (1978), reduced the period of sensorimotor asymmetry caused by unilateral microinfusions of the neurotoxin MPP+ into the neostriatum (Schallert, Hall, Bembenek, & Abell, unpublished data, 1987). As shown by the representative histological section in Fig 1.6, the MPP+ nonspecifically damaged cells throughout the neostriatum in one hemisphere. When tested with the home cage partway open, the lesioned rats in the nonrestricted feeding group failed to orient to somatosensory stimuli (von Frey hairs) presented contralateral to the damaged side (neglect). As shown in Table 1.1, this asymmetry appeared to be quite enduring, whereas in the restricted feeding group (which was rated as tamer and less agitated than the nonrestricted group when the home cage was opened), little or no dysfunction occurred. Under more familiar testing circumstances (i.e., cage closed), the deficit in the nonrestricted group was mild and lasted less than 1 week. It seems reasonable to propose that the slightly stressful/distracting testing situation (open cage) precipitated an otherwise unseen deficit in the rats that were not exposed to the preoperative restricted feeding regimen, and also that the level of stress/distraction when the cage was opened was far less in the restricted-feeding rats than it was in the nonrestricted rats.

A further observation was consistent with this idea. When a subgroup of these rats in the restricted-feeding group was left unhandled for 52 weeks (except for routine cage cleaning), they became quite agitated when the home cage was opened, as though they had lost the tameness acquired during the restricted feeding schedule one year earlier. Accordingly, sensorimotor testing (with the open cage) revealed severe contralateral neglect. Recall that severe impairment had not been observed in this group of rats under any environmental conditions during the period of testing immediately after surgery. The impairment was apparent only in the subgroup of animals that had not been handled over the 52-week period.

These data suggest that certain sensorimotor or other impairments observed after brain damage may be distraction-associated. Common anecdotal evidence from the study of brain-damaged people is consistent with this suggestion. That

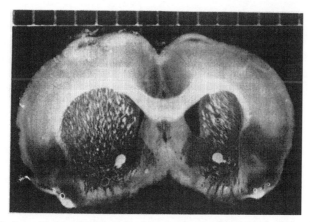

FIG. 1.6.   Unilateral lesion of the right caudate caused by infusion of 10 μg/μl of MPP+ into 3 different sites (restricted feeding group). Sham infusion of an equivalent volume of vehicle-only was delivered to the left hemisphere to control for cortical or other damage unrelated to MPP+ per se. This rat was killed more than 1 year after surgery (Schallert, Hall, Bembenek, & Abell, 1987).

is, the effects of brain damage are more severe when the patient is examined in an unfamiliar environment (Hall & Bigler, personal communication). One way that preoperative restricted feeding can attenuate the deficit may be by promoting tameness and familiarity with the testing situation, thereby permitting the expression of functions that in the absence of distraction are unimpaired.

TABLE 1.1

Mean (±S.E.) Latency (in secs) to Orient to Continuous (1 Hz) Stimulation of the Snout Contralateral to Unilateral Infusion of the Neurotoxin MPP+ in Rats That Were Either Undeprived or Were Subjected Preoperatively to a 17-Day Regimen of Intermittent Access to Food

	Food Restricted			Nondeprived		
	Day 2	Day 7	Day 365†	Day 2	Day 7	Day 365
Cage Closed	7.8 ± 2.4	<1.0	<1.0	9.8 ± 3.3	1.3 ± .4	<1.0
Cage Open	10.6 ± 3.1*	<1.0*	52.0 ± 6.3	56 ± 12.9	49.4 ± 8.4	44.7 ± 10.4

*Significantly faster to orient than nondeprived/cage open.

Note: Latency to respond to ipsilateral stimulation was <1 sec in all conditions. Sensorimotor procedures are detailed in Schallert & Hall, 1988. †Data at Day 365 are from subgroup of animals which were unhandled following surgery. For handled animals (who were given various food "treats" on a regular basis), the mean latency to orient = <1.0 sec. in both the closed cage and open cage conditions.

CONCLUSION

It is interesting but perhaps not surprising that a preoperative enriched environment or overtraining might help prepare an animal or person to perform more efficiently in complex tasks when motor or memory functions are compromised by brain damage (Hebb, 1949; Weinstein & Teuber, 1957). In contrast, preoperative intake schedules seem more mysterious because it is not obvious why a feeding or drinking regimen should impart such an enormous enhancing influence on sensorimotor responses. In this chapter we entertained three (not mutually exclusive) frameworks that might be helpful in accounting for these effects.

There appears to be some, but mainly indirect, evidence in support of the hypothesis that the preoperative events interact specifically with basic mechanisms involved in true recovery of function. For example, there may be a brief period immediately after brain damage during which compensatory processes involved in recovery are particularly sensitive to manipulation. It seems reasonable that preoperative changes might linger long enough transoperatively to influence these mechanisms.

The hypothesis that the preoperative treatment acts by changing baseline performance is supported principally by data indicating that sensorimotor reactivity improves in nonlesion groups. The degree of change has been such that one can expect such treatment to provide adequate resistance to the detrimental effects of brain damage in standard behavioral tests.

Finally, it was argued that a key effect of preoperative intake regimens has been to promote a high degree of tameness and to extend the range of testing "comfort" or familiarity that would permit optimal circumstances for sensorimotor performance in the postoperative period. Data were discussed that indicate that brain damage-specific dysfunctions can be precipitated by distraction or other conditions associated with testing in a novel environment.

ACKNOWLEDGMENTS

The experiments not previously published were supported by NIH grants NS17274 and NS23964. I thank T. Jones, S. Hall, and D. James for their help.

REFERENCES

Ahern, G. L., Landin, M. L., & Wolf, G. (1978). Escape from deficits in sodium intake after thalamic lesions as a function of preoperative experience. *Journal of Comparative & Physiological Psychology, 92,* 544–554.

Baker, R. A. (1955). The effects of repeated deprivation experience on feeding behavior. *Journal of Comparative & Physiological Psychology, 48,* 37–42.

Balagura, S., & Harrell, L. E. (1974). Lateral hypothalamic syndrome: Its modifications by obesity and leanness. *Physiology & Behavior, 13,* 345–347.

Balagura, S., Harrell, L., & Ralph, T. (1973). Glucodynamic hormones modify the recovery period after lateral hypothalamic lesions. *Science*, *182*, 59–60.

Barney, C. C., Homeister, J. W., Muiderman, A. K., Laman, T. G., & Crumbaugh, J. S. (1988). Prostaglandin E, hyperthermia in water or food deprived rats. *Brain Research Bulletin*, *20*, 183–188.

Barth, T. M., & Schallert, T. (1987). Somatosensory function of the superior colliculus, somatosensory cortex, and lateral hypothalamus in the rat. *Experimental Neurology*, *95*, 661–678.

Benjamin, R. M. (1959). Absence of deficits in taste discrimination following cortical lesions as a function of the amount of preoperative practice. *Journal of Comparative & Physiological Psychology*, *52*, 255–258.

Bolles, R. C. (1965). Consummatory behavior in rats maintained aperiodically. *Journal of Comparative & Physiological Psychology*, *60*, 239–243.

Bolles, R. C. (1968). Anticipatory general activity in thirsty rats. *Journal of Comparative & Physiological Psychology*, *65*, 511–513.

Boyeson, M. G., & Feeney, D. M. (1984). The role of norepinephrine in recovery from brain injury. *Society for Neuroscience Abstracts*, *10*, 68.

Carlson, J. N., Glick, S. D., Hinds, P. A., & Baird, J. L. (1988). Food deprivation alters dopamine utilization in the rat prefrontal cortex and asymmetrically alters amphetamine-induced rotational behavior. *Brain Research*, *454*, 373–377.

Crowne, D. P., Richardson, C. M., & Ward, G. (1983). Brief deprivation of vision after unilateral lesions of the frontal eye field prevents contralateral inattention *Science*, *200*, 527–530.

Dalrymple–Alford, J. C., & Kelche, C. R. (1985). Behavioral effects of preoperative and postoperative differential housing in rats with brain lesions: A review. In B. F. Will, P. Schmitt, & J. C. Dalrymple–Alford (Eds.), *Brain plasticity, learning, and memory*. New York: Plenum Press.

Davis, J. N., Crisostomo, E. A., Duncan, P. W., Propst, M., & Feeney, D. M. (1987). Amphetamine and physical therapy facilitate recovery from stroke: correlative animal and human studies. *The 15th Princeton Conference on Cerebrovascular Disease*. New York: Raven Press.

DeVietti, T. L., Pellis, S. M., Pellis, V. C., & Teitelbaum, P. (1985). Previous experience disrupts atropine-induced stereotyped "trapping" in rats. *Behavioral Neuroscience*, *99*(6), 1128–1141.

DiCara, L. V. (1970). Role of postoperative feeding experience in recovery from lateral hypothalamic damage. *Journal of Comparative & Physiological Psychology*, *72*, 60–65.

Donovick, P. J., Burright, R. G., & Bentsen, E. O. (1975). Presurgical dietary history and the behavior of control and septal lesioned rats. *Developmental Psychobiology*, *8*, 13–26.

Donovick, P. J., Burright, R. G., & Swidler, M. A. (1973). Presurgical rearing environment alters exploration, fluid consumption, and learning of septal lesioned and control rats. *Physiology & Behavior*, *11*, 543–553.

Einon, D. F., Morgan, M. F., & Will, B. E. (1980). Effects of post-operative environment on recovery from dorsal hippocampal lesions in young rats: Tests of spatial memory and motor transfer. *Quarterly Journal of Experimental Psychology*, *32*, 137–148.

Faugier–Grimaud, S., Frenois, C., & Stein, D. G. (1978). Effects of posterior parietal lesions on visually guided behavior in monkeys. *Neuropsychologia*, *16* 151–168.

Feeney, D. M., Bailey, B. Y., Boyeson, M. G., Hovda, D. A., & Sutton, R. L. (1987). The effect of seizures on recovery of function following cortical contusion in the rat. *Brain Injury*, *1*(1), 27–32.

Feeney, D. M., & Baron, J.-C. (1987). Diaschisis. *Stroke*, *17*, 817–830.

Feeney, D. M., Gonzales, A., & Law, W. A. (1982). Amphetamine, haloperidol, and experience interact to affect rate of recovery after motor cortex injury. *Science*, *217*, 855–857.

Feeney, D. M., & Sutton, R. L. (1987). Pharmacotherapy for recovery of function after brain injury. *CRC Critical Reviews in Neurobiology*, *3*, 135–197.

Feeser, H. R., & Raskin, L. A. (1987). Effects of neonatal dopamine depletion on spatial ability during ontogeny. *Behavioral Neuroscience*, *101*(6), 812–818.

Feldon, J., & Weiner, I. (1988). Long-term attentional deficit in nonhandled males: possible involvement of the dopaminergic system. *Psychopharmacology*, *95*, 231–236.

Finger, S., & Stein, D. G. (1982). *Brain damage and recovery: Research and clinical perspectives.* Academic Press: New York.

Gentile, A. M., Beheshti, Z., & Held, J. M. (1987). Enrichment versus exercise effects on motor impairments following cortical removals in rats. *Behavioral & Neural Biology*, *47*, 321–332.

Ghent, L. (1951). The relation of experience to the development of hunger. *Canadian Journal of Psychology*, *5*, 77–81.

Ghent, L. (1957). Some effects of deprivation on eating and drinking behavior. *Journal of Comparative & Physiological Psychology*, *50*, 172–176.

Glick, S. D., & Greenstein, S. (1972a). Facilitation of recovery after lateral hypothalamic damage by prior ablation of frontal cortex. *Nature (New Biology)*, *239*, 187–188.

Glick, S. D., & Greenstein, S. (1972b). Facilitation of survival following lateral hypothalamic damage by prior food and water deprivation. *Psychonomic Science*, *28*, 163–164.

Glick, S. D., Greenstein, S., & Zimmberberg, B. (1972). Facilitation of recovery by alpha-methyl-p-tyrosine after lateral hypothalamic damage. *Science*, *177*, 534–535.

Golani, I., Wolgin, D. L., & Teitelbaum, P. (1979). A proposed natural geometry of recovery from akinesia in the lateral hypothalamic rat. *Brain Research*, *164*, 237–267.

Greenough, W. T., Fass, B., & DeVoogd, T. (1976). The influence of experience on recovery following brain damage in rodents: Hypotheses based on development research. In R. Walsh & W. T. Greenough (Eds.), *Environments as therapy for brain dysfunction.* New York: Plenum Press.

Grijalva, C. V., & Lindholm, E. (1980). Restricted feeding and its effects on aphagia and ingestion-related disorders following lateral hypothalamic damage. *Journal of Comparative & Physiological Psychology*, *94*(1), 164–177.

Grijalva, C. V., Lindholm, E., Schallert, T., & Bicknell, E. (1976). Gastric pathology and aphagia following lateral hypothalamic lesions in rats: Effects of preoperative weight reduction. *Journal of Comparative & Physiological Psychology*, *90*, 505–519.

Harrell, L. E., & Balabura, S. (1974). The effects of dark and light on the functional recovery following lateral hypothalamic lesions. *Life Science*, *15*, 2079–2088.

Harrell, L. E., Raubeson, R., & Balagura, S. (1974). Acceleration of functional recovery following lateral hypothalamic damage by means of electrical stimulation in the lesioned areas. *Physiology and Behavior*, *12*, 897–899.

Hebb, D. O. (1949). *Organization of behavior.* New York: Wiley.

Held, J. M., Gordon, J., & Gentile, A. M. (1985). Environmental influences on locomotor recovery following cortical lesions in rats. *Behavioral Neuroscience*, *99*, 678–690.

Hernandez, T. D., Kiefel, J., Barth, T. M., Grant, M. L., & Schallert, T. (1988). Disruption and facilitation of recovery of function: Implication of the GABA/benzodiazepine receptor complex. In M. Ginsberg, & W. D. Dietrich (Eds.), *Sixteenth Princeton Conference on Cerebral Vascular Diseases.* New York: Raven Press.

Hernandez, T. D., & Schallert, T. (1988). Seizures and recovery from experimental brain damage. *Experimental Neurology*, *102*, 318–324.

Holeckova, E., & Fabry, P. (1959). Hyperphagia and gastric hypertrophy in rats adapted to intermittent starvation. *British Journal of Nutrition*, *13*, 260–266.

Hovda, D. A., & Feeney, D. M. (1984). Amphetamine with experience promotes recovery of locomotor function after unilateral frontal cortex injury in the cat. *Brain Research*, *298*, 358.

Hovda, D. A., Feeney, D. M., Salo, A. A., & Doyeson, M. G. (1983). Phenoxybenzamine but not haloperiodol reinstates all motor and sensory deficits in cats fully recovered from sensorimotor cortex albations. *Soc. Neurosci. Abstracts*, *9*, 1002.

Hsiao, S., Wang, C. H., & Schallert, T. (1979). Cholecystokinin, meal pattern, and the intermeal interval: Can eating be stopped before it starts? *Physiology and Behavior*, *23*, 909–914.

Hughes, K. R. (1965). Dorsal and ventral hippocampus lesions and maze learning: Influence of preoperative environment. *Canadian Journal of Psychology*, *19*, 325–332.

Hynes, M. D., Anderson, C. D., Gianutsos, G., & Lal, H. (1975). Effects of haloperidol, methyltyrosine, and morphine on recovery from lesions of the lateral hypothalamus. *Pharmacology Biochemistry & Behavior, 3,* 755–759.

King, B. M., & Gaston, M. G. (1973). The effects of pretraining on the bar-pressing performance of VMH-lesioned rats. *Physiology & Behavior, 11,* 161–166.

Keesey, R. E., Powley, T. L., & Kemnitz, J. W. (1976). Prolonging lateral hypothalamic anorexia by tube feeding. *Physiology & Behavior, 17,* 367–371.

Kelche, C., Dalrymple-Alford, J. C., & Will, B. E. (1988). Housing conditions modulate the effects of intracerebral grafts in rats with brain lesions. *Behavioural Brain Research, 28,* 287–295.

Kolb, B., Whishaw, I. Q., & Schallert, T. (1977). Aphagia, behavior sequencing and body weight set point following orbital frontal lesions in rats. *Physiology & Behavior, 19,* 93–109.

König, J. F. R., & Klippel, R. A. (1970). *The rat brain.* Huntington, NY: Kreiger. (Original work published 1963)

Krieger, D. T., Crowley, W. R., O'Donohue, T. L., & Jacobowitz, D. M. (1980). Effects of food restriction on the periodicity of corticosteroids in plasma and on monoamine concentrations in discrete brain nuclei. *Brain Research, 188,* 167–174.

Lindner, M. D., & Schallert, T. (1988). Aging and atropine effects on spatial navigation in the Morris water task. *Behavioral Neuroscience, 102,* 621–634.

Lonati-Galligani, M. (1988). Hypothalamus, frontal cortex, and lymphocyte β_2-adrenergic receptors in acute and chronic starvation in the rat. *Brain Research, 442,* 329–334.

Macht, M. B. (1950). Effects of D-amphetamine on hemi-decorticate, decorticate and decerebrate cats. *American Journal of Physiology, 163,* 731–732.

Marshall, J. F. (1984). Brain function: Neural adaptations and recovery from injury. *Annual Review of Psychology, 35,* 277–308.

Marshall, J. F. (1985). Neural plasticity and recovery after brain injury. In J. P. Smythies & R. J. Bradley (Eds.), *International Review Neurobiology* (Vol. 26). New York: Academic Press.

Marshall, J. F., Turner, B. H., & Teitelbaum, P. (1971). Sensory neglect produced by lateral hypothalamic damage. *Science, 174,* 523–525.

Masoro, E. J. (1988). Food restriction in rodents: An evaluation of its role in the study of aging. *Journal of Gerontology: Biological Sciences, 43,* B59–64.

McFarland, D. J. (1970). Recent developments in the study of feeding and drinking in animals. *Journal of Psychosomatic Research, 14,* 229–237.

Misantone, L. J., Schaffer, S. R., & Lombardi, L. (1980). Accelerated recovery from eating behavior deficits after sequential lesions of cortex and hypothalamus: Is dopamine involved? *Experimental Neurology, 70,* 236–259.

Morgan, M. J. (1974). Resistance to satiation. *Animal Behavior, 22,* 449–466.

Mori, M., Ishihara, H., & Iriuchijima, T. (1988). Water deprivation changes naloxone binding in the rat brain. *Neuroendocrinology, 47,* 290–293.

Neuringer, A. J. (1969). Animals respond for food in the presence of free food. *Science, 166,* 399–401.

Osborne, S. R. (1977). The free food (contrafreeloading) phenomenon: A review and analysis. *Animal Learning & Behavior, 5,* 221–235.

Perlmutter, L. S., Tweedle, C. D., & Hatton, G. I. (1985). Increased synaptic contacts in the hypothalamus with water deprivation. *Brain Research, 361,* 225–232.

Post, R. M. (1980). Intermittent versus continuous stimulation: Effect of time interval on the development of sensitization or tolerance. *Life Sciences, 26,* 1275–1282.

Powley, T. L., & Keesey, R. E. (1970). Relationship of body weight to the lateral hypothalamic feeding syndrome. *Journal of Comparative & Physiological Psychology, 70,* 25–36.

Robinson, T. E., & Whishaw, I. Q. (1974). Effects of posterior hypothalamic lesions on voluntary behavior and hippocampal electroencephalograms in the rat. *Journal of Comparative & Physiological Psychology, 86,* 768–786.

Rose, F. D., Davey, M. J., Love, S., & Dell, P. A. (1987). Environmental enrichment and recovery from contralateral sensory neglect in rats with large unilateral neocortical lesions. *Behavioural Brain Research, 24,* 195–202.

Rosenzweig, M. R. (1984). Experience, memory and the brain. *American Psychology, 39,* 365–376.

Rosenzweig, M. R., & Bennett, E. L. (1976). Enriched environments: facts, factors and fantasies. In J. L. McGaugh & L. Pentrinovich (Eds.), *Knowing, thinking and believing.* New York: Plenum.

Ruger, J., & Schulkin, J. (1980). Preoperative sodium appetite experience and hypothalamic lesions in rats. *Journal of Comparative & Physiological Psychology, 94,* 914–920.

Schallert, T. (1977). Reactivity to food odors during hypothalamic stimulation in rats not experienced with stimulation-induced eating. *Physiology & Behavior, 18,* 1061–1066.

Schallert, T. (1982). Adipsia produced by lateral hypothalamic lesions: Facilitation of recovery by preoperative restriction of water intake. *Journal of Comparative & Physiological Psychology, 96*(4), 604–614.

Schallert, T. (1983). Sensorimotor impairment and recovery of function in brain-damaged rats: Reappearance of symptoms during old age. *Behavioral Neuroscience, 97* (1), 159–164.

Schallert, T. (1987). Aging-dependent emergence of sensorimotor dysfunction in rats recovered from dopamine depletion sustained in early life. In J. A. Joseph (Ed.), *Central determinents of age-related declines in motor function.* Annals of the New York Academy of Sciences: New York.

Schallert, T., DeRyck, M., & Teitelbaum, P. (1980). Atropine stereotypy as a behavioral trap: A movement subsystem and electroencephalographic analysis. *Journal of Comparative & Physiological Psychology, 94,* 1–24.

Schallert, T., & Hall, S. (1988). "Disengage" sensorimotor deficit following apparent recovery from unilateral dopamine depletion. *Behavioural Brain Research* 30, 15–24.

Schallert, T., Hall, S., Bembenek, M., & Abell, C. (1987). Chronic behavioral effects of MPP+. In preparation.

Schallert, T., Hernandez, T. D., & Barth, T. M. (1986). Recovery of function after brain damage: Severe and chronic disruption by diazepam. *Brain Research, 379,* 104–111.

Schallert, T., Pendergrass, M., & Farrar, S. B. (1982). Cholecystokinin-octapeptide effects on eating elicited by "external" versus "internal" cues in rats. *Appetite: Journal for Intake Research, 3,* 81–90.

Schallert, T., Petrie, B., & Whishaw, I. Q. (in press). Spared and unspared sensorimotor functions following neonatal dopamine depletion, and effects of further dopamine depletion in adulthood. *Psychobiology.*

Schallert, T., & Teitelbaum, P. (1978). Unpublished data.

Schallert, T., & Whishaw, I. Q. (1978). Two types of aphagia and two types of sensorimotor impairment after lateral hypothalamic lesions: Observations in normal weight, dieted, and fattened rats. *Journal of Comparative & Physiological Psychology, 92,* 720–741.

Schallert, T., & Whishaw, I. Q. (1984). Bilateral cutaneous stimulation of the somatosensory system in hemidecorticate rats. *Behavioral Neuroscience, 98,* 518–540.

Schallert, T., & Whishaw, I. Q. (1985). Neonatal hemidecortication and bilateral cutaneous stimulation in rats. *Dev. Psychobiol., 18,* 501–514.

Schulkin, J. (1988). The effects of preoperative ingestive events on feeding and drinking behavior following brain damage. *Psychobiology, 16,* 185–195.

Schwartz, S. (1964). Effect of neocortical lesions and early environmental factors on adult rat behavior. *Journal of Comparative & Physiological Psychology, 57,* 72–77.

Sherrington, C. S. (1900). The spinal cord. In E. A. Schafer (Ed.), *Textbook of physiology* (Vol. 2). Edinburgh: Pentland.

Simansky, K. J., Bourbonais, K. A., & Smith, G. P. (1984). *Food-related stimuli increase the DOPAC/DA ratio in rat hypothalamus.* Paper presented at the annual meeting of the Eastern Psychological Association.

Singh, D. (1973). Effects of preoperative training on food-motivated behavior of hypothalamic hyperphagic rats. *Journal of Comparative & Physiological Psychology, 84,* 47–52.

Singh, D. (1974). Role of preoperative experience on reaction to quinine taste in hypothalamic hyperphagic rats. *Journal of Comparative & Physiological Psychology, 86*, 674–678.

Snyder, A. M., Stricker, E. M., & Zigmond, M. J. (1985). Stress-induced neurological impairments in an animal model of Parkinsonism. *Annals of Neurology, 18*(5), 544–551.

Stellar, E., & Morgan, C. T. (1943). The roles of experience and deprivation in the onset of hoarding behavior in the rat. *Journal of Comparative & Physiological Psychology, 36*, 47–55.

von Monakow, C. (translated and excerpted by G. Harris). (1969). "Diachisis," the localization in the cerebrum and functional impairment by cortical loci. In K. H. Pribam (Ed.), *Mood states and mind.* Baltimore: Penguin.

Watson, C. W., & Kennard, M. A. (1945). The effect of anticonvulsant drugs on recovery of function following cerebral cortical lesions. *Journal of Neurophysiology, 8*, 221–231.

Weingarten, H. P. (1985). Stimulus control of eating: Implications for a two-factor theory of hunger. *Appetite, 6*, 387–401.

Weinstein, S., & Teuber, H. L. (1957). The role of preinjury education and intelligence level in intellectual loss after brain injury. *Journal of Comparative & Physiological Psychology, 50*, 535–539.

Whishaw, I. Q., Nonneman, A. J., & Kolb, B. (1981). Environmental constraints on motor abilities used in grooming, swimming, and eating by decorticate rats. *Journal of Comparative & Physiological Psychology, 95*(5), 792–804.

Whishaw, I. Q., Sutherland, R. J., Kolb, B., & Becker, J. B. (1986). Effects of neonatal forebrain noradrenaline depletion on recovery from brain damage: Performance on a spatial navigation task as a function of age of surgery and postsurgical housing. *Behavioral & Neural Biology, 46*, 285–307.

Whishaw, I. Q., & Tomie, J. (1987). Cholinergic receptor blockade produces impairments in a sensorimotor subsystem for place nagivation in the rat: Evidence from sensory, motor, and acquisition tests in a swimming pool. *Behavioral Neuroscience, 101*(5), 603–616.

Whishaw, I. Q., Zaborowski, J. A., & Kolb, B. (1984). Postsurgical enrichment aids adult hemidecorticate rats on a spatial navigation task. *Behavioral & Neural Biology, 42*, 183–190.

White, N. M. (1986). Control of sensorimotor function by dopaminergic nigrostriatal neurons: Influence on eating and drinking. *Neuroscience and Biobehavioral Reviews, 10*, 15–36.

Will, B. E., & Kelche, C. R. (1979). Effects of different postoperative environments on the avoidance behavior of rats with hippocampal lesions: Recovery or improvement of functions? *Behavioral & Neural Biology, 27*, 96–106.

Will, B. E., Rosenzweig, M. R., & Bennett, E. L. (1976). Effects of differential environments on recovery from neonatal brain lesions, measured by problem-solving scores and brain dimensions. *Physiology and Behavior, 16*, 603–611.

Wolgin, D. L., & Teitelbaum, P. (1978). Role of activation and sensory stimuli in recovery from lateral hypothalamic damage in the cat. *Journal of Comparative & Physiological Psychology, 92*, 474–500.

Young, P. T. (1949). Food-seeking drive, affective processes, and learning. *Psychological Review, 56*, 98–121.

2

The Effects of Preoperative Alimentary Experiences on a Regulatory Neurobehavioral System

Jay Schulkin
Department of Anatomy and Institute of Neurological Sciences
University of Pennsylvania

INTRODUCTION

Salt hunger, or the appetite for salt, is a model neurobehavioral drive system (Wolf & Schulkin, 1980). In the rat the behavior is triggered by natriorexigenic, or salt appetite-producing hormones (e.g., Fluharty & Epstein, 1983). The behavior is simple to study and is easily elicited and well controlled (e.g., Wolf, 1969). In addition, animals will perform operants to obtain the salt (Denton, 1982; Schulkin, Arnell, & Stellar, 1985; Wolf, 1969). Therefore, one can gather insight into the basic mechanisms of motivated behavior (Miller, 1957; Stellar, 1954). Moreover, the mechanisms of body fluid homeostasis, in which sodium plays an important role, are intimately connected to cardiovascular regulation, and therefore the research is of medical import (Denton, 1982; Fitzsimons, 1979).

One important fact about the hunger for salt is that it is an innate appetite (Denton, 1982; Richter, 1956; Wolf, 1969). All, or almost all, other mineral and vitamin appetites are learned (e.g., Rozin, 1976); salt-hungry rats, within seconds after sampling a salty substance for the first time, ingest it immediately, before restorative consequences of the salt can have occurred.

Two brain regions, or systems, are considered essential for the expression of salt hunger. The first, the lateral hypothalamic (LH) region, contributes in the regulation of the drive; the second, the central gustatory system at the level of the caudal thalamic gustatory region, helps guide the ingestion through the identification of salt. Large lesions in either area abolish salt appetite (Wolf, 1967, 1968; Wolf & Schulkin, 1980). I will consider the central gustatory system first, because a protective effect was found there first.

21

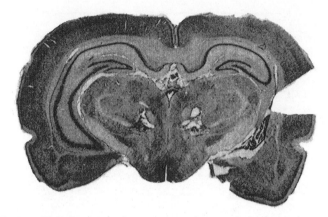

FIG. 2.1.   Photomicrograph of a representative lesion at the level of the caudal thalamic gustatory region.

CENTRAL GUSTATORY SYSTEM

In the laboratory of George Wolf, it was discovered that rats simply exposed preoperatively to the taste of salt were protected against the deficits in salt appetite that usually result from large lesions within the thalamic gustatory region (Ahern, Landin, & Wolf, 1978). Rats were either (1) exposed to 0.5 M NaCl with or without a hunger for salt, (2) made salt-hungry without the presence of salt for consumption, or (3) given control vehicle treatments. The method for eliciting the drive for salt was via a combination of natriuresis (sodium loss) and hormonal treatments (e.g., mineralocorticoids), which are known to elicit the ingestion of salt (e.g., Ahern et al., 1978). Rats were treated once weekly for 4 weeks. Following the last treatment, half the rats in each group were given large thalamic lesions and then allowed a month to recover from surgery.

A representative lesion for the following three studies is depicted in Fig. 2.1. The lesion is large and destroys, in addition to the thalamic taste region, the posterior intralaminer nuclei, the dorsomedial subthalamus and the rostral parts of the posterior nucleus and the reticular formation. In addition, there is damage to fiber systems including extralemniscal, noradrenergic, cerebellar, and cranial general sensory pathways. Most importantly, the lesion disconnects gustatory pathways enroute from the brainstem to the amygdala.

Figure 2.2 shows the behavioral result from the first study. Rats exposed to the salt preoperatively, with or without the drive for it, were protected against the lesion-induced deficits in salt appetite; rats with the salt drive experience

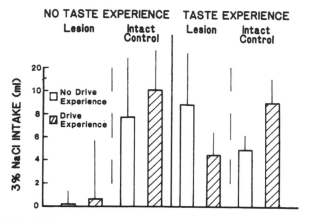

FIG. 2.2. Median increases of salt over baseline intake, with the interquartile range indicated. Unlike the two groups that tasted salt, the two lesion groups ingested significantly less salt than the intact groups ($p < .01$).

alone (or the vehicle treatments) were not protected. Thus, merely sampling the salt preoperatively was enough to protect them. Why does this protective effect occur?

We addressed this issue directly (Paulus, Eng, & Schulkin, 1984). Rats are able to recognize and remember where salt is located, even though they have never been salt-hungry. We know that they remember where salt is, or how to acquire it, or what it is associated with, because the first time they are rendered salt-hungry they return to where the salt was located, or labor to obtain it (Krieckhaus, 1970; Krieckhaus & Wolf, 1968; Rescorla, 1981). One critical aspect of the earlier study was that the salt solution was located in the same place both pre- and postoperatively. The rats may have been protected because they remembered tasting salt in a particular place. Thus, despite damage to gustatory sensibility the rats returned to the place, guided by the memory of salt and its location in space. This hypothesis was tested by changing the location of the salt solution postoperatively for one group of rats and keeping it the same for another group.

Figure 2.3 shows the placement of the salt solutions. Two groups of rats were preoperatively exposed to the salt solutions. They were given access to the 3% salt in either of the two positions depicted in Fig. 2.3 for 1 week *ad libitum*. Both groups had continuous access to water. Rats sampled the salt solution in both positions, but the amount ingested was negligible. A third group was given access to two bottles of water in both positions, thereby giving them experience drinking out of both positions. Rats then underwent central gustatory surgery. Following recovery (1 month postsurgery) they were tested for salt appetite with the salt source placed in Position A.

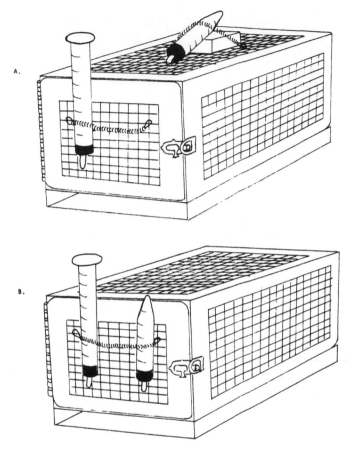

FIG. 2.3.   A: Position of salt and water tubes during preoperative experience for the same place group. This is also the position of two water tubes during preoperative experience for the water control group and the position of salt and water tubes during postoperative salt appetite test for all groups. B: Position of salt and water during tubes during preoperative experience for the different-place groups.

Figure 2.4 shows the behavioral data. The data are clear; Only those rats with the salt solution in the same place both pre- and postoperatively were protected. Therefore, place learning figured significantly in providing protection; rats with central gustatory damage remembered where the salt was located.

Salt-hungry rats remember where salt is located when not salt-hungry with minimal exposure to it: just 4–10 licks of 0.1 ml of NaCl over 2-5 min. was sufficient for such learning (Bregar, Strombakis, Allan, & Schulkin, 1983; Wirsig & Grill, 1982). We extended this line of research by determining

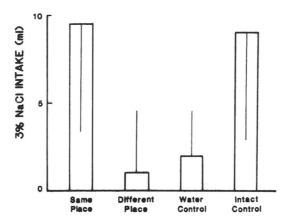

FIG. 2.4.   Median increases of salt over baseline intake, with the interquartile range indicated. Only the group that tasted salt in the same place was protected; the other two lesion groups manifested deficits in their salt intake, compared with the intact group ($p < .01$).

whether exposure to salt within seconds was enough to protect the central gustatory damaged animal (Hartzell, Paulus, & Schulkin, 1985).

Preoperatively, one group was given access to salt when thirsty for 30 seconds, a second group was given access to sucrose when thirsty, and a third group was a nonlesion control group. Following recovery from surgery rats were tested for salt appetite as described.

The behavioral data are shown in Fig. 2.5. Brief exposure to salt preoperatively was enough to protect rats postoperatively against deficits in regulatory salt-ingestive behavior.

In all the studies cited, the brain-damaged animals preoperatively exposed to the salt behaviorally appeared very much like normal animals postoperatively. In the first study they were exposed to the salt for 4 weeks, in the second study they were exposed to it for 1 week, and in the last study they were exposed to it

FIG. 2.5.   Median increases of salt over baseline intake, with the interquartile indicated. The group preoperatively exposed to the salt was protected. The other group manifested deficits in salt intake, compared with the intact group ($p < .01$).

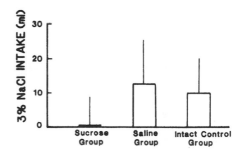

for only 30 seconds. Thus, the protective effect can be implemented with only a brief exposure to the salt. There is a precedent for these phenomena in other innate behavioral systems. For example, other innate systems such as language (Chomsky, 1968; Lenneberg, 1967), bird song or imprinting behavior (see Marler & Hamilton, 1966) or other sensory discriminations (e.g., Knudsen, Knudsen, & Esterly, 1984) require minimal exposure to the relevant biological signal in order to trigger behavioral competence.

HYPOTHALAMIC SYSTEM

In the next series of experiments we demonstrated that preoperative salt drive arousal would protect the LH-damaged animal.

In the first experiment (Ruger & Schulkin, 1980), rats either had or did not have preoperative arousal with salt drive (as described) once weekly for 4 weeks. All groups were allowed access to the 3% salt solution. About half the rats were subsequently lesioned in the LH, and the other half were not. Following recovery from surgery, all rats were given access to the salt solution. After several days, salt hunger was induced (as described).

Figure 2.6 depicts a representative LH lesion for the following three experiments. The lesion was centered within the tuberal region of the LH area. The most rostral lesion is at the anterior tip of the ventromedial nucleus and the most caudal lesion is centered just posterior to the ventromedial nucleus. In some, but not in most, there was damage to the ventral part of the zona incerta.

Figure 2.7 shows the salt ingestion. LH-damaged animals in whom the drive was aroused preoperatively demonstrated salt appetite postoperatively; LH rats with no history of drive arousal did not.

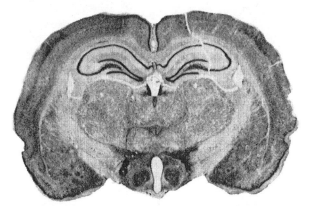

FIG. 2.6.   Photomicrograph of a representative lateral hypothalamic lesion. The lesion is centered at the level of the ventromedial hypothalamus and ventrolateral to the fornix.

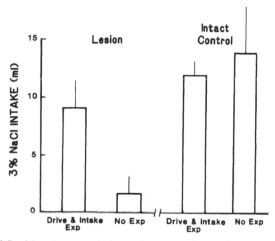

FIG. 2.7.   Mean increases of salt over baseline intakes, with the standard error indicated. Unlike the experienced group, the nonexperienced group showed a significant decrease in their salt intake, compared with intact controls ($p < .001$).

In the next two experiments, we sought to determine whether salt drive alone without ingestion would protect the LH animal. These studies are analogous to the experiment that showed that salt taste, but not salt drive, is what protects the central gustatory damaged animal. First, we replicated our earlier results that preoperative salt drive and ingestion reduced the deficits in salt appetite seen after LH damage, and we also found that salt drive alone without salt ingestion also protected the animals (Wolf, Schulkin, & Fluharty, 1983). But we discovered that thirsty rats ingesting isotonic saline preoperatively (0.15 M NaCl) also had reduced postoperative impairments in salt appetite. These results are shown in Fig. 2.8. Note first that the protective effects were less pronounced than in the first LH experiment. This fact can be accounted for; brain-damaged animals, and LH rats in particular, are notoriously worse in demonstrating ingestive competence than nonbrain-damaged animals in short-term tests (e.g., Stricker, Friedman, & Zigmond, 1975). This ingestion test lasted for 2 hours; recall that the first experiment measured the ingestion of salt over 24 hours. Despite this fact we were able to see protective effects in the short-term test.

But there were still unanswered questions. Since the group with thirst preoperative experiences was also protected, how specific must the preoperative manipulation be to see postoperative protection in salt appetite? Thirst and salt appetite are closely linked alimentary drives; water and salt ingestion are essential in the regulation of body fluid homeostasis (e.g., Denton, 1982; Epstein, Kissileff, & Stellar, 1973; Fitzsimons, 1979; Stricker, 1983). The ingestion of

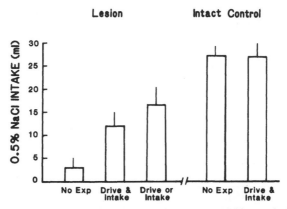

FIG. 2.8. Mean increases of salt over baseline intakes with the standard error indicated. The experienced groups ingested more salt than the nonexperienced group ($p < .01$), but all lesion groups ingested less salt than intact groups (p's < .05, < .01).

isotonic saline (which is the concentration of extracellular fluid) preoperatively in thirsty rats may have protected them because the drives are linked and the rats may have generalized the satisfaction of one drive with the other. Therefore, in the last experiment we analyzed separately the role of preoperative thirst and other drive experiences and their effects on salt appetite following LH damage.

This final experiment demonstrates conclusively that (1) preoperative salt drive (without ingestion) is both necessary and sufficient to protect the LH animal, (2) access to the taste of salt without the salt drive preoperatively is neither necessary nor sufficient to protect them, and (3) other alimentary preoperative drive experiences, such as hunger, and thirst (with the rats ingesting water), did not protect them postoperatively against lesion-induced deficits in salt appetite.

The results from this experiment are shown in Fig. 2.9. Only those LH rats preoperatively treated with salt drive (once weekly for 3 weeks as described) were protected. Rats that were exposed to the salt taste without the salt drive were not protected. Moreover, rats that were water-deprived daily and then given access to water 1 hr a day were also not protected. Nor were rats who were rendered hungry by insulin treatments protected. This treatment is known to reduce the aphagia and metabolic regulatory deficits in recovered LH-damaged animals (see Grijalva, this volume).

If, however, the means of eliciting the appetite was different pre- and postoperatively the protective effect was diminished (Fig. 2.10). Postoperatively we just used the mineralocorticoid to elicit the appetite for salt; preoperatively we had depleted these rats of sodium, which triggers the release of the natriorex-

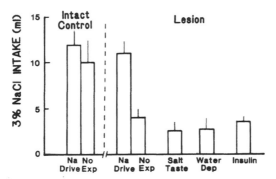

FIG. 2.9.   Mean increases of salt over baseline intakes, with the standard error indicated. Unlike the experienced group, the non-sodium-derived groups ingested significantly less salt than the intact groups ($p < .01$).

igenic hormones (e.g., angiotensin and aldosterone; Stricker, 1983). By administering just the mineralocorticoids postoperatively, angiotensin could play no role and there was less of a protective effect.

At a behavioral level of analysis, part of the explanation for the preoperative protective effect for the LH animal is that prior salt hunger treatments can increase the amount of salt that rats will subsequently ingest when they are rendered salt-hungry (Falk, 1966; Sakai, Fine, Frankmann & Epstein, 1987). In other words, the amount of salt that the LH animal will ingest may be elevated because of the preoperative salt drive arousal. The taste of salt becomes more rewarding, more palatable (Berridge, Flynn, Schulkin, & Grill, 1984; Denton, 1982). Therefore, the decrease in drive that results from the LH lesion is averted by the increase in the palatability of the salt.

At a neural-hormone level of analysis, the sodium depletion preoperative treatment releases the steroid hormone, aldosterone, which may produce steroid-induced organizational changes in critical brain regions (Arnold &

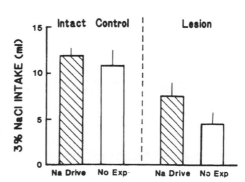

FIG. 2.10.   Mean increases of salt over baseline intakes, with the standard error indicated. Both lesion groups ingested less salt than the intact groups ($p < .005$).

Breedlove, 1985; Goy & McEwen, 1980), changing the subsequent long-term ingestion of salt. Thus, despite the reduced level of circulating aldosterone that may result from hypothalamic damage (Palkovits, deJong, & deWied, 1974), brain mineralocorticoid receptors may be altered by the regulatory challenges.

SUMMARY STATEMENT

Salt when coupled with place association, but not salt drive, protected the central gustatory-damaged animal: Preoperative salt drive was important to the hypothalamic-damaged animal. In addition, salt taste but not sucrose taste protected the central gustatory-damaged animal, while salt drive and not other alimentary drives protected the hypothalamic-damaged animal.

GENERAL CONSIDERATIONS

In both lesion preparations the amygdala may be crucial for the protective effects. First, the amygdala for some time has been implicated in the regulation of drives (Herrick, 1948). Second, the main taste-visceral projection to the ventral forebrain terminates in the central nucleus of the amygdala (Norgren, 1984). This pathway has long been thought, even before its actual discovery in a mammal (Herrick, 1948), to be a visceral-drive pathway (Pfaffmann, 1960). Third, the amygdala is anatomically tied to brain stem visceral regions, for example, solitary nucleus and the dorsal motor nucleus of the vagus nerve, in addition to preoptic-hypothalamic brain regions, which are known to be involved in appetitive behavior (Deolmos, Alheid, & Beltramino, 1985; Krettek & Price, 1978; Nauta, 1962; Simmerly & Swanson, 1986; Swanson & Mogenson, 1981). Fourth, preoperative effects of feeding and drinking behavior are abolished following amygdala damage (Fonberg, 1974; Kemble & Davies, 1981). That is, it appears that preoperative feeding and drinking experiences do not protect the amygdala-damaged rat against deficits in these two behaviors postoperatively, as they do for the hypothalamic-damaged animal. Fifth, rats retain salt taste associations following the removal of the entire neocortex (Wirsig & Grill, 1982), nor is the dorsal hippocampus or septum essential for the expression of salt hunger (Chiaraviglio, 1969; Marinos, Coirini, DeNicola, & McEwen, 1986) while damage to the amygdala disrupts salt hunger (Cox et al., 1977; Nachman & Asche, 1974; Schulkin, Marini, & Epstein, 1989; Zolovick, Avrith, & Jalowiec, 1977). Sixth, aldosterone, one of the principal hormones, is localized in the corticomedial region of the amygdala (McEwen, Lambin, Rainbow, & DeNicola, 1986), and angiotensin, the other principal hormone, has both fibers and cell bodies in both the central and medial nucleus of the amygdala (Gehlert, Speth, & Wamsley, 1986; Lind, Swanson, & Ganten,

1984). Seventh, therefore, all preoperative salt regulatory protective effects should be abolished following damage to the amygdala. And in fact unpublished observations of amygdala-damaged animals suggest just such a loss of pre-operative effects; that is, there appears to be no protective effects from pre-operative experience of either tasting salt or the drive for salt following amygdala damage (Schulkin, unpublished observations).

Consider this hypothesis about the amygdala's potential role for the protection a bit further. The central gustatory lesion at the level of the thalamic nucleus disconnects afferents en route to the central nucleus of the amygdala from the lower brainstem (Norgren, 1984; Paulus et al., 1984; Schulkin, Flynn et al., 1985). The damage results in the salt-hungry rat's not ingesting the salt, because the taste of salt has lost its significance to the animal. In fact damage along this taste visceral pathway results in the loss of the expression of salt hunger (Paulus et al., 1984; Schulkin, Flynn et al., 1985).

However, once the rat tastes salt preoperatively, the taste-visceral pathway is no longer necessary; the animal recalls where the salt was located and returns there. Transition zones of caudal amygdala and ventral hippocampus may mediate such taste–place associations. Thus, despite impairments in gustatory-related behaviors (Schulkin, Flynn et al., 1985), the brain compensates by remembering where the salt was located which require amygdala function (e.g., Mishkin & Appenzeller, 1987).

The hypothalamic animal may be protected because preoperative salt hunger treatments invoke organizational changes in critical brain regions similar to those in the formation of gender (Goy & McEwen, 1980). In fact, organizational effects occur in the medial nucleus of the amygdala (Nishizuka & Arai, 1983), which not only receives visceral input and concentrates natriorexigenic hormones but appears to be involved in mineralocorticoid-induced salt hunger (Schulkin, Marini, & Epstein, 1989). The kinds of changes in the medial nucleus may include morphological, synaptic organization, neural connectivity, the synthesis of new proteins in the form of neurotransmitters and an upregulation of mineralocorticoid binding sites.

In closing, note that neither central gustatory nor the LH region (or pathways into the ventral forebrain) are necessary for the expression of this behavior, once the appropriate information is conveyed (tasting salt and the drive for salt) to the amygdala. And, thus, despite the loss, or a reduction of sensory-visceral input, the behavior is still expressed because of the possible effects of the relevant preoperative experience on amygdala function.

REFERENCES

Ahern, G., Landin, M., & Wolf, G. (1978). Escape from deficits in sodium intake after thalamic lesions as a function of preoperative experience. *Journal of Comparative & Physiological Psychology, 92*, 544–554.

Arnold, A. P., & Breedlove, S. M. (1985). Organizational and activational effects of sex steroids on brain and behavior: A reanalysis. *Hormones and Behavior, 19,* 469–498.

Berridge, K. C., Flynn, F. W., Schulkin, J., & Grill, H. J. (1984). Sodium depletion enhances salt palatability in rats. *Behavioral Neuroscience, 98,* 562–660.

Bregar, R. E., Strombakis, R. H., Allan, R. W., & Schulkin, J. (1983). *Brief Exposure to a Saline Stimulus Promotes Latent Learning in the Salt Hunger System.* Society for Neuroscience.

Chiaraviglio, E. (1969). Effects of lesions in the septal area and the olfactory bulbs on sodium chloride intake. *Physiology and Behavior, 4,* 693–697.

Chomsky, N. (1968). *Language and mind.* New York: Harcourt Brace Jovanovich.

Coirini, H., Magarinos, A. M., DeNicola, A. F., Rainbow, T. C., & McEwen, B. S. (1985). Further studies of brain aldosterone binding sites employing new mineralocorticoid and glucocorticoid receptor markers in vitro. *Brain Research, 37,* 212–216.

Cox, J. C., Cruz, C. E., & Ruger, J. (1978). Effect of total amygdalectomy upon regulation of salt intake in rats. *Brain Research Bulletin, 3,* 431–435.

Denton, D. A. (1982). *The hunger for salt.* New York: Springer-Verlag.

Deolmos, J. D., Alheid, G. F., & Beltramino, C. A. (1985). Amygdala. In G. Pavinos (Ed.), *The rat neuron system.* New York: Academic Press.

Epstein, A. N., Kissileff, H. R., & Stellar, E. (1973). *The Neuropsychology of thirst: New findings and advances in concepts.* New York: Wiley.

Falk, J. L. (1966). Serial sodium depletion and NaCl solution intake. *Physiology and Behavior, 1,* 75–77.

Fitzsimons, J. T. (1979). *The physiology of thirst and sodium appetite.* Cambridge, England: Cambridge University Press.

Fluharty, S. J., & Epstein, A. N. (1983). Sodium appetite elicited by intracerebral ventricular infusions of angiotensin II: Synergistic interactions with systemic mineralocorticoids. *Behavioral Science, 97,* 746–758.

Fonberg, E. (1974). Amygdala functions within the alimentary system. *Acta Neurobiology Experimentalis, 34,* 435–466.

Gehlert, D. R., Speth, R. C., & Wamsley, J. K. (1986). Distribution of angiotensin binding sites in the rat brain: A qualitative autoradiographic study. *Neuroscience 18,* 837–856.

Goy, R. S., & McEwen, B. S. (1980). *Sexual differentiation of the brain.* Cambridge, MA: MIT Press.

Hartzell, A. R., Paulus, R. A., & Schulkin, J. (1985). Brief preoperative exposure to saline protects rats against behavioral impairments in salt appetite following central gustatory damage. *Behavioural Brain Research, 15,* 9–13.

Herrick, C. J. (1948). *The brain of the tiger salamander.* Chicago: University of Chicago Press.

Kemble, E. D., & Davies, V. A. (1981). Effects of prior environmental enrichment and amygdaloid lesions on consummatory behavior, activity, predation, and shuttlebox avoidance in male and female rats. *Physiological Psychology, 9,* 340–346.

Knudsen, E. R., Knudsen, P. F., & Esterly, S. D. (1984). A critical period for the recovery of sound localization accuracy following monaural occlusion in the barn owl. *Journal of Neuroscience, 4*(4), 1012–1020.

Krettek, J. E., & Price, J. L. (1978). Amygdaloid projections to subcortical structures within the basal forebrain in the rat and cat. *Journal of Comparative Neurology, 178,* 225–254.

Krieckhaus, E. E. (1970). "Innate recognition" aids rats in sodium regulation. *Journal of Comparative & Physiological Psychology, 73,* 117–122.

Krieckhaus, E. E., & Wolf, G. (1968). Acquisition of sodium by rats: Interactions of innate mechanisms and latent learning. *Journal of Comparative & Physiological Psychology, 65,* 197–201.

Lenneberg, E. H. (1967). *Biological foundations of language.* New York: Wiley.

Lind, R. W., Swanson, L. W., & Ganten, D. (1984). Organization of angiotensin II immunoreactive cells and fibers in the rat central nervous system. *Neuroendocrinology, 40,* 2–24.

Marinos, A. M., Coirini, H., DeNicola, A. F., McEwen, B. S. (1986). Mineralocorticoid regulation of salt intake is preserved in hippocampectomized rats. *Neuroendocrinology, 44*, 494–497.

Marler, P. R., & Hamilton, W. J. (1966). *Mechanisms of animal behavior.* New York: Wiley.

McEwen, B. S., Lambin, L. T., Rainbow, T. C., & DeNicola, A. F. (1986). Aldosterone effects on salt appetite in adrenalectomized rats. *Neuroendocrinology, 43*, 38–43.

Miller, N. E. (1957). Experiments on motivation; studies combining psychological, physiological, and pharmacological techniques. *Science, 126*, 1271–1278.

Mishkin, M., & Appenzeller, P. (1987). The anatomy of memory. *Scientific American.* May, 80–89.

Nachman, M., & Ashe, J. H. (1974). Effects of basolateral amygdala lesions of neopobia, learned taste aversions, and sodium appetite in rats. *Journal of Comparative & Physiological Psychology, 87*, 622–643.

Nauta, W. J. H. (1962). Neural associations of the amygdaloid complex in the monkey. *Brain, 85*, 505–520.

Nishizuka, M., & Arai, Y. (1981). Sexual dimorphism in synaptic organization in the amygdala and its dependence on neonatal hormone environment. *Brain Research, 212*, 31–38.

Norgren, R. (1984). *Central neural mechanisms of taste. Handbook of physiology:* Sect. 1. *The nervous system:* Vol. 3 *Sensory processes* (pp. 1087–1128). American Physiological Society, Washington DC.

Palkovitz, M., deJong, W., & deWied, D. (1974). Hypothalamic control of aldosterone production in sodium deficient rats. *Neuroendocrinology, 14*, 297–309.

Paulus, R. A., Eng, R., & Schulkin, J. (1984). Preoperative latent place learning preserves salt appetite following damage to the central gustatory system. *Behavioral Neuroscience, 98*, 146–151.

Pfaffmann, C. (1960). The pleasures of sensation. *Psychological Review, 67*, 253–268.

Rescorla, R. A. (1981). Simultaneous associations. In P. Harzen & M. D. Zeller (Eds.), *Predictability, correlation and contiguity.* New York: Wiley.

Richter, C. P. (1956). Salt appetite of mammals: Its dependence on instinct and metabolism. In Fondation Singer Polignac (Ed.), *L'instinct dans le comportement des animaux et de l'homme* (pp. 527–629). Paris: Masson.

Rozin, P. (1976). The selection of foods by rats, humans, and other animals. In J. S. Rosenblatt, R. A. Hinde, E. Shaw, & C. Beer (Eds.), *Advances in the Study of Behavior* (Vol. 6). New York: Academic Press.

Ruger, J., & Schulkin, J. (1980). Preoperative sodium appetite experience and hypothalamic lesions in rats. *Journal of Comparative & Physiological Psychology, 94*, 914–920.

Sakai, R. R., Fine, W. B., Frankmann, S., & Epstein, A. N. (1987). Salt appetite is enhanced by one prior episode of sodium depletion in the rat. *Behavioral Neuroscience, 101*, 724–731.

Schulkin, J., Arnell, P., & Stellar, E. (1985). Running to the taste of salt in mineralocorticoid-treated rats. *Hormones and Behavior. 19*, 413–425.

Schulkin, J., & Fluharty, S. J. (1985). Further studies on salt appetite following lateral hypothalamic lesions: Effects of preoperative alimentary experiences. *Behavioral Neuroscience, 99*, 929–935.

Schulkin, J., Flynn, F. W., Grill, H. J., & Norgren, R. (1985). Central gustatory lesions: Effects on salt appetite and taste aversion learning. *Neuroscience Abstracts*, 11:1259.

Schulkin, J., Marini, J., & Epstein, A. N. (1989). A role for the medial region of the amygdala in mineralocorticoid induced salt hunger. *Behavioral Neuroscience, 103*, 178–185.

Simmerly, R. B., & Swanson, L. W. (1986). The organization of neural inputs to the medial preoptic nucleus of the rat. *Journal of Comparative Neurology, 246*, 312–342.

Stellar, E. (1954). The physiology of motivation. *Psychological Review, 61*, 5–22.

Stricker, E. M. (1983). Thirst and sodium appetite after colloid treatment in rats: Role of the renin-angiotensin-aldosterone system. *Behavioral Neuroscience, 97*, 725–737.

Stricker, E. M., Friedman, M. I., & Zigmond, M. J. (1975). Glucoregulatory feeding by rats after intraventricular 6-hydroxydopamine or lateral hypothalamic lesions. *Science, 189,* 895–897.

Swanson, L. W., & Mogenson, G. J. (1981). Neural mechanisms for the functional coupling of autonomic, endocrine and somatomotor responses in adaptive behavior. *Brain Research Reviews, 3,* 1–34.

Wirsig, C. R., & Grill, H. J. (1982). Contribution of the rat's neocortex to ingestive control: 1. Latent learning for the taste of sodium chloride. *Journal of Comparative & Physiological Psychology, 96,* 615–627.

Wolf, G. (1967). Hypothalamic regulation of sodium intake: Relations to preoptic and tegmental function. *American Journal of Physiology, 213,* 1433–1438.

Wolf, G. (1968). Thalamic and tegmental mechanisms for sodium intake: Anatomical and functional relations to the lateral hypothalamus. *Physiology and Behavior, 3,* 997–1002.

Wolf, G. (1969). Innate mechanisms for regulation of sodium intake. In D. Pfaffman (Ed.), *Olfaction and taste.* New York: Rockefeller University Press.

Wolf, G., & Schulkin, J. (1980). Brain lesions and sodium appetite: An approach to the neurological analysis of homeostatic behavior. In M. Kare & M. J. Fregly (Ed.), *Biological and behavioral aspects of salt intake.* New York: Academic Press.

Wolf, G., Schulkin, J., & Fluharty, S. J. (1983). Recovery of salt appetite after lateral hypothalamic lesions: Effects of preoperative salt drive and salt intake experiences. *Behavioral Neuroscience, 97,* 506–511.

Zolovick, A. J., Avrith, D., & Jalowiec, J. E. (1977). Reversible colchicine-induced disruption of amygdaloid function in sodium appetite. *Brain Research Bulletin, 5,* 35–39.

3

Recovery of Function Following Lateral Hypothalamic Damage: The Influence of Preoperative Manipulations

Carlos V. Grijalva
Department of Psychology
Brain Research Institute, UCLA

Ernest Lindholm
Department of Psychology
Arizona State University

Barbara Roland
Department of Psychology
UCLA

INTRODUCTION

The lateral hypothalamic lesion (LH) syndrome, as originally described by Teitelbaum and Epstein (1962), has served not only as a valuable model for the study of ingestive behaviors but also as a very useful model for examining the processes potentially involved in recovery of function following brain damage. Within recent years, considerable attention has been given to the spectrum of disorders induced by LH damage that presumably underlie or contribute to the initial periods of postoperative aphagia and anorexia. The disorders thought to contribute to the initial feeding deficits include a lack of motivation (e.g., Epstein, 1971; Rodgers, Epstein & Teitelbaum, 1964; Teitelbaum & Epstein, 1962), motor dysfunctions (Baillie & Morrison, 1963; Morrison, 1968), somatic sensorimotor dysfunctions (Marshall & Teitelbaum, 1974; Marshall, Turner, & Teitelbaum, 1971), oral sensorimotor dysfunctions (Zeigler & Karten, 1974), activational deficits (Wolgin, Cytawa, & Teitelbaum, 1976), alterations in body weight set point (Powley & Keesey, 1970), and metabolic-visceral abnormalities, including stomach erosions (Grijalva, Lindholm, Schallert, & Bicknell, 1976; Lindholm, Shumway, Grijalva, Schallert, & Ruppel, 1975).

There is little doubt that any one of these disorders, and others as yet unidentified, can have disruptive effects on ingestive behaviors; however, the relative importance of each remains to be determined. One way to ascertain the relative degree of involvement of particular lesion-induced abnormalities to the initial ingestive deficits, or to the chronicity of dysfunctions that persist in the recovered animal, is to examine the effects that preoperative manipulations have on the syndrome that characterizes the LH-damaged animal. For example, adjustments in preoperative body weight or feeding experience, extrahypothalamic damage prior to LH lesions, or the preoperative administration of bioactive agents have been shown to either shorten or lengthen the periods of postoperative aphagia. Similarly, the extent to which a deficit is characterized as being permanent may depend on the experiences relevant to the deficit that the animal encounters prior to surgery. This chapter reviews some of the current literature indicating that preoperative experience can significantly and, in some cases, dramatically influence the postoperative effects of damage to the LH area.

THE LATERAL HYPOTHALAMIC
SYNDROME

Prolonged periods of aphagia and adipsia typically follow LH lesions and these may persist until death unless the animal is given special postoperative care (Anand & Brobeck, 1951; also see Epstein, 1971). Although the feeding deficits appear permanent, Teitelbaum and Stellar (1954) demonstrated that aphagic rats would eventually recover their feeding behavior if kept alive by intragastric tube feeding and then progressively weaned from highly palatable hydrated diets to ordinary laboratory food. In their landmark paper, Teitelbaum and Epstein (1962) extensively examined the effects of LH lesions in rats and concluded that there were four successive stages of recovery by which animals become more competent in fulfilling their nutritive requirements. In Stage I (aphagia and adipsia), animals refuse to eat or drink and will die of starvation or dehydration unless they are artificially maintained by gastric intubation. During this stage, rats show no interest in food and will actively resist any attempts to coax them to eat. Animals enter Stage II (anorexia and adipsia) when they accept food; however, eating is not accompanied by body weight regulation or caloric intake. During this stage of recovery, rats show interest only in wet, palatable, and odorous foods, which is taken to indicate that their acceptance of food depends on its orosensory qualities. Although these animals will sample hydrated foods they are adipsic, and it is typically necessary to continue the intubation procedure. In Stage III (adipsia with dehydration aphagia), the rats are still adipsic but are capable of regulating caloric intake on wet and palatable foods. Regulation is also maintained on dry foods if the animal is artificially hydrated or offered sweetened fluids. In Stage IV (recovery), the drinking of water returns and the animals are capable of regulating body weight on dry food and water. A photomicrograph of typical bilateral electrolytic LH lesions is shown in Fig. 3.1.

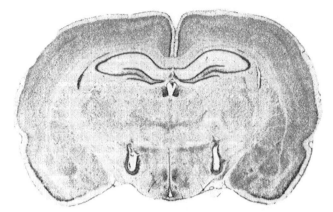

FIG. 3.1. Photomicrograph of typical bilateral LH lesions produced with elec-trolytic anodal current. Histological section taken from a rat 24 hours postopera-tively (Thionin stained). Reprinted with permission from [*Brain Research Bulletin*, 5(Suppl. 4), Grijalva, C. V., Novin, D., & Bray, G. A., Alterations in blood glucose, insulin, and free fatty acids following lateral hypothalamic lesions or parasagittal knife cuts], ©1980, Pergamon Press plc.

STAGE IV: RECOVERY?

It is clear that LH-damaged rats in a majority of experiments regain the ability to ingest standard laboratory chow and drink water to reach conditions of relative stability. It is only relative stability since they can survive without the nursing care of the experimenter but most certainly would not survive if subjected to severe physiological or environmental stressors. Epstein (1971) documented many of the deficits that tend to persist in Stage IV and they are briefly summa-rized here. Among their numerous deficits "recovered" rats drink water pran-dially (Kissileff, 1971; Kissileff & Epstein, 1969; Teitelbaum & Epstein, 1962), they have difficulty responding to hydrational challenges produced by cellular dehydration or extracellular hypovolemia (Stricker, 1976), and they fail to increase sodium intake following adrenalectomy (Wolf & Quartermain, 1967) or injections of desoxycorticosterone (Wolf, 1968). These animals also do not respond normally to particular stimuli which elicit feeding in the intact animal. For example, they do not typically increase their food intake in response to glucoprivation produced by the administration of insulin (Epstein & Teitel-baum, 1967) or 2-deoxy-D-glucose, an unmetabolizable glucose analog that decreases glucose utilization (Smith & Epstein, 1969; Wayner, Cott, Millner, & Tartagione, 1971). However, increases in feeding following glucoprivic chal-lenges can be induced in LH-lesioned rats if tested with palatable liquid diets as opposed to solid chow (Kanarek, Salomon, & Khadivi, 1981) or subjected to prolonged glucoprivation (Stricker, Friedman, & Zigmond, 1975). Recovered

LH animals are also thought to be more finicky eaters. In particular, they appear to be hyperresponsive to quinine adulteration of their food (Leach & Braun, 1976; Teitelbaum & Stellar, 1954). Rats in Stage IV do, however, respond normally to food deprivation and compensate for dilutions in caloric density (Epstein, 1971; Teitelbaum & Epstein, 1962), and will adjust their food intake to short-term changes in ambient temperature (Epstein & Teitelbaum, 1967). Nevertheless, LH-damaged rats display impairments in feeding behavior and body weight maintenance when subjected to prolonged cold exposure (Snyder & Stricker, 1985). Given the numerous persistent deficits, the "recovered" lateral animal is recovered only in the sense that it has regained sufficient homeostatic balance to survive in the sheltered laboratory environment.

PROPOSALS FOR INITIAL FEEDING DEFICITS

Although considerable research efforts have unveiled a spectrum of short- and long-term disorders in LH-damaged animals, the reasons for the initial aphagia and subsequent recovery of ingestive behaviors have yet to be firmly established. It is known that the period of aphagia is a function of the size and locus of the brain damage. Animals with unilateral or asymmetrical LH lesions recover more quickly than those with bilateral symmetrically placed lesions. Furthermore, large lesions produce prolonged periods of aphagia, which frequently necessitate gastric intubations to prevent death from inanition while small lesions produce temporary aphagia, which gives way to anorexia or hypophagia within a few days. Since animals with LH damage do recover their capacity to consume food and regulate body weight, the variables contributing to the initial feeding deficits and the possible mechanisms underlying functional recovery have received considerable attention.

Motivational Deficits. Teitelbaum and Epstein (1962) initially proposed that LH lesions interfere with motivational processes which underlie consummatory behaviors. According to their view, LH damage produces an apathetic animal which finds food and water aversive during the initial stages of recovery. The duration of the stages of recovery was said to be dependent on the locus and extent of brain damage, and the recovery process was thought to be mediated by surrounding undamaged tissue. Indeed, Teitelbaum and Epstein showed that aphagia and adipsia could be reinstated in otherwise recovered laterals by subjecting them to additional destruction of tissue adjacent to the initial lesions, and subsequent recovery was frequently prolonged and often incomplete. The possibility that recovery is based on spared neural tissue was further supported by Harrell, Raubeson, and Balagura (1974), who showed that the period of aphagia following mechanical LH lesions produced by chronically implanted macroelectrodes could be shortened by electrical stimulation through the same electrodes. These findings basically support the idea that recovery is mediated by intact neural tissue, although it is unclear whether recovery is the result of remaining intact LH neurons or due to regional changes in the functioning of adjacent axonal pathways (Grossman, 1979).

Motor Deficits.   Morrison (Baillie & Morrison, 1963; Morrison, 1968) interpreted the feeding deficits as the consequence of motor dysfunctions, proposing that the LH animal is motivated to eat but is unable, because of apraxia produced by the lesion. These investigators found that rats with LH lesions would not ingest food orally but would press a lever to obtain intragastric injections of food. Although there is general agreement that LH damage can produce transient motor dysfunctions, Rodgers, Epstein, and Teitelbaum (1965) subsequently showed that the syndrome could not be explained by motor deficits alone. When given a choice between orally consuming highly palatable foods or obtaining a liquid diet by intragastric injections, LH-damaged rats accepted the palatable foods before bar pressing for intragastric feedings. Rodgers and colleagues argued that Baillie and Morrison (1963) used a diet of minimal palatability to test feeding by mouth which would tend to reflect finickiness rather than LH aphagia. Others have also found little or no relationship between general motor disabilites and periods of aphagia or anorexia observed in animals given LH lesions (Balagura, Wilcox, & Coscina, 1969; Grijalva & Lindholm, 1980; Karli & Vergnes, 1964).

Sensory Neglect and Loss of Endogenous Activation.   Although the initial feeding deficits induced by LH lesions are not reliably associated with specific motor impairments, considerable evidence suggests that sensorimotor dysfunctions contribute to the periods of aphagia and anorexia. Marshall (Marshall & Teitelbaum, 1974; Marshall, Turner, & Teitelbaum, 1971) showed that LH damage in rats produces deficits in orientation to visual, olfactory, and tactile stimuli associated with food and that the transition from Stage I (aphagia) to Stage II (anorexia) occurs with the return of orientation to olfactory stimuli and whisker touch. The sensorimotor dysfunctions and ingestive deficits produced by LH damage have been attributed to disruption of the pallidofugal fiber system and, in particular, dopaminergic nigrostriatal projections (Marshall, Richardson, & Teitelbaum, 1974; Morgane, 1961a, 1961b; see also Stricker & Zigmond, 1976; Ungerstedt, 1971; White, 1986). The importance of facial and orosensory reflexes have also been emphasized by Zeigler and Karten (1974), however, they viewed the consummatory deficits attributed to LH lesions as being the result of damage to trigeminal pathways which course through adjoining diencephalic areas.

In addition to the possible contribution of sensory neglect or related sensorimotor dysfunctions to LH aphagia, the loss of endogenous activation also has been implicated (Wolgin, Cytawa, & Teitelbaum, 1976). Rats with large LH lesions display somnolence, catalepsy, and akinesia (Balagura et al., 1969; Levitt & Teitelbaum, 1975; Marshall & Teitelbaum, 1974). During the early stages of recovery this display of deficits in wakefulness and spontaneity is believed to be related to damage to the reticular activating system which courses through the LH area (Wolgin et al., 1976). This interpretation is supported by the findings that intense stimuli such as pain or cold (Levitt & Teitelbaum, 1975; Marshall, Levitan, & Stricker, 1976) or stimulant drugs such as amphetamines (Wolgin et al., 1976; also see Stricker & Zigmond, 1976) elicit eating in anorexic (Stage II) rats. These manipulations are believed to have a strong effect on the remaining intact reticular system.

The sensory neglect-loss of endogenous activation explanations are reminiscent of motor deficit hypothesis, but shifts the emphasis away from the inability to make motor responses. Instead, these explanations focus on the animal's inability to utilize sensory cues signaling the availability of food and the lack of background activation necessary to sustain feeding behavior.

Change in Body Weight Set Point.   Powley and Keesey (1970) proposed that LH damage alters the set point for body weight regulation and that the reinstatement of eating is a function of a new, lowered set point induced by the damage. Two findings in particular support the set point hypothesis. First, several investigations have demonstrated that animals with LH lesions maintain chronically lowered body weight levels relative to controls, and that the new, lowered levels are actively defended when the animal is calorically challenged (e.g., Keesey, Boyle, Kemnitz, & Mitchel, 1976; Keesey & Corbett, 1984). Secondly, animals subjected to approximately a 20% reduction in body weight by restricting their food intake prior to surgery show a dramatic attenuation in the period of aphagia after LH lesions (Balagura & Harrell, 1974; Grijalva, Lindholm, Schallert, & Bicknell, 1976; Mufson & Wampler, 1972; Powley & Keesey, 1970; Schallert & Whishaw, 1978). According to Powley and Keesey's original hypothesis, animals will either eat or not eat to attain their new body weight set points established by the lesions. Consequently, animals preoperative reduced in body weight will already approximate their new set points and should therefore display little, if any, aphagia. Furthermore, the loss in body weight will be proportional to the amount of LH damage; consequently, more extensive damage will lead to lower "target weights" and longer periods of aphagia.

Visceral Abnormalities.   Changes in visceral and metabolic functions have been shown to occur following various diencephalic manipulations. In particular, stimulation or destruction of the LH and adjoining areas can produce pronounced gastrointestinal changes (see Grijalva & Lindholm, 1982; Grijalva, Lindholm, & Novin, 1980; Powley, Opsahl, Cox, & Weingarten, 1980). In

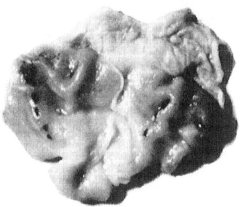

FIG. 3.2. Representative rat stomach exhibiting erosions of the glandular mucosa 24 hours after bilateral LH lesions. Reprinted with permission from [Brain Research Bulletin, 10(4), Grijalva, C. V., Tordoff, M. G., Geiselman, P. J., & Novin, D., Gastric mucosal damage induced by lateral hypothalamic lesions in rats: The potential contribution of bile], ©1983, Pergamon Press plc.

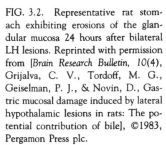

their initial studies on feeding behavior after LH lesions, Teitelbaum and Epstein (1962) noted in postmortem examinations of rats that had died following a period of aphagia, some showed massive stomach ulceration and hemorrhage. Although the gastric ulcers reported by them may have been related to the effects of starvation induced by the brain lesions, Lindholm and colleagues (1975) subsequently showed that stomach erosions were a direct consequence of hypothalamic damage. Rats with LH lesions developed gastric mucosal erosions within 24 hours postoperatively and the severity of the erosions increased during a 4-day observation period. Furthermore, these effects could not be accounted for by food or water deprivation, or damage to regions of the overlying thalamus. These results lead to the speculation that gastrointestinal dysfunctions or other viscerometabolic disorders induced by LH damage could have disruptive effects on subsequent feeding, and that the rate of initial postoperative recovery may be related to the severity of the viscerometabolic abnormalities. A representative stomach taken from an LH-lesioned rat 24 hours postoperatively is shown in Fig. 3.2.

Summary

Several hypotheses have been advanced to account for the feeding deficits which result from LH damage and the mechanisms involved recovery of function. In contrast to the persistent deficits noted in Stage IV, the visceral, sensorimotor, and activational disorders appear to be temporary, since the transition from Stage I to Stage II coincides with the decrease in the severity of these disorders.

Obviously, LH damage severely disrupts but does not abolish ingestive behaviors. The reinstatement of feeding behaviors may reflect the active process of attaining a new lowered body weight set point rather than recovery per se (Powley & Keesey, 1970). Conversely, the fact that animals can regain some capacity to regulate caloric intake after near-total destruction of the LH proper strongly suggests that extrahypothalamic influences are involved in the recovery process. Undoubtedly, the LH syndrome involves a complex interaction of physiological and behavioral disorders in which each stage or recovery is a function of the relative severity of these disorders and certain compensatory changes that occur both centrally and peripherally.

One general approach in evaluating the possible mechanisms involved in recovery of function following LH damage has been to examine the effects that certain preoperative manipulations have on the early stages of the LH syndrome.

PREOPERATIVE INFLUENCES ON FUNCTIONAL RECOVERY

Recovery Based on Neurochemical or Morphological Changes.   The far-lateral aspect of the LH lacks cellular uniformity and is known to be comprised primarily of a large number of ascending and descending neural pathways having their origin in extrahypothalamic structures. Of these systems the nigrostriatal bundle, which contains catecholaminergic neurons, has received considerable attention. Numerous studies have shown that persistent aphagia and adipsia can be produced by intracerebral injections of 6-hydroxydopamine (6-HDA), a neurotoxin which markedly depletes brain catecholamines, dopamine (DA), and norepinephrine (NE). Additionally, marked depletions in these catecholamines occur following LH lesions which produce aphagia and anorexia. Based on these and related findings, Stricker and Zigmond (1976) proposed a neurochemical model for the LH syndrome. Briefly, LH damage or the administration of certain neurotoxins, such as 6-HDA, produces less than total damage to central catecholamine-containing neurons and fibers. Immediately after the lesion there is a reduction in the net amount of catecholamine (CA) release which is proportional to the number of remaining undamaged neurons. The decreases in CA release, coupled with reduced receptor activation, causes an increase in the turnover and synthesis of CA in the residual neurons. Increases in CA are reflected by increased biosynthesis of tyrosine hydroxylase, a necessary enzyme for CA production. Likewise, increased enzymatic activity increases the capacity of residual cells to sustain elevated CA turnover. According to Stricker and Zigmond (1976) functional recovery is thus promoted to the elevation in CA turnover, the induction of supersensitivity of postsynaptic receptors, possibly eventual axonal sprouting, and compensatory functional adjustments in other neural systems which utilize other transmitter substances.

As appealing as the neurochemical model is in accounting for the feeding and drinking deficits and functional recovery associated with the LH syndrome, various lines of evidence question the central role that the nigrostriatial dopamine system is presumed to play in ingestive behaviors. It has been reported that LH lesions which deplete striatal DA levels by 50%–60% produce persistent aphagia and adipsia followed by serious long-term regulatory deficits, and these effects are not mimicked by intraventricular injections of 6-HDA unless striatal DA is depleted by 95% or more (Grossman, 1979). Additionally, rats treated with 6-HDA show some but not all components of the LH syndrome and the results are variable (cf. Fig. 5, Stricker & Zigmond, 1976). Furthermore, it has been shown that damage to striatal nondopaminergic neurons produced by intracaudate injections of kainic acid leads to periods of aphagia and adipsia, as well as other behavioral abnormalities, similar to those seen following lesions in the dopaminergic nigrostriatal bundle (Pettibone et al., 1978). Similar depressions in food and water intake have been shown to occur following the peripheral administration of the DA antagonist, domperidone, which does not cross the blood-brain barrier (Willis, Smith, & Kinchington, 1983). Thus, damage of the nigrostriatal dopaminergic system can undoubtedly disrupt ingestive behaviors and effect homeostatic processes, but the LH syndrome cannot be fully accounted for on this basis.

With regard to functional recovery, one possible mechanisms underlying the recovery process of LH-damaged rats, which has gained popular support in recent years, is that of supersensitivity. Supersensitivity is a well-known phenomenon in the peripheral nervous system (Sharpless, 1964), although denervation and pharmacological supersensitivity-like responses also have been described to occur in the central nervous system (for a recent review, see Marshall, 1984). Briefly, supersensitivity refers to an increase in responsiveness of an end organ or neuron after denervation, decentralization, or the administration of certain drugs. Both presynaptic and postsynaptic events are thought to occur. First, under normal circumstances, presynaptic terminals act to remove exogenous transmitter substance by their potent uptake mechanism. When these presynaptic terminals are partly denervated or pharmacologically blocked with an antagonist drug, they no longer are functional in the uptake process, thus making more transmitter substance available to the postsynaptic site. Secondly, the elimination of the transmitter substance by total (decentralization) or neartotal denervation or pharmacological blockade is believed to produce supersensitivity by increasing the sensitivity of the postsynaptic terminal. Basically, increased sensitivity of the postsynaptic site (receptor supersensitivity) is a pharmacological concept which implies a shift of agonist dose–response curves to lower concentrations. It has been suggested that the chemical changes occurring during increased sensitivity may act as a stimulus to elicit collateral sprouting in remaining intact axons adjoining the denervated neurons (Glick, 1974; Goldberger, 1974).

Supersensitivity has been advanced as a possible mechanism leading to enhanced LH recovery following the administration of various agents. Glick (Glick & Greenstein, 1974; Glick, Greenstein, & Zimmerberg, 1972) reported

that intraperitoneal injections of alpha-methyl-para-tyrosine (AMT) either pre-
or postoperatively facilitated recovery following LH lesions. Because AMT reduces brain levels of DA and NE it was proposed that AMT induces pharmacological supersensitivity of remaining neurons subserving recovery. Similarly,
Balagura, Harrell, and Ralph (1973) found that the period of LH aphagia could
be lengthened by preoperative subcutaneous glucagon injections or shortened by
insulin injections. The mechanisms underlying the effects of glucagon on the
prolongation of the feeding deficits in LH lesioned rats are not known. On the
other hand, insulin has been shown to alter adrenal levels of both tyrosine
hydroxylase and dopamine-beta hydroxylase, two enzymes necessary in the con-
version of tyrosine to NE (Weiner & Mosimann, 1970). Based on this finding,
Balagura and colleagues suggested that insulin, like AMT, facilitates recovery of
feeding behaviors by inducing a pharmacological denervation supersensitivity in
noradrenergic systems in the brain. Compatible with this view, studies have
generally reported a facilitation of recovery after LH damage when agents which
inhibit the activity of central catecholaminerigic receptors are administered
preoperatively over a course of several days (e.g., Hynes, Anderson, Gianutsos,
& Lal, 1975).

The contribution of NE to the recovery of feeding behavior has been implicated by Berger, Wise, and Stein (1971). They injected NE into the lateral
ventricles of LH-damaged rats recovering from anorexia (Stage II). This caused
an immediate feeding response, sometimes followed by overeating. Intraventricular injections of dopamine did not significantly facilitate feeding, suggesting that recovery after LH lesions coincides with recovery of adrenergic
function. In an extension of their previous work, Berger and colleagues (Berger,
Wise, & Stein, 1973) demonstrated that intraventricular administration of
nerve-growth factor (NGF), a protein structurally similar to insulin, also has a
facilitating effect on recovery. In their study two groups of rats were given
bilateral LH lesions and simultaneous implants of a cannula into the lateral
ventricle. Following the implant one group received an intraventricular injection of NGF while the other received an injection of saline. Rats treated with
NGF initially lost more weight than saline treated animals, but by the second
postoperative week their weight gains surpassed those of controls. During the
third week of recovery, intraventricular injections of NE into saline-treated LH
animals facilitated eating, but similar NE injections into NGF-treated LH rats
caused them to eat twice as vigorously. Berger et al. (1973) proposed that NGF
might temporarily interfere with input to remaining LH neurons and thus facilitate the development of supersensitivity during the initial postoperative periods.
During later stages of recovery NGF might promote the regeneration of reversi-
bly damaged noradrenergic neurons, as previously demonstrated by others
(Björklund & Stenevi, 1972).

Recovery Based on Preoperative Body Weight.   Powley and Keesey (1970)
were the first to show that the period of aphagia following LH lesions in rats

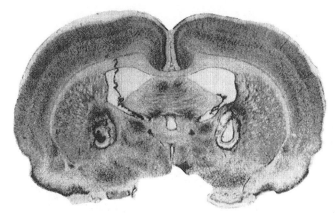

FIG. 3.3. Photomicrograph of representative bilateral globus pallidus lesions (Thionin stained).

could be dramatically shortened by gradually reducing their body weights prior to surgery. As mentioned earlier, this was taken as evidence for a reduced body weight set point following LH damage. However, it now appears that neither the chronic postoperative reductions in body weight nor the facilitatory influence of preoperative weight reduction on recovery are unique to the LH syndrome. For example, Grijalva (1980a) reduced two groups of rats to 80% of their initial body weight by restricting food intake (dieting) over a 2-week period. Two additional groups were maintained at normal weight by allowing them to feed *ad libitum* during the same period. One dieted and one normal weight group received bilateral electrolytic lesions of the globus pallidus (GP), an example of which is shown in Fig. 3.3. The remaining dieted and normal weight groups were given control operations. As represented in Fig. 3.4, preoperative dieting significantly shortened the period of aphagia induced by the brain lesions. The GP lesion-dieted group was aphagia for a mean of 2.4 days while the GP lesion-normal weight group was aphagic for 5 days. Both groups, however, were anorexic for about 2 or 3 days. Two months following surgery, both the dieted and normal weight groups with GP lesions were approximately 20% lower in body weight relative to both control-operated groups. In a manner similar to that seen in LH-damaged rats, dieting attenuated the period of aphagia following GP lesions and did not alter body weight maintenance, which was chronically reduced. These results generally support the view that certain aspects of the LH syndrome may be due to interruption of catecholaminergic fibers originating in the globus pallidus or other structures of the corpus striatum.

Kolb, Whishaw, and Schallert (1977) examined the effects of preoperative dieting or fattening in rats given ablations of the orbital frontal neocortex. They found that animals preoperatively dieted to 80% body weight did not exhibit a significant facilitation of recovery; however, those fattened to 120% body

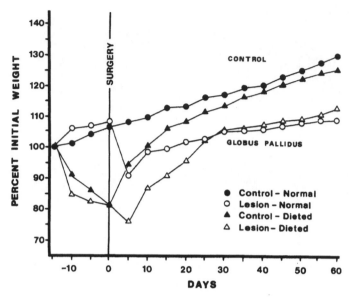

FIG. 3.4.   Mean percentage of body weight following globus pallidue lesions or control operations on dieted and normal weight rats ($n = 8$ per group).

weight displayed feeding deficits that were more pronounced than either normal weight or dieted animals. Nevertheless, preoperatively normal, dieted, or fattened rats all maintained a chronically reduced body weight level that was approximately 25% lower than controls.

The potential importance of extrahypothalamic influences and body weight level to the expression of the LH syndrome has also been demonstrated in studies employing multiple lesions. Glick and Greenstein (1972a) bilaterally ablated the frontal neocortex and the LH of rats simultaneously or ablated the frontal neocortex 10 or 30 days prior to LH lesions. They found that simultaneous LH and neocortical lesions produced terminal aphagia and adipsia equaling that of LH lesions alone (7 to 8 days with no recovery). Rats that were given frontal neocortical lesions 10 days prior to LH lesions were likewise aphagic and adipsic for about 8.5 days and also did not recover; however, their weight loss was significantly slower than those given either LH lesions alone or simultaneous LH and neocortical ablations. In contrast, animals given neocortical ablations 30 days prior to LH lesions were aphagic and adipsic for only 1 to 5 days. Furthermore, posterior neocortical ablations given 30 days prior to LH lesions did not facilitate recovery. According to Glick and Greenstein, ablation of the frontal neocortex 30 days prior to LH lesions may have facilitated recovery by inducing a time-dependent denervation supersensitivity in remaining intact LH neurons following the removal of noradrenergic input in LH area, or possibly that sprouting of intact input to the remaining LH had occurred. On the other hand, it is will documented that ablations of the frontal neocortex in rats produce a reduction in food intake and body weight (Braun, 1975; Glick, 1971; Grijalva, Kiefer, Gunion, Cooper, & Novin, 1985; Kolb & Nonneman, 1975; Kolb et al., 1977), and may therefore mimic the effects of preoperative dieting. Some support for the latter idea was obtained by Kolb, Nonneman, and Whishaw (1978). In their study, orbital frontal neocortical ablations were followed by aphagia, adipsia, and chronically reduced body weight to approximately 85% of controls. In agreement with previous findings (Glick & Greenstein, 1972a), rats given LH lesions exhibited a shortened period of postoperative aphagia if they had sustained frontal neocortical ablations several weeks prior. However, facilitation of recovery after LH damage did not occur if the reductions in body weight induced by prior orbital frontal neodecortications were prevented by allowing the animals to eat fattening diets. Interestingly, facilitation of recovery was also observed when the surgical procedures were reversed, that is, LH lesions given several weeks prior to frontal neocortical damage, so long as the animals were not fattened prior to the second brain operation. They further showed that unilateral lesions of either the orbital frontal neocortex or LH had little effect of food intake, but unilateral ablations of the frontal neocortex combined with a contralateral unilateral LH lesions produced feeding and drinking deficits similar to bilateral damage to either of these two structures alone.

Although the findings of Kolb and colleagues (1978) suggest that the facilitation of recovery from LH lesions induced by prior extrahypothalamic damage may be partly related to some body weight regulatory process, Misantone, Schaffer, and Lombardi (1980) showed that recovery from LH damage in rats could be enhanced by prior neocortical lesions without significant alterations in body weight. These researchers produced unilateral ablations of the rostral neocortex in groups of rats and then subjected them to either an ipsilateral or a contralateral unilateral LH lesion 30 days later. Body weights of rats with unilateral neocortical ablations were not significantly different from intact controls on the day prior to LH lesions. Rats given a unilateral neocortical ablation prior to an ipsilateral LH lesion recovered feeding behavior and body weight more rapidly than those given a unilateral neocortical ablation plus a unilateral contralateral LH lesion, or a unilateral LH lesion alone. When the sequence of the lesions was reversed, that is, a unilateral LH lesion followed 30 days later by either an ipsilateral or contralateral neocortical ablation, no facilitation of recovery occurred. In agreement with earlier findings (Kolb et al., 1978), Misantone and colleagues (1980) found that rats were more deficient in their feeding behaviors and showed greater weight losses when given a unilateral ablation of the rostral neocortex and a contralateral LH lesion, in either order. In some respects, the additive effects of unilateral contralateral LH-frontal neodecortical lesions are compatible with the view that recovery from LH damage is based on re-encephalization as described by Teitelbaum (1971). However, the re-encephalization hypothesis can not fully account for the findings that prior bilateral frontal neodecortications actually facilitate recovery from subsequent LH damage rather than retard it, so long as sufficient time elapses between surgeries (Glick & Greenstein, 1972a; Kolb et al., 1978), unless one assumes that undamaged neocortical areas remaining after the ablations take over the regulation of feeding in a manner similar to the mass action, equipotentiality phenomenon described by Lashley (1929).

While the results of Misantone and coworkers (1980) indicate that LH recovery can be facilitated by prior neocortical ablation without altering body weight levels, there are some notable differences between their study and that of Kolb et al. (1978). For example, Kolb, Nonneman, and Whishaw examined the effects of bilateral LH lesions and bilateral neocortical ablation placed in the region of the rhinal sulcus in male rats, whereas, Misantone's group employed unilateral LH lesions plus unilateral neocortical ablations placed more dorsally in female rats. In addition to the differences in brain damage between these two studies, it is well known that female rats regulate body weight quite differently from males and, hence, may exhibit a different pattern of ingestion-related deficits and recovery processes following LH damage. It is also interesting to note that although the nigrostriatal dopamine system has been strongly implicated in the LH syndrome (e.g., Stricker & Zigmond, 1976), and the frontal neocortex receives projections from this system (Fallon & Moore, 1978; Lindvall, Björklund, & Divac, 1978), the acceleration of recovery in unilaterally LH lesioned rats could not be accounted for by an increase in DA content in the neostriatum following unilateral neocortical damage (Misantone et al., 1980). Although there appears to be no significant increase in brain DA levels following rostral neocortical lesions (Misantone et al., 1980), other compensatory mechanisms involving either dopaminergic or nondopaminergic systems, such as increased transmitter turnover rates, supersensitivity, or axonal sprouting, may partly contribute to the subsequent enhancement in LH recovery. On the other hand, damage to the anterolateral neocortex, a receptive field for nigrostriatal dopaminergic projections, tends to spare rats of most of the chronic regulatory impairments seen after LH lesions (Grijalva et al., 1985), and these findings imply that the nigrostriatal projections to this region of the neocortex plays a relatively minor role in the regulation of ingestion.

The studies presently highlighted emphasize the relationship between preoperative experience, body weight levels, and neurochemical or morphological changes in the recovery process following brain damage. Consideration of these factors might be adequate for generalized theories on recovery of function but do not take into account the fact that, unlike most other behaviors, ingestive behaviors and energy balance involve complex interactions between central and peripheral mechanisms. Given the fact that visceral and metabolic processes are major components of consummatory behaviors, it is surprising just how little attention has been given to the role of peripheral mechanisms in functional recovery of feeding behaviors following brain damage. Indeed, recent studies suggest that viscero-metabolic disorders produced by LH damage may strongly contribute to the initial feeding deficits, and that the early stages of recovery may be based on *peripheral* as well as central mechanisms.

Recovery Based on Peripheral Processes.   Interest in visceral malfunctions produced by brain damage spans several decades and has been the subject of recent reviews (Grijalva, 1985; Grijalva, Lindholm, & Novin, 1980; Henke, 1979, 1982). Of particular interest for the present discussion are the effects of LH lesions on visceral and metabolic functions and their relationship to feeding behavior. As previously mentioned, Lindholm and colleagues (1975) demonstrated that ulceration of the stomach in rats is a direct consequence of LH damage, and they raised the possibility that gastric pathology contributes to the periods of aphagia and anorexia. In a subsequent study (Grijalva et al., 1976) the relationship between gastric pathology and aphagia produced by LH lesions was further examined. Previous reports had shown that if the body weight of rats was preoperatively reduced to 80% of normal weight by restricting the amount of daily food ration (dieting), LH lesions did not produce aphagia (e.g., Powley & Keesey, 1970). Grijalva et al. reasoned that, if gastric ulcers produced by LH lesions are importantly involved in feeding behavior, it must follow that preoperative dieting must somehow prevent ulcer formation since preoperative dieting prevents aphagia. The results were confirmatory (Grijalva et al., Experiment 1). Preoperative dieting not only dramatically shortened the period of postoperative aphagia but also dramatically truncated the appearance of gastric erosions (see Fig. 3.5). In a second experiment, the authors again reduced preoperative body weight to 80% of normal, but by two different methods. One method was the dieting regimen employed in the first experiment, but the second method was to reduce body weight by withholding all food but not water for 6 days (fasting). This was an attempt to discriminate between the set point hypothesis and the hypothesis that gastric pathology contributes importantly to aphagia. That is, a strict interpretation of the set point hypothesis would predict that rats reduced to 80% body weight by whatever means, should not be aphagic postoperatively since their body weights are below the new, postoperative set point. The "ulcer hypothesis," on the other hand, would predict that body weight per se is not important for the initiation of feeding, but that the condition of the stomach is important. Again, the results supported that latter hypothesis: Preoperatively fasted animals displayed longer periods of aphagia and greater gastric pathology than preoperatively dieted animals.

The importance of the method of weight reduction versus absolute body weight level to the initial recovery from LH damage was investigated further by Grijalva and Lindholm (1980). These investigators found that reductions in

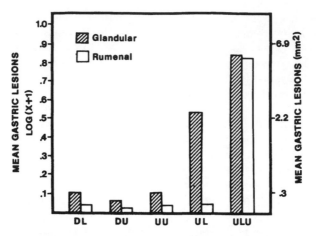

FIG. 3.5. Mean gastric lesions expressed as total area of damage (right ordinate), and as transformed scores used in statistical analysis (left ordinate) in groups of LH-lesioned or nonlesioned rats that were either at normal body weight (undieted) or preoperatively dieted to 80% of normal weight. Abbreviations: DL, dieted-LH lesion; DU, dieted-unoperated; UU, undieted-unoperated; UL, undieted-LH lesion; ULU, undieted-LH lesion-unyoked. Rats in groups DL, DU, UU, and UL were yoked, so that when an animal in either Group DL or UL first accepted food, it was sacrificed along with a rat of comparable pretreatment body weight in each of the other three groups. This was done so that stomachs could be evaluated at a time when aphagia terminated. Rats in Group ULU were not yoked to animals in any other group and were sacrificed when they independently accepted food, reached 65% body weight, or appeared close to death. Following a 20-hr postoperative deprivation period, rats in Group DL ($n = 10$) were aphagic for a mean of 7 hr. Of rats in Group ULU ($n = 10$), 5 were aphagic for a mean of 54 hr., 4 did not recover after several days of aphagia and were sacrificed because death was imminent, the remaining rat was prematurely sacrificed and eliminated from the study (adapted from Grijalva et al., 1976).

body weight to 95%, 85%, or 75% of normal weight by restricting food intake over a 2- or 3-week period, similarly shortened the period of postoperative aphagia, reduced the incidence of gastric pathology, and prevented the hyperthermia. Furthermore, animals preoperatively reduced in body weight displayed less pronounced deficits associated with tactile stimulation following LH lesions, but other motor and sensorimotor dysfunctions remained relatively unaltered. These results are in general agreement with the previous findings of Schallert and Whishaw (1978).

These results demonstrate a close correspondence between the presence of gastric pathology and the presence of aphagia, but it is unlikely that gastric pathology alone "causes" aphagia. Schallert, Whishaw, and Flannigan (1977) varied lesion locus and size and reported that the presence of gastric pathology produced by brain damage was not necessarily associated with aphagia. Additionally, Ruppel and Lindholm (unpublished observations, 1975) intubated anesthetized rats with a solution of HCl sufficiently dilute to produce gastric erosions comparable to that seen following LH damage. A control group was intubated with a similar volume of saline, and food intake and body weight were tracked for several days. The rats intubated with saline ate normal amounts of food and showed no change in their body weight functions, but rats intubated with HCl were typically hypophagic (not aphagic) and lost weight for about 2 days, then resumed normal food intake and regained body weights to control levels. These results in conjunction with those of Schallert et al. suggest that gastric pathology is not necessary for the appearance of aphagia, but may be sufficient for the appearance of hypophagia.

The mechanisms underlying the facilitation of recovery induced by restricted feeding regimens are not presently known; however, various possibilities might be suggested. For example, neurochemical changes in the brain produced by several days of food deprivation may influence the rate of recovery from LH damage (Balagura, Harrell, & DeCastro, 1978; Isaacson, 1974). Undernourished infant rats have reduced levels of NE in the brain (Sereni, Principi, Perletti, & Sereni, 1966; Shoemaker & Wurtman, 1971). In turn, lowered levels of NE are assumed to induce supersensitivity. Compatible with this notion, Glick and Greenstein (1972b) discovered that rats deprived of food and water for 2 days prior to surgery tended to survive longer and lose less body weight following LH lesions than animals not deprived. However, it is presently not known whether 2 days of starvation produced sufficient reductions in brain catecholamines to induce supersensitivity. On the other hand, recent findings indicate that restricted feeding regimens can alter the pattern of plasma corticosterone secretion and levels of monoamines in various limbic structures (Krieger, Crowley, O'Donohue, & Jacobowitz, 1980), although the significance of these alterations to the rate of recovery in LH-damaged animals remains unknown.

Alternatively, restricted feeding regimens produce adjustments in metabolic processes associated with increased efficiency in the absorption and utilization of nutrients (Chakrabarty & Leveille, 1968; Leveille, 1970; Wiley & Leveille, 1970), and reduced energy expenditure as reflected by a decrease in oxygen consumption (Keesey, Corbett, Hirvonen, & Kaufman, 1984), suggesting a possible physiological basis for the dieting effect (Grijalva & Lindholm, 1980; Grijalva et al., 1976). Immediately following LH lesions, rats display gastric pathology (Grijalva, Deregnaucourt, Code, & Novin, 1980; Lindholm et al., 1975), abnormally high metabolic rates with concomitant increases in body temperature and accelerated weight loss (Grijalva & Lindholm, 1980; Harrell, DeCastro, & Balagura, 1975; Keesey et al., 1984; Lindholm et al., 1975; Morgane, 1961a; Schallert & Whishaw, 1978; Stevenson & Montemurro, 1963), hypersalivation (Grijalva, Deregnaucourt et al., 1980; Schallert, Leach, &

Braun, 1978) and abnormal lacrimation (Grijalva, Deregnaucourt et al., 1980; Grijalva, Novin, & Bray, 1980). The antecedents of these abnormalities are not understood, but there is a tendency for them to wane at about the same time that voluntary ingestion of food reappears. Interestingly, preoperative restricted feeding dramatically retards, and in some cases totally prevents, the occurrence of the viscerometabolic disorders induced by LH damage, leading to the hypothesis that the generalized reduction in metabolic rate associated with restricted feeding regimens may form the physiological basis for its prophylactic effect.

Peripheral involvement in the initial stages of the LH syndrome is implicated further in studies demonstrating enhanced recovery of feeding behaviors produced by treatments that do not employ direct preoperative adjustments in feeding behavior or body weight. For example, Balagura and colleagues (1973) showed that the period of aphagia following LH lesions could be significantly shortened by pretreating rats with insulin. Grijalva (1980b) replicated this general finding; however, he reported that the administration of insulin also attenuated the occurrence of gastric pathology, but did not prevent the development of hyperthermia or reduce the severity of sensorimotor dysfunctions following LH lesions. Thus, it was shown that the initiation of feeding behaviors could occur in the presence of pronounced sensorimotor dysfunctions, and that recovery could be accelerated without alterations in preoperative body weight. These results were in contradiction to the sensorimotor deficit hypothesis and the set point hypothesis, and it appeared that the reinstatement of eating corresponded best with a reduction in the severity of gastric pathology. Grijalva (1980b) argued, therefore, that although insulin may influence recovery by preoperatively altering brain neurochemical processes, as suggested by Balagura et al. (1973), part of its protective effects could also be based on alterations in viscerometabolic functions that may parallel those induced by restricted feeding regimens.

A more convincing demonstration of the potential involvement of peripheral factors in the early stages of the LH syndrome was presented by Grijalva, Novin, and Cooper (1980). In this study, immediately prior to LH lesions, groups of rats received either a single subcutaneous injection of saline or propantheline bromide, an anticholinergic that does not readily cross the blood-brain barrier. Rats receiving saline injections were aphagic for a mean of 6.6 days and 6 of 9 rats in this group never actively ate. In contrast, propantheline-treated rats were aphagic for only a mean of 2 days and, as shown in Fig. 3.6, began to regulate body weight by Day 4 or 5 postoperatively.

These results are striking in view of the fact that recovery was dramatically facilitated by a single injection administered at the time of surgery and can not be accounted for by traditional explanations. For example, current theories of recovery of function after LH damage emphasize the role of body weight, neurochemical changes associated with denervation supersensitivity, morphological changes involving neuronal regenerative processes, or other compensatory

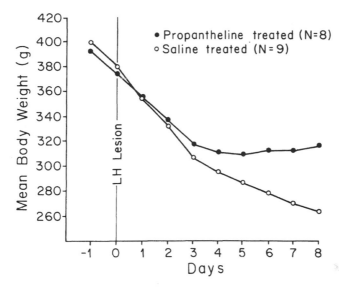

FIG. 3.6.   Mean postoperative body weight following propantheline treatment in LH-lesioned rats. Reprinted with permission from [*Brain Research Bulletin*, 5 (5), Grijalva, C. V., Novin, D., & Cooper, P. H., Facilitation of recovery by propantheline bromide after lateral hypothalamic damage], ©1980, Pergamon Press plc.

mechanisms involving central mechanisms, exclusively. Because rats were not reduced in body weight prior to surgery, it is clear that the set point hypothesis is inadequate to explain the results obtained with propantheline. Furthermore, the time course generally thought to be required for the induction of denervation supersensitivity or neuronal regeneration does not coincide with the rapid recovery of feeding behaviors seen in propantheline-treated animals, although recent studies indicate that the initial onset of pharmacological supersensitivity of DA receptors following intracerebral 6-HDA administration can take place within 1.5 to 3 days and reaches near maximal levels within 2 weeks (Neve, Kozlowski, & Marshall, 1982). Even so, it is unclear how a peripherally acting anticholinergic could induce supersensitivity centrally of a sufficient magnitude to induce a behavioral change (i.e., increased eating) within 1 to 2 days. A more parsimonious explanation is that propantheline facilitates recovery by preventing the occurrence of many of the viscerometabolic disorders induced by LH damage (Grijalva, Novin, & Cooper, 1980). Compatible with this view, Grijalva, Deregnaucourt et al., (1980) showed that similar injections of propantheline blocked the occurrence of stomach erosions, hypersalivation, and excessive tearing caused by LH lesions in rats. Thus, one could view the initial stages of the LH syndrome as a state of general debilitation and "ill health" brought about by an abrupt, severe disruption in autonomic or metabolic processes which are normally involved in the maintenance of homeostasis (Grijalva, Deregnacourt et al., 1980; Grijalva & Lindholm, 1980; Grijalva, Novin, & Cooper, 1980; Tordoff et al., 1984). By preventing the onset of viscerometabolic abnormalities, by whatever means, animals with LH damage would be more inclined to initiate a meal postoperatively in the presence of other behavioral deficits (e.g., motor, sensorimotor, activational) associated with the damage and, as a consequence, reduce the likelihood of further debilitation associated with subsequent starvation.

Recovery Based on Preoperative Experience.   As highlighted in the previous sections, considerable evidence has accumulated in support of the involvement of both central and peripheral factors in the rate of recovery of ingestive behaviors following LH damage. For the most part, research efforts have been concentrated on either the initial feeding and drinking deficits and the possible underlying causes, or on the identification of permanent deficits in animals that have recovered sufficiently to ingest food and water on their own. However, recent studies examining various aspects of the LH syndrome indicate that the manner in which certain short-term and long-term abnormalities are expressed is greatly dependent on the postoperative testing procedures as well as the preoperative experiences an animal has acquired that are relevant to the abnormality in question. Exactly when an animal begins to accept water, food, or both mixed together is a function not only of lesion size but of the palatability of the offered substances. Sweetened water is accepted before plain water, and foods high in carbohydrates (e.g., pulverized chocolate chip cookies, nutritive liquid diets such as human infant formulas) are accepted before standard laboratory chow. However, the extent to which animals are initially accepting of these atypical diets postoperatively is dependent on whether or not they were exposed to the diets prior to surgery (DiCara, 1970). Thus, how one initially quantifies aphagia and adipsia is greatly dependent on the test procedures as well as the novelty and palatability of the ingestant.

The importance of preoperative experience to the duration of LH aphagia is well illustrated by studies employing manipulations of body weight and feeding schedules; however, recent findings indicate that the severity of postoperative adipsia as well as the manifestation of various "chronic" deficits may also depend heavily on the type of experiences the animal has encountered prior to surgery. For example, Schallert (1982) found that the adipsia typically induced by LH lesions in rats could be significantly attenuated or completely eliminated by exposing the animals to a restricted daily water regimen for approximately 2 weeks prior to surgery. Furthermore, he reported that total water deprivation for 48–72 hours prior to surgery did not provide protection against the postoperative adipsia. These results are quite similar in nature to the differential effects of dieting and fasting on feeding behaviors of LH-lesioned rats (Grijalva et al.,

1976). Schallert (1982) suggested that the facilitation of recovery induced by restricted intake regimens may be related to some form of behavioral conditioning, in which the animals become increasingly aware of and responsive to the periodic availability of the substance being restricted (i.e., food or water).

The potential importance of behavioral conditioning to the rate of recovery of ingestive behaviors is implicated further by other lines of research. Weingarten (1984) demonstrated that meal initiation in normal animals could be controlled by internal signals of energy depletion as well as by externally learned food-related cues. In Weingarten's study, rats were given six daily meals which were preceded by a 4.5-min light- and buzzer-conditioned stimulus. In other cases, animals were presented with a pure tone that was never paired with food delivery. Food-related cues were found to have a strong influence on the initiation of a meal which, in turn, appeared independent of the depletion state of the animal. A somewhat similar conditioning paradigm was recently used with LH-damaged rats to test the influence of preoperative food-related cues on the rate of postoperative recovery. Roland, Grijalva, and Dess (1986) dieted one group of rats to 85% normal body weight by giving them one restricted meal per day preceded by a 4-min buzzer. Two additional normal weight groups were included, one which was fed *ad libitum* and exposed to a random presentation of the buzzer, and the other fed two daily meals, each preceded by the presentation of the buzzer. Following a 10-day conditioning period, all three groups were given LH lesions and then tested postoperatively for feeding in the presence of the buzzer. Roland et al. found that there was a greater tendency for the normal weight group preoperatively exposed to the contingent food-buzzer pairing to initiate a meal in the presence of the buzzer, although this was not sufficient to facilitate recovery of feeding significantly.

In some respects these results support the idea that motivational and behavioral processes are activated by prior states of partial deprivation and potentiated by environmental cues associated with presentation of food and water. These cues may be purposely introduced, as in the case of the Roland et al. study, or inadvertently introduced by particular conditions of the experiment which arouse an animal's anticipation of food or water (e.g., entry of the researcher into the experimental room at meal times, preparation of diets in the presence of the animal, feeding or watering consistently occurring on a predictable schedule, etc.). Following surgery these external ingestion-related cues may serve as an appropriate prompt signifying the availability of the highly rewarding food or fluid. The findings of Welle and Coover (1979) provide additional support for this idea. They showed that rats placed on a restricted feeding regimen for a 2-week period displayed reduced plasma corticosterone levels within 10 min of meal onset, and that similar reductions occurred when these animals were merely placed in the chambers where they previously had been fed. Furthermore, LH lesions did not disrupt the decreases in corticosterone levels associated with meals. Interestingly, reductions in plasma corticosterone levels have been taken as an indication of positive emotional states (Welle & Coover, 1979). If so, this would strengthen the idea that meals are particularly rewarding to animals placed on restricted feeding schedules and would indicate that LH lesions do not diminish the rewarding properties of food. These findings may help to explain why preoperatively dieted LH rats show a facilitation of recovery of feeding behaviors, whereas normal weight or preoperatively fasted animals do not (Grijalva et al., 1976). For example, normal-weight rats are allowed free access to food and are generally not highly motivated to eat. Consequently, these animals may not form strong associations with external food-related cues. On the other hand, fasted rats are highly motivated to eat, but because all food is withheld over a period of several days, external food-related cues are never associated with eating. Dieted rats are typically fed once daily and are also strongly motivated to eat, however, because of the regularity of the feeding schedule and reduced caloric intake, they become particularly responsive to external food-related cues. Postoperatively, these cues may be sufficient to activate an adaptive behavioral sequence initially that was preoperatively conditioned.

Preoperative experience is not only relevant to initial stages of the LH syndrome, but is also important in the extent to which animals display persistent deficits during later stages of the syndrome. It was long presumed that LH lesions produce a permanent deficit in the ability to eat to glucoprivic challenges (Epstein, 1971); however, it was later discovered that rats with LH damage could increase their food intake in response to glucoprivic challenges as long as glucoprivation was moderately induced over a prolonged period (Stricker et al., 1975), or if the animals were postoperatively tested with palatable liquid diets rather than standard laboratory chow (Kanarek et al., 1981). Recently, Kanarek and Konecky (1985) showed that feeding behaviors following glucoprivation could be significantly enhanced in recovered LH rats by preoperative experience with insulin. In this study, groups of rats were injected once a week for 4 weeks with either insulin or saline. Approximately 2 weeks after the last injection, pretreated groups were given either bilateral LH lesions or control operations, recovered for 3 weeks postoperatively, and then tested for ingestive behaviors in response to glucoprivic challenges. Of particular interest were the findings that LH-damaged rats subjected to insulin injections preoperatively, increased food intake in response to either insulin or 2-DG in a manner similar to nonlesioned controls. In contrast, animals preoperatively injected with saline failed to show this response.

It also appears that hydrational deficits induced by LH damage may not be as persistent as previously believed. Ruger and Schulkin (1980) showed that LH-damaged rats preoperatively experienced in drinking saline solutions in response to sodium deficits displayed a significant sodium appetite in response to the administration of deoxycorticosterone and furosemide postoperatively. In agreement with earlier studies, this response was not seen in nonexperienced LH animals. In a subsequent study, Schulkin and Fluharty (1985) found that LH rats acquiring preoperative experience with sodium deficiency, salt taste, water deprivation, or insulin treatments all exhibited postoperative increases in water ingestion in response to salt hunger treatments; however, saline intake was increased only in those animals which had preoperatively experienced sodium deficiencies. Thus, prior experience with salt drive is necessary for the protection of LH rats against subsequent deficits in salt appetite.

SUMMARY AND CONCLUSIONS

Over the past 35 years, various hypotheses have been advanced to account for the initial feeding and drinking deficits following LH damage and the possible mechanisms underlying functional recovery of these behaviors. Although each hypothesis receives some measure of support from existing data, it is clear that no single explanation can fully account for all features of the LH syndrome. It is apparent that how one quantifies various components of the syndrome is greatly dependent on the precise extent and location of the brain damage, the experiential history of the animal, and the particular parameters being measured. Brain manipulations, particularly those involving the hypothalamus, produce complex effects involving the endocrine system, the autonomic nervous system, the gastrointestinal system, and neural systems involved in sensory, motor, or activational processes. Furthermore, how these various systems are ultimately affected by hypothalamic damage may determine not only how a particular dysfunction is expressed but also the relative importance of certain mechanisms potentially involved in postoperative recovery. In many cases, a simple measurement of a particular set of transient disorders or the quantification of persistent deficits may not accurately reflect the true effects of the brain damage or the adaptive capabilities of the animal in overcoming the abnormalities in question. For example, the literature is filled with arguments emphasizing any one of a number of disorders as being the primary cause for the aphagia or hypophagia produced by LH damage, ranging from motivational, motor, sensorimotor, activational, or visceral abnormalities, to alterations in body weight set point. Yet, by simply manipulating the preoperative experience of the animal it has been shown that eating can occur in a manner that is incongruent with any one of these explanations.

The same appears to be true for arguments in favor of particular mechanisms underlying functional recovery of ingestive behaviors. It is generally accepted that if a dysfunction is caused by damage to a particular brain structure; then it must follow that functional recovery related to that dysfunction must be based on mechanisms occurring in the brain. These mechanisms might include an alteration in neurotransmitter release and uptake functions, the induction of supersensitivity, or the regeneration of neuronal processes specifically related to the neural system initially damaged, or the compensatory takeover of function by different undamaged systems in a vicarious or redundant fashion (Marshall, 1984). Since damage to various brain structures can produce consummatory deficits which are alleviated, given adequate time and postoperative care, there is little doubt that readjustments in central mechanisms (by whatever means) are involved in long-term functional recovery. However, there is evidence suggesting that the rate at which *initial* recovery occurs depends importantly on peripheral mechanisms. In this respect, one result can be recognized as more "critical" than others because it stands alone by not fitting comfortably into the pattern formed by other results taken together. In this sense, the facilitated recovery of feeding behaviors induced by propantheline treatments in LH-damaged rats (Grijalva, Novin, & Cooper, 1980) can be viewed as a critical result. This result raises two immediate questions. First, is this consistent with hypotheses stressing only central mechanisms (e.g., set point changes, sensory neglect, motivational impairment, neurochemical or morphological alterations in dopaminergic systems)?, To which the answer appears, at least at present, to be no. The second question is, can this result be explained by an analysis of visceral events or metabolic processes? Here, the answer is probably yes, but only by a broadening of perspective. It is necessary to adopt the view that LH lesions produce far-ranging and severe malfunctions of the entire brain-visceral relation and that serious consideration be given to the host of postoperative metabolic-visceral abnormalities which appear relevant to an understanding of ingestive behaviors (Frohman, 1980; Grijalva & Lindholm, 1982; Grijalva, Lindholm et al., 1980; Powley et al., 1980).

In this chapter we have reviewed several lines of research showing that preoperative manipulations can dramatically alter both the short-term and long-term effects of LH damage. This approach has been very useful in identifying the potential involvement of central, peripheral, and experiential factors in the expression of the LH syndrome, and the role that these factors play in the recovery process. While the syndrome has served as a useful model for the study of the neurology of ingestive behaviors as well as recovery of function, it is clear that more complete understanding of either one of these processes requires the integration of knowledge regarding both central nervous system mechanisms as well as peripheral functions.

REFERENCES

Anand, B. K., & Brobeck, J. R. (1951). Hypothalamic control of food intake in rats and cats. *Yale Journal of Biology and Medicine, 24,* 123–140.

Baillie, P., & Morrison, S. D. (1963). The nature of the suppression of food intake by lateral hypothalamic lesions in rats. *Journal of Physiology (London), 165,* 227–245.

Balagura, S., & Harrell, L. E. (1974). Lateral hypothalamic syndrome: Its modification by obesity and leanness. *Physiology and Behavior, 13,* 345–347.

Balagura, S., Harrell, L. E., & DeCastro, J. M. (1978). Organismic states and their effect on recovery from neurosurgery: A new perspective with implications for a general theory. *Brain, Behavior, and Evolution, 15,* 19–40.

Balagura, S., Harrell, L., & Ralph, T. (1973). Glucodynamic hormones modify the recovery period after lateral hypothalamic lesions. *Science, 182,* 59–60.

Balagura, S., Wilcox, R. H., & Coscina, D. V. (1969). The effect of diencephalic lesions on food intake and motor activity. *Physiology and Behavior, 4,* 629–633.

Berger, D. B., Wise, C. D., & Stein, L. (1971). Norepinephrine: Reversal of anorexia in rats with lateral hypothalamic damage. *Science, 172,* 281–284.

Berger, D. B., Wise, C. D., & Stein, L. (1973). Nerve growth factor: Enhanced recovery of feeding after lateral hypothalamic damage. *Science, 180,* 506–508.

Björklund, A., & Stenevi, U. (1972). Nerve growth factor: Stimulation of regenerative growth of central noradrenergic neurons. *Science, 175,* 1251–1253.

Braun, J. J. (1975). Neocortex and feeding behavior in the rat. *Journal of Comparative & Physiological Psychology, 89,* 507–522.

Chakrabarty, K., & Leveille, G. (1968). Influence of periodicity of eating on the activity of various enzymes in adipose tissue, liver, and muscle of the rat. *Journal of Nutrition, 96,* 76–82.

DiCara, L. (1970). Role of post-operative feeding experience in recovery from lateral hypothalamic damage. *Journal of Comparative & Physiological Psychology, 72,* 60–66.

Epstein, A. N. (1971). The lateral hypothalamic feeding syndrome: Its implications for the physiological psychology of hunger and thirst. In E. Stellar & J. M. Sprague (Eds.), *Progress in physiological psychology* (Vol 4, pp. 263–317). New York: Academic Press.

Epstein, A. N., & Teitelbaum, P. (1967). Specific loss of hypoglycemic control of feeding in recovered lateral rats. *American Journal of Physiology, 213,* 1159–1167.

Fallon, J. H., & Moore, R. Y. (1978). Catecholamine innervation of the basal forebrain. IV. Topography of the dopamine projection to the basal forebrain and neostriatum. *Journal of Comparative Neurology, 180,* 545–580.

Frohman, L. A. (1980). Hypothalamic control of metabolism. In P. J. Morgane & J. Panksepp (Eds.), *Handbook of the hypothalamus: Physiology of the hypothalamus* (Vol. 2, pp. 519–555). New York: Marcel Dekker.

Glick, S. D. (1971). Modulation of food and water intake by frontal cortex in the rat. *Communications in Behavioral Biology, 5,* 365–370.

Glick, S. D. (1974). Changes in drug sensitivity and mechanisms of functional recovery following brain damage. In D. G. Stein, J. J. Rosen, & N. Butters (Eds.), *Plasticity and recovery of function in the central nervous system* (pp. 339–372). New York: Academic Press.

Glick, S. D., & Greenstein S. (1972a). Facilitation of recovery after lateral hypothalamic damage by prior ablation of frontal cortex. *Nature New Biology, 239,* 187–188.

Glick, S. D., & Greenstein, S. (1972b). Facilitation of survival following lateral hypothalamic damage by prior food and water deprivation. *Psychonomic Science, 28,* 163–164.

Glick, S. D., & Greenstein, S. (1974). Facilitation of lateral hypothalamic recovery by postoperative administration of alpha-methyl-para-tyrosine. *Brain Research, 73,* 180–183.

Glick, S. D., Greenstein, S., & Zimmerberg, B. (1972). Facilitation of recovery by alpha-methyl-para-tyrosine after lateral hypothalamic damage. *Science, 177,* 534–535.

Goldberger, M. E. (1974). Recovery of movement after CNS lesions in monkeys. In D. G. Stein, J. J. Rosen, & N. Butters (Eds.), *Plasticity and recovery of function in the central nervous system* (pp. 265–337). New York: Academic Press.

Grijalva C. V. (1980a). Alterations in feeding behavior and body weight following globus pallidus lesions in rats. *Society for Neuroscience Abstracts, 6,* 129.

Grijalva, C. V. (1980b). Aphagia, gastric pathology, hyperthermia, and sensorimotor dysfunctions after lateral hypothalamic lesions: Effects of insulin pretreatments. *Physiology and Behavior, 25,* 931–937.

Grijalva, C. V. (1985). Experimental ulceration after lateral hypothalamic lesions. In H. Weiner

(Moderator), Neurobiologic and psychobiologic mechanisms in gastric function and ulceration. *Western Journal of Medicine, 143*, 212–215.

Grijalva, C. V., Deregnaucourt, J., Code, C. F., & Novin, D. (1980). Gastric mucosal damage in rats induced by lateral hypothalamic lesions: Protection by propantheline, cimetidine, and vagotomy. *Proceedings of the Society for Experimental Biology and Medicine, 163*, 528–533.

Grijalva, C. V., Kiefer, S. W., Gunion, M. W., Cooper, P. H., & Novin, D. (1985). Ingestive responses to homeostatic challenges in rats with ablations of the anterolateral neocortex. *Behavior Neuroscience, 99*, 162–174.

Grijalva, C. V., & Lindholm, E. (1980). Restricted feeding and its effects of aphagia and ingestion-related disorders following lateral hypothalamic damage. *Journal of Comparative & Physiological Psychology, 94*, 164–177.

Grijalva, C. V., & Lindholm, E. (1982). The role of the autonomic nervous system in hypothalamic feeding syndromes. *Appetite, 3*, 111–124.

Grijalva, C. V., Lindholm, E., & Novin, D. (1980). Physiological and morphological changes in the gastrointestinal tract induced by hypothalamic intervention: An overview. *Brain Research Bulletin, 5*(Suppl. 1), 19–31.

Grijalva, C. V., Lindholm, E., Schallert, T., & Bicknell, E. J. (1976). Gastric pathology and aphagia following lateral hypothalamic lesions in rats: Effect of preoperative weight reduction. *Journal of Comparative & Physiological Psychology, 90*, 505–519.

Grijalva, C. V., Novin, D., & Bray, G. A. (1980). Alterations in blood glucose, insulin, and free fatty acids following lateral hypothalamic lesions or parasagittal knife cuts. *Brain Research Bulletin, 5*, (Suppl. 4), 109–117.

Grijalva, C. V., Novin, D., & Cooper, P. H. (1980). Facilitation of recovery by propantheline bromide after lateral hypothalamic damage. *Brain Research Bulletin, 5*, 525–529.

Grijalva, C. V., Tordoff, M. G., Geiselman, P. J., & Novin, D. (1983). Gastric mucosal damage induced by lateral hypothalamic lesions in rats: The potential contribution of bile. *Brain Research Bulletin, 10*, 441–444.

Grossman, S. P. (1979). The biology of motivation. *Annual Review of Psychology, 30*, 209–242.

Harrell, L. E., DeCastro, J. M., & Balagura, S. (1975). A critical evaluation of body weight loss following lateral hypothalamic lesions. *Physiology and Behavior, 15*, 133–136.

Harrell, L. E., Raubeson, R., & Balagura, S. (1974). Acceleration of functional recovery following lateral hypothalamic damage by means of electrical stimulation in the lesioned areas. *Physiology and Behavior, 12*, 897–899.

Henke, P. G. (1979). The hypothalamus-amygdala axis and experimental gastric ulcers. *Neuroscience and Biobehavioral Reviews, 3*, 75–82.

Henke, P. G. (1982). The telencephalic limbic system and experimental gastric pathology: A review. *Neuroscience and Biobehavioral Reviews, 6*, 381–390.

Hynes, M. D., Anderson, C. D., Gianutsos, G., & Lal, H. (1975). Effects of haloperidol, methyltyrosine, and morphine on recovery from lesions of the lateral hypothalamus. *Pharmacology, Biochemistry, & Behavior, 3*, 755–759.

Isaacson, R. I. (1974). *The limbic system.* New York: Plenum Press.

Kanarek, R. B., & Konecky, M. S. (1985). Preoperative experience with insulin enhances glucoprivic feeding in rats with lateral hypothalamic lesions. *Physiology and Behavior, 34*, 987–994.

Kanarek, R. B., Salomon, M., & Khadivi, A. (1981). Rats with lateral hypothalamic lesions do eat following acute cellular glucoprivation. *American Journal of Physiology, 241*, R362–R369.

Karli, P., & Vergnes, M. (1964). Dissociation expérimentale du comportement d'aggression interspécifique rat-souris et du comportemente alimentaire. *Comptes Rendus des Séances de la Société de Biologie, 158*, 650–653.

Keesey, R. E., Boyle, P. C., Kemnitz, J. W., & Mitchel, J. S. (1976). The role of the lateral hypothalamus in determining the body weight set point. In D. Novin, W. Wyrwicka, & G. A. Gray (Eds.), *Hunger: Basic mechanisms and clinical implications* (pp. 243–255). New York: Raven Press.

Keesey, R. E., & Corbett, S. W. (1984). Metabolic defense of body weight set-point. In A. J. Stunkard & E. Stellar (Eds.), *Eating and its disorders* (pp. 87–96). New York: Raven Press.

Keesey, R. E., Corbett, S. W., Hirvonen, M. D., & Kaufman, L. N. (1984). Heat production and body weight changes following lateral hypothalamic lesions. *Physiology and Behavior, 32,* 309–317.

Kissileff, H. R. (1971). Acquisition of prandial drinking in weanling rats and in rats recovering from lateral hypothalamic lesions. *Journal of Comparative and Physiological Psychology, 77,* 97–109.

Kissileff, H. R., & Epstein, A. N. (1969). Exaggerated prandial drinking in the "recovered lateral" rat without saliva. *Journal of Comparative and Physiological Psychology, 67,* 301–308.

Kolb, B., & Nonneman, A. J. (1975). Prefrontal cortex and the regulation of food intake in the rat. *Journal of Comparative & Physiological Psychology, 88,* 806–815.

Kolb, B., Nonneman, A. J., & Whishaw, I. Q. (1978). Influence of frontal neocortical lesions and body weight manipulation on the severity of lateral hypothalamic aphagia. *Physiology and Behavior, 21,* 541–547.

Kolb, B., Whishaw, I. Q., & Schallert, T. (1977). Aphagia, behavior sequencing, and body weight set point following orbital frontal lesions in rats. *Physiology and Behavior, 19,* 93–103.

Krieger, D. T., Crowley, W. R., O'Donohue, T. L., & Jacobowitz, D. M. (1980). Effects of food restriction on the periodicity of corticosteroids in plasma and monoamine concentrations in discrete brain nuclei. *Brain Research, 188,* 167–174.

Lashley, K. S. (1929). *Brain mechanisms and intelligence.* Chicago: University of Chicago Press.

Leach, L. R., & Braun, J. J. (1976). Dissociation of gustatory and weight regulatory responses to quinine following lateral hypothalamic lesions. *Journal of Comparative & Physiological Psychology, 90,* 978–985.

Leveille, G. A. (1970). Adipose tissue metabolism: Influence of periodicity of eating and diet composition. *Federation Proceedings, 29,* 1294–1301.

Levitt, D. R., & Teitelbaum, P. (1975). Somnolence, akinesia, and sensorimotor activation of motivated behavior in the lateral hypothalamic syndrome. *Proceedings of the National Academy of Sciences of the United States of America, 72,* 2819–2823.

Lindholm, E., Shumway, G. S., Grijalva, C. V., Schallert, T., & Ruppel, M. (1975). Gastric pathology produced by hypothalamic lesions in rats. *Physiology and Behavior, 14,* 165–169.

Lindvall, O., Björklund, A., & Divac, I. (1978). Organization of catecholamine neurons projecting to the frontal cortex in the rat. *Brain Research, 142,* 1–24.

Marshall, J. F. (1984). Brain function: Neural adaptations and recovery from injury. *Annual Review of Psychology, 35,* 277–308.

Marshall, J. F., Levitan, D., & Stricker, E. M. (1976). Activation-induced restoration of sensorimotor functions in rats with dopamine-depleting brain lesions. *Journal of Comparative and Physiological Psychology, 90,* 536–546.

Marshall, J. F., Richardson, J. S., & Teitelbaum, P. (1974). Nigrostriatal bundle damage and the lateral hypothalamic syndrome. *Journal of Comparative and Physiological Psychology, 87,* 808–830.

Marshall, J. F., & Teitelbaum, P. (1974). Further analysis of sensory inattention following lateral hypothalamic damage in rats. *Journal of Comparative and Physiological Psychology, 86,* 375–395.

Marshall, J. R., Turner, B. H., & Teitelbaum, P. (1971). Sensory neglect produced by lateral hypothalamic damage. *Science, 174,* 523–525.

Misantone, L. J., Schaffer, S. R., & Lombardi, L. (1980). Accelerated recovery form eating deficits after sequential lesions of cortex and hypothalamus: Is dopamine involved? *Experimental Neurology, 70,* 236–257.

Morgane, P. J. (1961a). Medial forebrain bundle and "feeding centers" of the hypothalamus. *Journal of Comparative Neurology, 117,* 1–25.

Morgane, P. J. (1961b). Altration in feeding and drinking behavior in rats with lesions of globi pallidi. *American Journal of Physiology, 201,* 420–428.

Morrison, S. D. (1968). The relationship of energy expenditure and spontaneous activity to the aphagia of rats with lesions in the lateral hypothalamus. *Journal of Physiology (London), 197,* 325–343.

Mufson, E. J., & Wampler, R. S. (1972). Weight regulation with palatable food and liquids in rats with lateral hypothalamic lesions. *Journal of Comparative & Physiological Psychology, 80,* 382–392.

Neve, K. A., Kozlowski, M. R., & Marshall, J. F. (1982). Plasticity of neostriatal dopamine receptors after nigrostriatal injury: Relationship to recovery of sensorimotor functions and behavioral supersensitivity. *Brain Research, 244,* 33–44.

Pettibone, D. J., Kaufman, L. N., Scally, M. C., Meyer, E., Jr., Ulus, I., & Lytle, L. D. (1978). Striatal nondopaminergic neurons: Possible involvement in feeding and drinking behavior. *Science, 200,* 1175–1177.

Powley, T. L., & Keesey, R. E. (1970). Relationship of body weight to the lateral hypothalamic feeding syndrome. *Journal of Comparative & Physiological Psychology, 70,* 25–36.

Powley, T. L., Opsahl, C. A., Cox, J. E., & Weingarten, H. P. (1980). The role of the hypothalamus in energy homeostasis. In P. J. Morgane & J. Panksepp (Eds.), *Handbook of the hypothalamus: Behavioral studies of the hypothalamus* (Vol. 3, pt. A, pp. 211–298). New York: Marcel Dekker.

Rodgers, W. L., Epstein, A. N., & Teitelbaum, P. (1965). Lateral hypothalamic aphagia: Motor failure or motivational deficit? *American Journal of Physiology, 208,* 334–342.

Roland, B., Grijalva, C. V., & Dess, N. (1986). External activation of ingestive motivational behavior in rats with lateral hypothalamic lesions. *Society for Neuroscience Abstracts, 12* (Pt. 2), 1553.

Ruger, J., & Schulkin, J. (1980). Preoperative sodium appetite experience and hypothalamic lesions in rats. *Journal of Comparative and Physiological Psychology, 94,* 914–920.

Schallert, T. (1982). Adipsia produced by lateral hypothalamic lesions: Facilitation of recovery by preoperative restriction of water intake. *Journal of Comparative and Physiological Psychology, 96,* 604–614.

Schallert, T., Leach, L. R., & Braun, J. J. (1978). Saliva hypersecretion during aphagia following lateral hypothalamic lesions. *Physiology and Behavior, 21,* 461–463.

Schallert, T., & Whishaw, I. Q. (1978). Two types of aphagia and two types of sensorimotor impairment after lateral hypothalamic lesions: Observations in normal weight, dieted, and fattened rats. *Journal of Comparative and Physiological Psychology, 92,* 720–741.

Schallert, T., Whishaw, I. Q., & Flannigan, K. P. (1977). Gastric pathology and feeding deficits induced by hypothalamic damage in rats: Effects of lesion type, size, and placement. *Journal of Comparative and Physiological Psychology, 91,* 598–610.

Schulkin, J., & Fluharty, S. J. (1985). Further studies on salt appetite following lateral hypothalamic lesions: Effects of preoperative alimentary experiences. *Behavioral Neuroscience, 99,* 927–935.

Sereni, F., Principi, N., Perletti, L., & Sereni, L. P. (1966). Undernutrition and the developing rat brain. *Biologia Neonatorum, 10,* 254–265.

Sharpless, S. K. (1964). Reorganization of function in the nervous system: Use and disuse. *Annual Review of Physiology, 26,* 357–388.

Shoemaker, W. J., & Wurtman, R. J. (1971). Perinatal undernutrition: Accumulation of catecholamines in rat brain. *Science, 171,* 1017–1019.

Smith, G. P., & Epstein, A. N. (1969). Increased feeding in response to decreased glucose utilization in the rat and monkey. *American Journal of Physiology, 217,* 1083–1087.

Snyder, G. L., & Stricker, E. M. (1985). Effects of lateral hypothalamic lesions on food intake in rats during exposure to cold. *Behavioral Neuroscience, 99,* 310–327.

Stevenson, J. A. F., & Montemurro, D. G. (1963). Loss of weight and metabolic rate of rats with lesions in the medial and lateral hypothalamus. *Nature, 198,* 92.

Stricker, E. M. (1976). Drinking by rats after lateral hypothalamic lesions: A new look at the lateral hypothalamic syndrome. *Journal of Comparative & Physiological Psychology, 90,* 127–143.

Stricker, E. M., Friedman, M. I., & Zigmond, M. J. (1975). Glucoregulatory feeding by rats after intraventricular 6-hydroxydopamine or lateral hypothalamic lesions. *Science, 189,* 895–897.

Stricker, E. M., & Zigmond, M. J. (1976). Recovery of function after damage to central catecholamine-containing neurons: A neurochemical model for the lateral hypothalamic syndrome. In J. M. Sprague & A. N. Epstein (Eds.), *Progress in psychobiology and physiological psychology* (Vol. 6, pp. 121–188). New York: Academic Press.

Teitelbaum, P. (1971). The encephalization of hunger. In E. Stellar & J. M. Sprague (Eds.), *Progress in physiological psychology* (Vol. 4, pp. 319–350). New York: Academic Press.

Teitelbaum, P., & Epstein, A. N. (1962). The lateral hypothalamic syndrome: Recovery of feeding and drinking after lateral hypothalamic lesions. *Psychological Review, 69,* 74–90.

Teitelbaum, P., & Stellar, E. (1954). Recovery from the failure to eat produced by hypothalamic lesions. *Science, 120,* 894–895.

Tordoff, M. G., Grijalva, C. V., Novin, D., Butcher, L. L., Walsh, J. H., Pi-Sunyer, F. X., & VanderWeele, D. A. (1984). Influence of sympathectomy on the lateral hypothalamic lesion syndrome. *Behavioral Neuroscience, 98,* 1039–1059.

Ungerstedt, U. (1971). Stereotaxic mapping of the monoamine pathways in the rat brain. *Acta Physiologica Scandinavica, 367* (Suppl. 1) 1–49.

Wayner, M. J., Cott, A., Millner, J., & Tartagione, R. (1971). Loss of 2-deoxy-d-glucose induced eating in recovered lateral rats. *Physiology and Behavior, 7,* 881–884.

Weingarten, H. P. (1984). Meal initiation controlled by learned cues: Basic behavioral properties. *Appetite, 5,* 147–158.

Weiner, N., & Mosimann, W. F. (1970). The effect of insulin on the catecholamine content and tyrosine hydroxylase activity of cat adrenal glands. *Biochemical Pharmacology, 19,* 1189–1199.

Welle, S., & Coover, G. P. (1979). Meal-induced decreases in serum corticosterone in the lateral hypothalamic syndrome. *Physiology and Behavior, 23,* 547–555.

White, N. W. (1986). Control of sensorimotor function by dopaminergic nigrostriatal neurons: Influence on eating and drinking. *Neuroscience and Biobehavioral Reviews, 10,* 15–36.

Wiley, J. H., & Leveille, G. A. (1970). Significance of insulin in the metabolic adaptation of rats to meal ingestion. *Journal of Nutrition, 100,* 1073–1080.

Willis, G. L., Smith, G. C., & Kinchington, P. C. (1983). Peripheral DA receptor blockade facilities behavioural recovery from nigrostriatal damage. *Brain Research Bulletin, 11,* 15–19.

Wolf, G. (1968). Effect of dorsolateral hypothalamic lesions on sodium appetite elicited by desoxycorticosterone and acute hyponatremia. *Journal of Comparative and Physiological Psychology, 58,* 519–530.

Wolf, G., & Quartermain, D. (1967). Sodium chloride intake of adrenalectomized rats with lateral hypothalamic lesions. *American Journal of Physiology, 211,* 113–118.

Wolgin, D. L., Cytawa, J., & Teitelbaum, P. (1976). The role of activation in the regulation of food intake. In D. Novin, W. Wyrwicka, & G. A. Bray (Eds.), *Hunger: Basic mechanisms and clinical implications* (pp. 179–191). New York: Raven Press.

Zeigler, H. P., & Karten, H. J. (1974). Central trigeminal structures and the lateral hypothalamic syndrome in the rat. *Science, 186,* 636–638.

4

Preoperative Manipulation and Ventromedial Hypothalamic Syndrome (VMH)

Devendra Singh
Department of Psychology
University of Texas, Austin

INTRODUCTION

Damage to the ventromedial hypothalamic (VMH) area produces a multitude of disorders affecting eating, adiposity, activity level, affective behavior, thermal regulation, and metabolic functions. This constellation of disorders has been commonly referred to as the VMH syndrome. A great deal of research effort, historically, has been devoted to determine whether the nature of primary disorder caused by VMH damage is behavioral or metabolic. That metabolic and behavioral factors could be of equal importance has been rarely considered. Furthermore, historically there is a clear cyclical trend for favoring one explanation over the other. Early investigators chose the metabolic explanation. Then the behavioral explanation became preferred. Recently, the metabolic explanation has come back into vogue (see Powley, Opsahl, Cox, & Weingarten, 1980, for an excellent summary of this historical trend).

Early clinical and experimental studies assumed primary deficit caused by VMH damage to be metabolic. These studies ignored overeating and affective disorders caused by VMH damage and concentrated on adiposity and pathological obesity. The trend changed when Ranson and associates (e.g., Hetherington & Ranson, 1942) demonstrated that hyperphagic behavior of VMH-damaged rats was influenced by palatability of diet. The metabolic explanation was seriously weakened when Brobeck (1946) proposed that the VMH damage produced primary disorders in eating behavior and that metabolic disorders were secondary. The final event which nearly eclipsed the metabolic explanation were the classical studies of Miller, Bailey, and Stevenson (1950) and Teitelbaum (1955). Expounding on the proposal of Brobeck, these investigators

65

suggested that behavioral factors (deficit in satiety and hunger motivation) could account for hyperphagic behavior of the VMH-lesioned animals.

Most studies during the 1950s through early 1970s focused on the behavioral problems of satiety, hyperreactivity to sensory properties of food, and strength of hunger motivation in animals with VMH damage. The majority of these studies were directly or indirectly influenced by the findings of Miller and Teitelbaum and were largely designed to validate or refute the explanations offered by these investigators (Grossman, 1979; King, 1980). Such bias effectively precluded any significant attempt to ascertain the relative contribution of metabolic factors in the development and maintenance of VMH syndrome. Presently, the trend has been to pursue and stress metabolic factors to account for VMH syndrome. Once again, the behavioral factors, rather than being integrated with metabolic factors and treated as of equal importance, are considered as secondary consequences of metabolic factors (Bray & York, 1979; LeMagnen, 1983).

The purpose of this brief historical review was to show that prevalent theoretical bias has determined which element of the VMH syndrome was explored and which was ignored. Such bias has hindered the understanding of the functional role of the VMH areas. The notion of syndrome assumes a relatedness of various elements which covary with each other and are supposedly produced by a unitary cause (Powley et al., 1980). Therefore, it is critical to examine all the elements of the syndrome and ascertain their interrelatedness. It is possible that while some elements of the syndrome are highly correlated with many other elements, others are only partly correlated. Furthermore, it could be that some elements are extremely rigid, while others are quite plastic and respond to various experiential factors. One of the disorders produced by VMH damage is hyperemotionality, which has been rarely measured or systematically examined. Wheatley (1944) was first to demonstrate a "rage" syndrome caused by VMH damage and suggested that such animals were hyperreactive to their environment. The clinical literature also reported invariable occurrences of hyperemotionality with hyperphagia in humans (e.g., Reeves & Plum, 1969). In spite of these findings, very few investigators in this field pursued the role of emotionality or attempted to integrate it with other elements of the VMH syndrome (for exception, see Grossman, 1966).

Emotionality induced by neural damage can be significantly modified by pharmacological agents as well as by experiential factors. Its magnitude has been shown to depend on various programs of experiences, such as rearing condition and preoperative experience. Thus, the factor of emotionality can be experientially manipulated and its effects on other disorders produced by VMH damage can be examined to evolve a more accurate description of VMH function. Furthermore, it is quite probable that other elements of VMH syndrome, such as thermal regulation, may turn out to be quite plastic and can be modified by preoperative experience. The influence of preoperative experience on the nature and magnitude of neural injury has been extensively studied for various cortical functions. The investigations by Greenough, Fass, and DeVoogd, (1976) and Rosenzweig (1986) have demonstrated that the preoperative experience can overcome or minimize the effect of neural damage. Such systematic investigations of preoperative experience on VMH function have been rarely conducted.

In this chapter, I will attempt to demonstrate that preoperative experience significantly determines the nature and magnitude of various disorders induced by VMH damage and that the further use of this manipulation can help in formulating better targeted questions to understand the functional role of VMH area.

Prior to examining relevant studies in this area, I will briefly describe the classical VMH syndrome and discuss variables that may confound the experimental findings reported after VMH damage. Isolating potential confounding variables may provide a perspective within which many conflicting, and often contradictory, findings can be meaningfully explained.

THE VMH SYNDROME

Damage to the VMH area in rats produces hyperphagia and, if maintained on *ad libitum* regular rat chow, leads to excessive body weight gain and obesity (Miller et al., 1950; Teitelbaum, 1955, 1961). The effects of the lesions are manifested in three sequential stages: acute, dynamic, and static. Immediately after lesions are made, animals exhibit a burst of uncontrolled eating and hyperactivity which lasts approximately 24 hours (Balagura & Devenport, 1970; Harrell & Remley, 1973). No behavioral research is available on this acute stage, since most of the investigators routinely remove food for 24 hours after lesion to prevent food-induced suffocation (Hoebel, 1975). After this initial bout of overeating, the dynamic phase of lesion starts, during which animals eat two to three times more food than nonlesioned animals and the rate of body weight gain becomes much greater than that of control animals. Finally, after 2 to 3 months of *ad libitum* feeding, lesioned animals enter the static phase, during which their food intake and rate of body weight gain approximate that of unlesioned animals (Teitelbaum, 1961).

During both dynamic and static stages, animals also exhibit finickiness and reduced hunger motivation. Finickiness refers to overreactivity to both negative and positive aspects of the palatability (sensory properties such as texture, taste, and flavor) of food. Reduced hunger motivation is inferred from lack of willingness to work in order to obtain food and the reduction in food intake when required to tolerate electrical shock to obtain food (Miller et al., 1950; Teitelbaum, 1961). Finickiness and reduced hunger motivation are exhibited during the dynamic stage but are greatly pronounced during the static stage, suggesting an interactive role played by obesity and VMH damage.

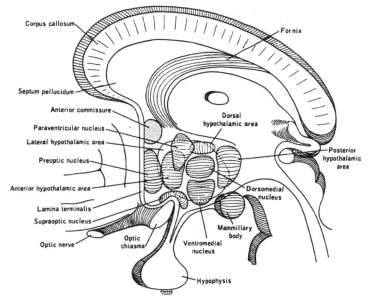

FIG. 4.1.   Three-dimensional reconstruction of the hypothalamus (from House & Pansky, 1960).

ANATOMICAL DESCRIPTION OF
VMH AREA

Fig. 4.1 shows a three-dimensional reconstruction of the hypothalamic area within which the ventromedial area is located. The hypothalamus on each side of the third ventricle is traversed by the fornix (terminating in the mammillary body), thereby dividing each half of the hypothalamus into a medial and lateral zone. Commonly, the ventromedial area refers to that part of medial hypothalamus which contains ventromedial hypothalamic nuclei and is bordered laterally and dorsally by the fornix. The degree of hyperphagia and obesity as well as finickiness depend on the location of damage within this area. Significant parts of this area can be damaged without causing hyperphagia if the damage is restricted to medial aspects. Hyperphagia and obesity have been reported in the rat when lesions were restricted to arcuate nuclei and the VMH nuclei was intact (Valenstein, Cox, & Kakolewski, 1969). Graff and Stellar (1962) were the first to demonstrate that hyperphagia and finickiness are regulated by independent, although overlapping, neural mechanisms. Thus, it is possible to place selective lesions in the VMH area which produce only hyperphagia, only finickiness, or both. Many authors (Hoebel, 1975; Sclafani, 1976) suggest that finickiness can be disassociated from overeating and that finickiness most readily occurs when lesions destroy the subfornical region lateral to ventromedial nuclei. Similarily, parasagittal knife cuts placed lateral to the plane of the fornix produce enhanced finickiness. The lateral extent of VMH damage, not medial damage, is the important factor influencing motivational effects (see Sclafani & Kirchgessner, 1986). Thus the precise location of the damage within the VMH area is critical in the manifestation of *total* VMH syndrome.

FACTORS IN DEFICITS AFTER
VMH DAMAGE

Unlike many other cortical and subcortical areas, the effects of VMH damage are greatly influenced by age, sex, strain difference as well as the technique used to induce neural damage. The involvement of so many factors in determining the nature and magnitude of deficits after VMH damage make comparing the findings of various studies extremely difficult. I will briefly discuss the role of some of these factors to underscore that caution is needed when comparing various studies.

Age and Sex Differences

The most prominent effect of VMH damage pertains to disorder of feeding behavior. However, the feeding behavior even in neurologically intact animals depends on age and sex differences (Nance, Gorski, & Panksepp, 1976; Nisbett, Braver, Jusela, & Kezur, 1975).

Kennedy (1969) has suggested that functioning of VMH in normal animals deteriorates from sexual maturity to old age, and therefore, older neurologically intact animals should exhibit feeding behavior similar to young VMH-lesioned animals. Although no studies have been conducted specifically to compare VMH-lesioned rats with older normal animals, Nisbett et al. (1975) systematically investigated the behavior of young and old animals for "VMH mediated behavior." One of the relevant findings was that older male rats (7½ months) prefer more oily food than younger rats (3½ months); such age-dependent preference was not evident for female rats. Finally, weaning rats with VMH damage not only do not exhibit hyperphagia, they have growth retardation (Bernardis, 1971; Bernardis & Bellinger, 1976).

The sex differences play a significant role in regulating in feeding behavior. Kennedy (1969) has suggested that neurologically intact males regulate their feedings more like VMH-lesioned rats than do normal female rats. First, female rats show much more extreme dinurnal distributions of feeding (Panksepp, 1976). Second, some investigators have reported greater sweet intake in female than male rats (Nance et al., 1976). Third, female rats differ from male rats in food-induced thermogenesis as well as in responses to a starvation diet (Hoyenga

& Hoyenga, 1982). Fourth, female rats (Wistar) are more reactive to quinine-adulterated food than male rats and reject higher concentrations of quinine sulfate-adulterated water (0.1%) than male rats.

Sex differences in feeding behavior have also been demonstrated after VMH damage (Singh, 1970; Singh & Meyer, 1968; Valenstein et al., 1969). These authors have shown that after anodal electrolytic lesion, female rats show greater weight gain than male rats. Furthermore, male VMH-lesioned rats react more to cellulose-adulteration of the diet than do female VMH rats (Singh & Meyer, 1968). Grossman (1976) also found greater hyperphagia and obesity in female rats than in male rats with coronal cuts behind the VMH area. Recently King and Frohman (1986) have shown that female lesioned rats gain more weight than male rats.

Species and Strain Differences

The basic effect of VMH damage on hyperphagia and obesity has been demonstrated for humans, (Bray, 1984) monkeys, rabbits, hamsters, cats, dogs, and birds (King, 1980; Powley et al., 1980).

However, there are no systematic studies comparing various strains of rats or other species. Typically, various investigators have used albino (Holtzman, Sprague–Dwaley, Charles River, Wistar) or black and white Long–Evans rats. There have been reports showing differences in emotionality between albino and Long–Evans rats. Jacobs and Sharma (1969) report that normal Charles River rats eat much greater amounts of food than Holtzman and Wistar, and they suggest that Charles River rats can be described as "obese hyperphagic."

Another species which has been extensively studies is mice. However, most studies using mice have exclusively used gold thioglucose (GTG) injection for damaging the VMH area. The use of GTG injected in mice studies confound the species comparison since it is difficult to ascertain whether observed behavioral deficit are due to GTG technique or species differences. Nevertheless, GTG-treated mice also exhibit sex differences in obesity (females become more obese) and male and female reject quinine adulterated food (Singh, Lakey, & Sanders, 1974; Sanders, Lakey, & Singh, 1973), and do not work harder to obtain food than normal mice at an increasingly demanding work schedule (Sclafani, 1976; Singh et al., 1974). However, unlike VMH-lesioned rats, when given .14% saccharin-mixed diets or 12.5% cellulose-mixed diets, GTG mice do not reduce in their food intake and consume as much as untreated mice (Sanders et al., 1973). VMH-lesioned monkeys work as hard as unoperated-on monkeys to obtain food (but see the section on the effect of pretraining on food-motivated behavior), and eat as many quinine-mixed food pellets as unoperated-on monkeys (Hamilton & Brobeck, 1964). VMH-lesioned hamsters become obese only when they are given sunflower seeds but do not gain much weight when fed lab chow diet (Marks & Miller, 1972). Balinska (1963) has reported that dynamic hyperphagic rabbits pull a ring to obtain food more often and much faster than normal rabbits.

This brief review should make it eminently clear that investigators are bound to obtain contradictory results in regulation of feeding behavior, reactivity to taste and texture of diet, and strength of hunger motivation, even when using the same species, if factor of sex and strain differences are not controlled. Inclusion of a sham group cannot solve this problem of confounding, as these factors may have an interactive effect with VMH damage.

Neural Damage Technique

Finally, unlike any other brain area, the technique used to produce VMH damage significantly determines the nature and magnitude of observed disorder. Historically, VMH lesions were produced by electrolytic anodal direct current, (Kennedy, 1969; Miller et al., 1950) and this technique remains the most frequently used. Another technique, parasagittal knife cuts (Gold, Kapatos, & Carey, 1973; Sclafani, 1971) has been popular since, unlike electrolytic lesion, it can selectively destroy fiber connections. In this technique a guide shaft containing a wire is lowered to the brain and an inner wire is extended to cut fibers between the LH and VMH nuclei, or between other areas. Less popular techniques are radio frequency (rf), which produces damage by electrocauterization, and cathodal electrolytic (direct current) lesion, which invariably produces larger and more irregular lesions than anodal lesions (Singh, 1975). Finally, chemical lesions have been produced by procaine injections in rats (Berthoud & Jeanrenaud, 1979; Larkin, 1975) and by goldthinoglucose (GTG) injection in mice (Weipkema, 1968).

Many of these techniques produce different behavioral and metabolic dysfunctions associated with VMH damage. For example, when VMH lesions are produced by electrolytic cathodal current, rats gain only about 65% of body weight during a 30-day *ad libitum* period, compared with rats that receive electrolytic anodal current lesions (King & Frohman, 1985). Furthermore, rats with cathodal current lesions, unlike the rats with electrolytic anodal lesions, do not exhibit basal or postabsorptive hyperinsulinemia. Finally, while rats with anodal current lesions exhibit hyperemotionality, rats with cathodal current lesions do not (King & Frohman, 1985). In a recent study King and Frohman (1986) compared the effect of radio frequency lesion with electrolytic (anodal) lesion to re-examine an early controversy regarding whether radio frequency-lesioned rats exhibit hyperphagia and obesity (Hoebel, 1965; Reynolds, 1965). These authors found that both male and female rats gain significantly less body weight when the VMH areas were damaged by radio frequency than rats with electrolytic lesions. King and Frohman (1986) argue that electrolytic anodal lesions (using stainless steel electrodes) leave metallic ion deposits and produce irritative lesions, while the use of cathodal electrolytic lesion and radio frequency (using

TABLE 4.1
Comparison of Dysfunctions Produced by Electrolytic and Knife-Cut Damage

Nature of Dysfunction	Electrolytic Lesion	Knife Cut
acute dynamic stage of lesion	present[7]	absent[7]
gonadal atrophy	yes[2]	no[4]
hyperinsulinemia	yes[3]	no(yes only after overeating)[8]
hypovolemic thrust challenge	not impaired[4]	impaired[9]
hyperemotionality	yes-chronic[5]	no-transient[6]
spontaneous activity	decreased[6]	partial decrease[6]
activity cycle	abolished[6]	no effect[6]

[1]Balagura and Devenport (1970); [2]Valenstein et al., (1969); [3]King and Frohman (1985); [4]King and Grossman (1977); [5]Singh (1969); [6]Sclafani (1971); [7]Powley et al., (1980); [8]Bray, Sclafani, and Novin (1982); [9]Sclafani, Berner, and Maul (1975)

platinum electrodes) leave fewer metallic ions and therefore produce nonirritative lesions (Gold, 1975; King & Frohman, 1985). Typical obesity, hyperinsulinemia, and hyperemotionality are found only in animals with irritative lesions.

Since the technique used in destroying the VMH area significantly determines the nature and magnitude of behavioral, endrocrinological, and metabolic disorders, many contradictory findings in the literature could be due to this factor alone. A comparison of two most popularly used techniques, electrolytic (anodal) and parasagittal knife cuts clearly justifies this conclusion (see Table 4.1).

It is obvious that these factors singularly or interactively can confound results and render many comparisons between studies using knife cuts and electrolytic lesions useless at best and confusing at worst.

This brief review of various factors which can influence observed behavior after VMH damage was intended to show that many studies in this area are not comparable. This may account for some of the contradictory inferences drawn by some investigators. While investigating the effects of preoperative manipulation on VMH syndrome, it is critical to control these factors to assure valid inferences.

Within the confines of these cautions, the effect of preoperative experience on VMH damage in animals will be examined. To date, the effect of preoperative events and experiences have been demonstrated for hyperphagia, emotionality, bitter taste, bait shyness, and behaviors motivated by food and water.

HYPERPHAGIA AND OBESITY

One explanation for hyperphagia observed after VMH damage is that lesions affect the body weight set point, and therefore animals overeat to defend the new body set point. Once lesioned animals gain enough body weight, they regulate their eating to maintain an obese body weight (Teitelbaum, 1961). This explanation can readily account for near-normal food intake and rate of weight gain in lesioned animals during static phase of lesion. A direct test of this hypothesis was conducted by Hoebel and Teitelbaum (1966). In this classical study, female Sherman rats were injected with long-acting insulin (Protamine Zinc insulin) every day for 4 months. Such treatment induces these animals to eat excessively (powdered Purina rat chow) due to hypoglycemia and to become obese. When VMH lesions (electrolytic anodal) are produced in these obese rats, no hyperphagia is observed. The magnitude of hyperphagia and weight gain depends on prelesioned weight levels of these rats; the greater the prelesion body weight, the lesser the hyperphagia and rate of weight gain. Thus, preoperative obesity inhibits hyperphagia which is normally evident after VMH damage.

The effect of presurgical weight reduction on the degree of hyperphagic response after VMH damage in rats has also been investigated (Sclafani, 1977). Conceptually, this study investigates the opposite end of the Hoebel and Teitelbaum study. Sclafani (1977) used female Charles River rats which were divided into two groups: either ad libitum food (Purina rat chow) or restricted food intake to induce 80% ad libitum body weight. After 15 days, VMH knife cuts were made, and ad libitum food intake and body weight recorded for all animals during 13 consecutive days. On the basis of the previous findings that prior obesity inhibits hyperphagia, one would expect that below-normal body weight prior to the lesion would enhance hyperphagia. The results of the study, however, show that presurgical body weight reduction does not cause increased food intake. All VMH-damaged rats, whether normal or below-normal body weight were equally hyperphagic. It should be pointed out that Sclafani did not investigate the role of the experience of starvation per se. It could be that the experience of starvation prior to VMH damage, rather than the body weight level, is more critical in determining the magnitude of postoperative hyper-phagia. On the basis of the two studies conducted in this area, it seems that a preoperative increase in obesity has an effect on overeating after VMH lesion, but a complementary effect of weight reduction prior to surgery on hyperphagia is not found.

The degree of hyperphagia and obesity can also be affected by abdominal vagotomy. It has been demonstrated that a complete surgical cut of vagus nerves (subdiaphragmatic vagotomy) eliminates hyperphagia and obesity in both male and female VMH-lesioned rats (Powley & Opsahl, 1976). The elimination of hyperphagia is more pronounced if rats are fed regular rat pellets; those fed a high fat diet continue to exhibit slight hyperphagia and weight gain (Powley & Opsahl, 1976; Sclafani, Aravich, & Landman, 1981). Furthermore, vagotomy does not alter food intake in neurologically intact obese (genetic, ovarietomy or dietary induced obesity) rats (Gold, Sawchenko, DeLuca, Alexander, & Eng, 1980; Powley & Opsahl, 1976).

Powley (1977) has argued that VMH damage produces a functional disorder of the vagus nerve as evident from hyperinsulinemia and gastric hyperacidity in such animals. Subdiaphragmatic vagatomy normalizes these disorders and thereby eliminates hyperphagia and obesity in VMH-lesioned rats. Many other investigators, however, argue that vagotomy induced normalization of overeating and obesity may be due to some other factors (Grossman, 1984; Inoue & Bray, 1977; King & Frohman, 1982). Vagotomy produces difficulty in swallowing and a multitude of gastrointestinal disorders, including gastric distention, dehydration, and rapid gastric emptying of liquid food.

Given the fact the VMH-lesioned rats are also hyperemotional, King, Carpenter, Stamoutsos, Frohman, & Grossman (1977b) argue that VMH-lesioned rats overreact to the aversive consequence of vagotomy and reduce their food intake; if so, preoperative adaptation to the effect of vagotomy may eliminate or attenuate typical effects found in VMH-lesioned rats. Findings support this reasoning. Specifically, those rats (female Long Evans) which received vagotomy first and 70 days later received VMH lesions, and were fed regular rat chow, exhibited hyperphagia and obesity. However, when the sequence of vagotomy and lesion was reversed, VMH-lesioned rats lost weight, and reduced food intake similar to vagotomized rats. These results can not be explained on the basis of regeneration of vagus nerve since control vagotomized rats do not increase their food intake during a 70-day period. King, Phelps, and Frohman (1980) replicated these findings with VMH lesions made 150 days after vagotomy.

In summary, preoperative manipulations which increase body weight can eliminate hyperphagia while preoperative vagotomy can maintain hyperphagia induced by VMH damage. It should be pointed out that diet palatability per se can maintain hyperphagia in vagotomized VMH-lesioned rats. Furthermore, highly palatable diet can induce obesity (dietary obesity) in neurologically intact rats. It is thus quite probable that had Hoebel and Teitelbaum (1966) used a highly palatable diet, presurgically made obese VMH-lesioned rats might have exhibited hyperphagia.

HYPEREMOTIONALITY AND HYPERREACTIVITY

Damage to the VMH area induces marked changes in affective behavior. VMH animals exhibit hyperemotionality and attack viciously when attempts are made to handle and capture them (Brooks, Lockwood, & Wiggins, 1946; Hetherington & Ranson, 1942; Singh, 1969). These animals also exhibit an increased sensitivity to pain, appear to be less fearful, and exhibit an increase in pain-elicited fighting (Grossman, 1972). The most commonly utilized test to infer affective changes in these animals are: rating scale, passive avoidance, and active avoidance tests.

Rating scale

Most investigators rate emotionality level by observing the behavior of the animal in response to handling, capture, vocalization, and a tap on the back (see Brady & Nauta, 1953). Based on such rating, VMH-lesioned rats exhibit hyperemotionality right after recovery from surgery. The hyperemotionality of VMH lesion persists through the static stage without any attenuation. In addition, these animals do not habituate to daily handling in capture (Singh, 1969). Rats with knife cuts also exhibit hyperemotionality; however, unlike electrolytically lesioned rats, there is a decline in reactivity over time (Sclafani, 1971). Similarly, rats made obese by using nonirritative lesion do not show hyperemotionality (King & Frohman, 1985) nor do the rats with lesion in the paraventricular hypothalamic are (PVH) which leads to obesity (Weingarten, Chang, & McDonald, 1985). Apparently, obesity per se does not induce hyperemotionality or hyperreactivity, since dietary and genetically obese rats and mice do not exhibit these syndromes (Singh et al., 1974).

Passive Avoidance Test

In this type of test, animals are required to suppress either a punished, consummatory, or nonconsummatory response. VMH-lesioned rats require a greater number of punished trials than control to suppress response on this test (Sclafani & Grossman, 1971; Singh, 1973b). The problem with using consummatory response for a passive avoidance test is that the deficit could be due to increased drive level, emotionality, or both. Many studies, however, have shown the passive avoidance deficit in VMH rats in a wide variety of nonconsummatory tasks (Colpaert & Wiepkema, 1976; King, Carrington, & Grossman, 1978).

It should be pointed out that while obesity per se does induce passive avoidance deficit, obese VMH-lesioned rats show less deficit than dynamic-lesioned rats. This difference in performance between obese and lean VMH-lesioned rats cannot be ascribed to differential sensitivity to electric shock, since lean and obese rats do not differ in latencies to escape shock (King et al., 1978).

Active Avoidance Test

In this test, unlike passive avoidance task animals, have to engage in specific behavior in order to avoid or escape the shock. This is a much more complex test in which many test situational demands can affect performance—for example, difference in the type of response required (bar pressing, wheel turning, running) and whether the onset of the shock is signaled (discriminated avoidance) or unsignaled (nondiscriminated avoidance). Finally, the intensity of the shock employed can affect performance. Most of the earlier studies demonstrated that VMH lesions facilitate acquisition of discriminated active avoidance task (Grossman, 1966; Levine & Soliday, 1960; Weisman & Hamilton, 1972). Since many parameters can modify the outcome in active avoidance task, it is impressive that so many studies using different procedures had similar results. King and Gaston (1976b) were the first investigators to use nondiscriminated active avoidance task and found that VMH-lesioned rats perform worse than control rats. This contradictory finding led King and Grossman to delineate systematically various factors which may affect the learning and performance of these animals in the active avoidance test (King, Alheid, & Grossman, 1977a; King & Grossman, 1978). The following factors play a critical role: (1) Pre-operative habituation to the test apparatus affects the escape latencies of VMH-lesioned rats; when habituated to the test apparatus, no difference in escape latencies are found between lesioned and control rats; (2) The degree of obesity affects the performance; obese rats do not perform as well as lean VMH and, unlike lean VMH-lesioned rats, do not show improvement over testing session. However, this performance deficit in obese rats is not due to their activity level, as they emit equal or more responses than control rats; (3) The shock intensity used affects performance; when low or moderate shock intensities are used, control animals perform better than obese lesioned rats. However, when high shock intensities are used, the performance of obese as well as lean rats is better than control rats. It should be noted that at higher shock intensities, the performance of control rats is impaired and therefore, by comparison, VMH lesioned rats are found to perform better.

The only study which has investigated the role of preoperative training on active avoidance is that of King and Gaston (1976b). In their first experiment, female Long–Evans hooded rats were trained in operant chambers to avoid (.03-sec duration) shock by lever pressing. Three shock levels (0.8, 1.6, and 3.2 m) were used. Rats were tested for 10 consecutive days on the avoidance schedule with 30-sec response–shock (r–s) and a 10 sec shock–shock (s–s) interval for 2 hr a day. Under this schedule a rat was shocked every 10 sec unless it bar pressed (shock was then postponed for 30 sec) or the rat could avoid shock entirely by pressing a bar at least every 30 sec. In this type of avoidance VMH-lesioned (anodal electrolytic) rats received significantly more shocks and made fewer responses than control rats for all shock levels throughout 10 days of testing.

In the second experiment, the effect of pretraining was investigated. VMH lesions were produced in the control rats used in the first experiment. After surgery, all rats were given four additional sessions (2 hr) at the same shock intensity at which they were previously tested. The preoperative training (10 sessions) combined with 4 additional postoperative training sessions greatly facilitated the performance of these animals, although they never performed at their preoperative level. To infer the protective effect of pretraining, it is crucial to compare the performance of preoperatively trained with nonpretrained VMH-lesioned rats. Authors King and Gaston (1976b) report that pretrained VMH-lesioned rats made significantly more responses and received less shock than VMH-lesioned rats without pretraining.

I am not aware of any study investigating the effect of preoperative training on other measures of emotionality, such as passive avoidance or shock-elicited fighting in VMH-lesioned animals. The only other study investigating the effect of pretraining is on the magnitude of frustration effect in VMH-lesioned rats (Beatty, Vilberg, Shirk, & Siders, 1975). These investigators, however, failed to replicate earlier findings of a greater frustration effect in VMH-lesioned rats than control rats.

The facilitative effect of preoperative training found in avoidance test is significant since VMH damage induces persistent hyperemotionality which shows no abatement over time. The procedure of daily handling of the animals reduces hyperemotionality in septal-lesioned rats, but such procedure does not affect the hyperemotionality in VMH-damaged rats (Singh, 1969). It would be useful to investigate the specificity and the degree of effectiveness that preoperative training produces. For example, would tranquilizers facilitate the performance of VMH-lesioned rats on avoidance task to the same, more, or less degree that preoperative training does. Finally, it should be ascertained whether the effects of preoperative training are task-specific or global. Would such training, for example, affect the intake of quinine adulterated diet in VMH-lesioned rats?

DIET PALATABILITY AND FINICKINESS

Both increases and decreases in food consumption can be induced in VMH-lesioned rats by manipulating texture, taste, flavor, and caloric density of the diet. This exaggerated response to the positive and negative sensory properties of the food (palatability) is referred to as finickiness. Rats with VMH damage have been shown classically to exhibit greater degree of finickiness to food quality than normal rats. This phenomenon of finickiness in VMH-damaged animals has aroused a great deal of controversy and research. There appear to be two basic issues. Is the finickiness due to exaggerated orosensory responding as classically proposed (Corbit & Stellar, 1964; Teitelbaum, 1955), or is it due to some metabolic postingestive and postabsorptive consequence of diet? While the early investigators tended to emphasize primarily sensory factors, later investigators have stressed ingestive consequences of diet (Powley, 1977). The second issue refers to the role of obesity in determining finickiness. Some investigators have maintained that damage to VMH area is critical (Franklin & Herbert, 1974; Peters & Gunion, 1980). Those favoring the role of obesity point to the fact that both negative and positive finickiness can be more readily demonstrated in the static than the dynamic phase of VMH lesions. Further, dietary obese rats also exhibit finickiness similar to VMH-lesioned rats. The opposite camp cites the studies showing that finickiness can be demonstrated during dynamic phase (Peters & Gunion, 1980; Weingarten, Chang, & Jarvie, 1983), that VMH-lesioned rats maintained on quinine-adulterated food drastically reduce their food intake (Ferguson & Keesey, 1975), and those lesioned rats that exhibit little hyperphagia on a powder diet increase their food intake when offered the same diet in pelleted form (Corbit & Stellar, 1964; Grossman & Grossman, 1971). Finally, the fact that the genetically obese rats (Greenwood, Quartermain, Johnson, Cruce, & Hirsch, 1974), and ovariectomized obese rats (Gale & Sclafani, 1977) do not exhibit finickiness, weakens the argument for the role of obesity. It seems that finickiness at least in VMH-damaged animals is affected by lesions as well obesity and that the two factors work synergistically to maximize it.

The technique of sham feeding permits the isolation of the role played by orosensory factors as well as that of obesity in the manifestation of finickiness. In sham feeding procedure, ingested food and liquid drains out of the alimentary tract through a gastric cannula and does not activate gastrointestinal feeding control mechanisms (Kraly, Carty, & Smith, 1978). Furthermore, since the amount of food ingested by the animal can be regulated, its body weight can be more reliably controlled. Weingarten (1982), using a sham feeding situation, has reported greater sucrose solution consumption in male VMH-lesioned rats (maintained at the same body weight as control animals) than control rats. Recently Cox and Smith (1986) have replicated these findings in female VMH-lesioned rats and have demonstrated that VMH-lesioned and vagotomized rats sham feed more on a milk diet than control vagotomized rats. Thus, sensory factors greatly affect the positive finickiness shown by VMH-lesioned rats. These authors also report that female Zuker obese rats, while consuming as much as VMH-lesioned rats during normal feeding consume less than half as much as VMH-lesioned rats during sham feeding. Cox and Smith suggest that "exaggerated sham feeding is specific to the VMH syndrome, which is consistent with a proposal that a disturbance of orosensory reactivity underlies VMH hyperphagia" (1986, p. 59).

The role of preoperative training in sham feeding has not yet been investigated.

Effect of Quinine Adulteration

Quinine adulteration of food or water produces a sharp reduction in intake in both VMH-lesioned and rats with knife cuts. The degree of rejection of quinine-adulterated diet, however, depends on the diet composition as well as the vehicle (solid vs. liquid) used. Jacob and Sharma (1969) reported that normal deprived rats show *decreased* quinine tolerance when mixed in a stock diet, but show *increased* quinine tolerance when presented in liquid base. Normal rats also show a consistent preference for sucrose solution over crystalline form when presented in same strength (Young & Greene, 1953). In rats with VMH lesions, finickiness can be demonstrated when rats are fed .2% quinine sulfate, mixed in rat chow mash; however, when presented with .4% quinine mixed in a high fat diet (two-thirds powdered rat chow with one-third Crisco oil), VMH-lesioned rats eat more than control rats (Gunion & Peters, 1979).

Arguing that adding quinine in food not only changes the palatability of food but also its postingestive and postabsorptive consequences, Sclafani, Aravich, and Schwartz (1979), suggested that the rejection of quinine is based on toxic consequences rather than taste factors. To support this inference, these authors have demonstrated that while VMH knife-cut rats reject quinine-adulterated food, they do not reject equally bitter sucrose octa acetate (SOA) which has no known aversive postingestive effect.

Weingarten, Chang, & Jarvie, (1983) have investigated this problem further, using sham feeding situation. These authors offered male Long–Evans VMH-lesioned rats, maintained at 90% of their *ad libitum* body weight, a 30% sucrose solution mixed with quinine (.001%, .002%, and .005%). The VMH-lesioned rats consumed less of adulterated solution compared to their intake of 30% unadulterated sucrose solution. Similarly, when given .05% quinine mixed wet mash, during normal feeding VMH-lesioned rats reduced intake by 35 g and control rats by an average of 15 g. These authors note that although quinine adulteration leads to greater suppression in intake of VMH-lesioned rats, in both normal and sham feeding situation they continue to consume more adulterated food and liquid than control rats. The authors, therefore, suggest that only when within group comparisons are made, do VMH-lesioned rats exhibit negative finickiness.

The effect of preoperative experience on quinine-adulterated water in VMH-lesioned rats has been investigated by Singh (1974). The basic design of this experiment consisted of providing rats quinine water solution for 30 days before surgery (electrolytic anodal lesions) and comparing their postoperative intake with VMH-lesioned rats which had no such preoperative experience. Female Holtzman rats were maintained on *ad libitum* Purina chow and were given .12% quinine–sulfate mixed water for 21 consecutive days if they were assigned to a preoperative experience condition (adapted group). After surgery, the adapted VMH group was tested along with a nonadapted VMH group (nonpreoperative training) for another 21 days. The daily fluid intake (the only water available was quinine-adulterated) along with food intake was recorded for each animal. The findings are shown in Fig. 4.2. As is evident from the figure, nonpretrained, VMH-lesioned rats (nonadapted VMH group) showed a marked reduction in fluid intake in keeping with reported findings (Corbit, 1965; Mook & Blass, 1968). Increased reactivity to quinine taste was not evident in preoperatively adapted VMH group; they consumed as much quinine-mixed water as control-adapted and nonadapted rats. The effect of preoperative adaption persists, albeit markedly reduced, even after 45 days of *ad libitum* food and plain water, which produced significant body weight gain in VMH-lesioned rats (400 g vs. 280 g in control groups). The adapted and nonadapted group not only had comparable VMH lesions, they displayed identical hyperemotionality and consumed identi-

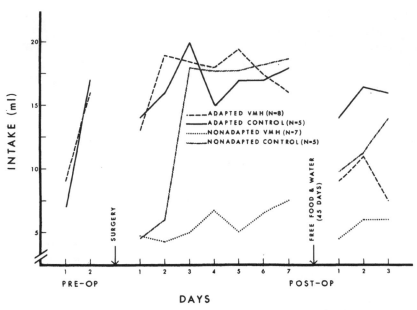

FIG. 4.2.   Mean quinine-adulterated water intake by experimental and control groups. (Each block consists of 3 days. Preoperative Data 2 represents the last 3 days (Preoperative Days 28–30) of the adaptation period.) © American Psychological Association, 1974.

cal amounts of 3% dextrose-mixed water. Thus, preoperative experience was quite specific and affected only the consumption of quinine-adulterated water.

Bait-Shyness

When ingestion of a diet with a distinct flavor or taste is followed by noxious gastrointestinal distress or illness, animals subsequently avoid that diet. This phenomenon of bait-shyness or taste aversion learning has been demonstrated in both animals and humans. Typically, the bait-shyness paradigm requires the animal to avoid a highly palatable (i.e., sucrose, saccharin) liquid or food. The fact that VMH-lesioned rats overreact to the palatability of diet and exhibit hyperemotionality have led some investigators to examine the development of bait-shyness in VMH-lesioned rats. The reported passive avoidance deficit and failure to suppress punished responses in VMH-lesioned rats suggest that VMH-lesioned rats would be retarded in acquiring bait-shyness. Gold and Proulex (1972) were the first to report impaired bait-shyness acquisition in VMH-lesioned rats using saccharin water. Peters and Reich (1973) replicated these findings, using sucrose pellets, although these authors argued that impaired aversive conditioning in VMH-lesioned rats is due to their increased hunger motivation. Notwithstanding the mechanism involved, these studies indicate that impaired taste aversion learning in VMH-lesioned rats can be demonstrated using thirst as well as hunger motivation. There are, however, two studies that report enhanced acquisition of taste aversion learning in VMH-lesioned rats (Thomas & Smith, 1975; Weisman, Hamilton, & Carlton, 1972). A closer examination reveals significant problems with these two studies.

In Weisman et al.'s study, VMH-lesioned rats had *lower* milk intake than control rats during conditioning session (prior to bait-shyness training) and were not *hyperphagic*. Similarly, VMH-lesioned rats in Thomas and Smith (1975) experiments consumed less water than control rats prior to bait-shyness training. The reduced intake of VMH-lesioned rats prior to and during conditioning sessions in both of these studies cast serious doubts on the validity of their reported findings.

The study by Gold and Proulex (1972) is of special importance since these authors also examined the effect of pretraining experience on the bait-shyness in VMH-lesioned rats. These researchers reported that rats which had acquired bait-shyness before lesioning (electrolytic anodal) behave similarly to control rats; when required to learn after VMH damage, rats show retarded learning, compared with control rats. Specifically, Gold and Proulex, trained water-deprived female (Carworth CFE) rats to consume 0.1% solution of saccharin water during a 15 min drinking session. Immediately after this session, rats were given i.p. injection of apomorphine Hcl. Every third day, the saccharin-and-injection procedure was repeated until a combination of 50% suppression (mean intake of saccharin was 50% below the mean water intake during 15-min session) was reached. Rats then were placed on extinction, during which drug injection was replaced by saline injection. The extinction criterion was the point at which the intake of saccharin was no less than 90% of intake of water. The VMH-lesioned rats without preoperative training took significantly more trials to avoid saccharin water than control rats and achieved extinction criterion in fewer trials than control rats. Thus, VMH lesions not only retarded acquisition of bait-shyness but facilitated the extinction of learned responses as well. However, rats in which VMH lesions are made before training exhibit bait-shyness equal to that exhibited by control rats and extinguish at the same rate as control rats.

Thus, while the lack of preoperative training retards the acquisition of bait-shyness habit, preoperative training with bait-shyness is retained by VMH-damaged rats and their performance is comparable with that of control rats.

HUNGER AND THIRST
MOTIVATED BEHAVIOR

The most common technique used to infer the strength of hunger and thirst drive is to observe the willingness of the animal to work to obtain the goal object. Earlier studies found that VMH-lesioned rats are less willing to work to obtain food than control rats and hence inferred that VMH damage induces reduced hunger motivation (Miller et al., 1950; Teitelbaum, 1955). Later studies have questioned the validity of this inference and have attempted to isolate factors which may account for earlier classical findings. It appears that reinforcement schedule (work schedule), test duration, type of reinforcement used, level of deprivation, degree of obesity, and preoperative training significantly affect the motivated behavior of VMH-lesioned rats (King, 1980). The two factors which have been most extensively investigated and affect the motivated behavior of VMH-lesioned rats pertain to the effect of body weight (manipulated by level of food deprivation) and preoperating training.

The earliest study reporting the facilitative effect of preoperative training on food-motivated performance was that of Hamilton and Brobeck (1964; also see, Falk, 1961); although these authors choose an explanation based on species difference for their findings. In this study, male rhesus monkeys were preoperatively trained on an ascending fixed ratio (reward to number of response ratio) schedule (6 days of FR1, 2 days each at FR4, 8 and 16, 6 days at FR32 and 8 days at FR64) to obtain food reinforcement. After VMH damage, both obese and dynamic hyperphagic monkeys obtained significantly greater reinforcement than normal monkeys up to FR64; however, for ratios on which monkeys were not pretrained (FR 128, 256, 512, and 1024), lesioned and normal monkeys did not differ in their performance. In another study, (Singh, 1972), rats were preoperatively trained on a two-chambered box; on one side, food could be obtained by working (bar pressing on FR1, 3, or 11) while on the other side food pellets could be obtained without any food-contingent response (freeloading). All animals (female Holtzman) received 500 reinforcements respectively in both work and "free" side before surgery. After surgery, (anodal electrolytic), all rats were additionally trained for 6 days before preference testing began. For preference testing, the rats were placed in the middle of the box (divider removed) and could choose to either work or freeload. The preference test (15-min session) was conducted for 8 successive days. For the first 4 days, both sides of the chamber provided regular 45-mg pellets; for the remaining 4 days, the freeloading side provided 50% cellulose mixed 45-mg pellets while the work side provided regular 45-mg pellets. Both VMH-lesioned and normal rats preferred to obtain pellets by working (85%–90%) rather than freeloading, regardless of FR schedule. Furthermore, preference to work was maintained by VMH-lesioned rats even when the pellets obtained by working were adulterated (55%–75%) and regular pellets were available on freeloading side. Unlike VMH-lesioned rats, normal rats switch their preference and (30%–45% by working) consumed more food on freeloading side.

Thus, it appears that after preoperative training, VMH-lesioned rats, in a choice situation, are not only willing to work to obtain food, but do not exhibit typically reported aversion to cellulose mixed food. Unfortunately, in this study a nonpreoperatively trained group was not used, so there was no determination of the behavior of VMH-lesioned rats in a choice situation. It could be that in choice situations, all VMH-lesioned rats, whether preoperatively trained or not, would have worked for their food reinforcement.

In the next study (Singh, 1973a), performance of preoperatively trained VMH-lesioned rats was compared with VMH-lesioned rats without pretraining on successively increasing FR schedules. All rats assigned to preoperative training conditions were trained 4 hours a day for 4 consecutive days on successively increasing FR ratios of 1, 4, 16, 64, and 256. Total food intake was restricted to reinforcement obtained on FR schedule plus 10 mg of purina rat chow given after half of an hour of daily session. Rats assigned to nonpreoperative training were identically trained and treated, except that the FR training was initiated after a 10-day postoperative recovery. The performance of all the groups on FR 256 is shown in Fig. 4.3. The preoperatively trained VMH-lesioned rats perform as well as control rats, while nonpretrained VMH-lesioned rats perform as poorly as reported in the classical study of Teitelbaum (1955). The effect of pretraining persisted even during static stages when all rats were tested again after 2 months of ad libidem food and water. The obese nonpretrained VMH-lesioned rats made fewer than 2,000 responses, while preoperatively trained obese VMH-lesioned rats made more than 7,000. Similar effects of pretraining in obese rats is evident in extinction session. Thus, while pretraining had a facilitative effect on the performance of obese rats, it did not obliterate the effect of obesity on performance.

King and Gaston (1973) similarly found that preoperative training on FR schedule attenuated the performance deficit in VMH-lesioned rats. In a later study they demonstrated facilitative effects of preoperative training on FR 128 (highest ratio used in both the studies) by VMH-lesioned rats when tested without a period of ad libidem feeding and retraining on lower ratios (King & Gaston, 1976a). Beatty et al. (1975) also reported facilitative effects of pretraining on the performance of VMH-lesioned rats on FR 128.

The other factor that facilitates the performance of VMH-lesioned rats is the level of deprivation. When VMH-lesioned and normal rats are compared under identical food deprivation (percentage of body weight loss) condition, VMH-lesioned rats perform as well as normal rats (Kent & Peters, 1973; Marks & Remley, 1972; Porter & Allen, 1977; Sclafani & Kluge, 1974). The fact that both identical deprivation and preoperative training facilitate the performance of VMH-lesioned rats has led some investigators to evaluate the respective role played by these factors (King & Gaston, 1976a; Porter & Allen, 1977). Both of these studies employed a factorial design to assess the contribution of identical deprivation and preoperative training variable. Testing rats on a FR schedule (FR 128 was the highest ratio), King and Gaston (1976a) found that the performance of preoperatively trained lean as well as obese VMH-lesioned rats was comparable with that of normal rats; identical deprivation alone, on the other hand, had minimal effects.

Porter and Allen (1977), using a VI 1-min (rats are required to respond on

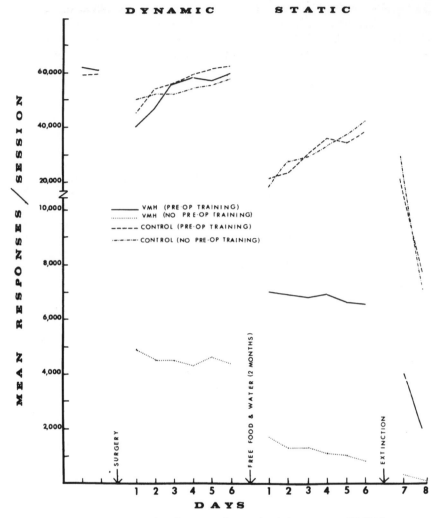

FIG. 4.3.   Mean number of responses during 4-hr. daily sessions on FR-256 by experimental and control groups during successive stages of testing. © American Psychological Association, 1973.

the average of one response per min), found that neither identical deprivation nor pretraining facilitate the performance of VMH-lesioned rats. The inconsistent results of these two studies are probably due to different schedules of reinforcement used. The FR and VI schedule are not comparable in amount of work required (number of bar presses) to obtain reinforcement and lead to differential performance when the same rats are tested on these two schedules (Sclafani & Kluge, 1974).

The facilitative role of preoperative training has also been demonstrated in a thirst-motivated situation (King & Gaston, 1976a). These authors used a factorial design involving identical deprivation and preoperative training as two factors to investigate the performance VMH-lesioned rats on a FR schedule for water reinforcement. All rats were maintained on 22-hr water deprivation (*ad libitum* food throughout testing sessions) and were tested in 90-min sessions for 2 days at FR 1, 4, 8, 16, 32, 64, 96, 128. After a testing session, rats were given *ad libitum* water for 30 min. While preoperative training greatly facilitated performance of VMH-lesioned rats, identical deprivation had no effect on the performance.

Furthermore, preoperative training was found to facilitate the performance of VMH-lesioned rats more on higher FR ratios than control rats. Thus, preoperative training facilitates the performance of VMH-lesioned rats on both hunger- and thirst-motivated task when a taxing work schedule (FR schedule) is used.

The facilitative effect of preoperative training only on the taxing schedule could be due to habituation to stress induced by the schedule itself. The demanding work schedule (FR 128 requires animal to make 128 bar presses to obtain one pellet of food), by definition, is more stressful than less taxing schedule (VI 1-min requires the animal to respond on the average of 1 min per min) of work. It could be that during pretraining, the animal becomes habituated to stress induced by demanding schedules, which in turn facilitates performance postoperatively. The less demanding task does not induce stress and hence no facilitative effect is observed postoperatively. Another factor, in addition to stress habituation, could be the development of response efficiency. It would appear that when the task is demanding, the animal engages in various response topographies to discover the most efficient response. The response variability required to discover the most efficient response would be more readily available to a neurologically intact animal than an animal with neural damage. This practiced response variability would enable the preoperatively trained animal to retain some of the response strategies after neural damage which, in turn, could facilitate its behavior postoperatively.

CONCLUSION

A variety of preoperative experiences, ranging from environmental conditions in which animals are raised to specific training on the task, as well as some nonspecific experience appear to provide protection against later deficit caused by neural damage. I will briefly describe these various programs of preoperative experience to establish that protective effects of prelesion experience are not artifactual and can be reliably induced by various manipulations.

Enriched and Complex Environment

In this type of manipulation animals are raised in complex group environment as exemplified by classical studies of Rosenzweig's group (1986) and Greenough et al., (1976). Such rearing conditions have been shown to enhance the performance of normal neurologically intact rats in a variety of learning situations. Such rearing conditions also appear to overcome or minimize the effect of neural damage in later life. For example, rats raised in such complex environments and later subjected to septal or hippocampal damage do not exhibit all of the typical behavioral disorders associated with damage to these areas (Greenough et al., 1976). It is indeed very impressive that nonspecific preoperative training can induce protective effect against specific behavior disorders caused by neural damage.

Nonspecific Experience

There is also evidence that some nonspecific preoperative experiences in adult animals can minimize the effect of neural injury. For example, Harrell and Balagura (1974) report that rats maintained for 5 days in darkness prior to lateral hypothalamic damage (LH) exhibit less impairment on typical motor deficit associated with such damage than rat without such experience; also, such experience with lighting conditions postoperatively has no effect. The mechanism responsible for such facilitative effect of nonspecific experience on specific disorders is not clear (for possible mechanism, see Greenough et al., 1976).

Specific or Related Experience

Unlike the two preoperative manipulations mentioned herein, in this type of situation animals are extensively trained prior to surgery on the task to be used postoperatively. Most of the studies described here fall in this category. The mechanism responsible for the survival of preoperative training after neural damage is not known. There are also a few studies in which animals are pre-operatively exposed to an experience which is related to, but is not specific to, postoperative task. For example, Schallert (1982) found that preoperative experience with restricted water intake attenuates adipsia in the rats with LH damage. Similarly, preoperative insulin injection facilitates recovery from LH damage in rats (Balagura, Harrell, & Ralph, 1973).

Thus, it seems that a variety of specific and nonspecific preoperative experiences can affect the nature and magnitude of disorders observed after neural damage. Attenuation of behavioral disorders caused by neural damage by preoperative experience have been reported in this volume for various areas of the brain. Furthermore, the preoperative experience is not restricted to certain functions or types of behavior; the effects of preoperative experience has been observed in behavior ranging from basic appetitive to complex acquired behaviors. Taken together, these findings establish the legitimacy and potency of preoperative experience.

The use of preoperative manipulation can be extremely useful in elucidating the nature of functional disorders for regulatory systems such as VMH and LH areas where the damage is presumed to produce a syndrome. As stated before, the notion of syndrome assumes some degree of relatedness among various elements and are supposedly produced by a unitary cause. Notwithstanding the validity of such an idea, damage to both VMH and LH areas does produce a constellation of behavioral and physiological effects. An intriguing question is whether the preoperative manipulation on one element would generalize to all or, at least, some other elements of the constellation. For example, would the preoperative experience with restricted water intake which attenuates adipsia in the LH-damaged rats, also affect diet finickiness and sensory neglect as well in these LH-damaged rats? Similarly, if rats are raised in varying environmental temperature preoperatively, would such experience affect their thermal regulation as well as dietary finickiness and hunger motivation (willingness to work) after VMH damage? It may be that the effect of the preoperative experience is more global for those brain areas which produce a syndrome, compared with areas where the damage, for example, occipital cortex, does not produce a broad range of diverse disorders. It is, therefore, extremely critical that the preoperative experience manipulation experiments measure as many elements of the LH and VMH syndrome as possible to ascertain the extent of, or lack of, protective effect of experimental factors.

Furthermore, it is quite possible that the nature and the magnitude of the preoperative experience determines whether the effects are global or specific. We do not know what minimal training is needed to produce protective effects. The amount of training necessary to induce protective effect for various functions may be different, yet unknown. It may turn out that for some behavior mere habituation to the test situation is sufficient, whereas for other behavior an extended and specific training may be necessary to demonstrate protective effect after brain damage. While a large body of research dealing with the effect of overtraining on sparing of the function exists (e.g., Finger & Stein, 1982), there are no studies specifically investigating the nature of the training on sparing of a function after brain damage.

Finally, the mechanisms responsible for preoperative experience are not clear (however, see Greenough et al., 1976). The protective effects could be due to either an associative (animal learning various adaptive strategies) or a nonassociative (reduction in fear, altered drive strength) mechanism. Either of these mechanisms, singularly or jointly, can affect the nature and magnitude of observed behavior. Isolating the relative roles played by each of the mechanisms is critical in our understanding of the protective function of preoperative experience.

The main advantage of using preoperative manipulation to elucidate the nature of disorders produced by VMH damage is that it does not favor either metabolic or behavioral explanation, but it provides a means to examine the interrelatedness of various disorders cause by VMH damage. The investigation of preoperative experience, its limitation, and its mechanisms may enable researchers to develop a more accurate description and understanding of neurobehavioral relationship.

REFERENCES

Balagura, S., & Devenport, L. D. (1970). Feeding patterns of normal and ventromedial hypothalamic lesioned male and female rats. *Journal of Comparative & Physiological Psychology, 71*, 357–364.

Balagura, S., Harrell, L., & Ralph, T. C. (1973). Glucodynamic hormones modify the recovery period after lateral hypothalamic lesions. *Science, 182*, 59–60.

Balinska, H. (1963). Food preference and conditioned reflex type activity in dynamic hyperphagic rabbits. *Acta Biologae Experimentalis, 23*, 33–44.

Beatty, W. W., Vilberg, T. R., Shirk, T. S., & Siders, W. A. (1975). Pretraining: Effects on operant responding for food, frustration, and reactiveness to food-related cues in rats with VMH lesions. *Physiology & Behavior, 15*, 577–584.

Bernardis, L. L. (1971). Growth retardation following ventromedial hypothalamic lesions current. *Growth, 35*, 137–143.

Bernardis, L. L., & Bellinger, L. L. (1976). Production in weanling rat of ventromedial and dorsomedial hypothalamic syndromes by electrolytic lesions with platinum-cridium electrode. *Neuroendocrinology, 22*, 99–106.

Berthoud, H. R., & Jeanrenaud, B. (1979). Changes of insulinemia, glycemia and feeding behavior induced by VMH-procainization in the rat. *Brain Research, 174*, 184–187.

Brady, J. V., & Nauta, W. J. H. (1953). Subcortical mechanisms in emotional behavior: Affective changes following septal forebrain lesions in the albino rat. *Journal of Comparative & Physiological Psychology, 46*, 339–346.

Bray, G. A. (1984). Syndromes of hypothalamic obesity in man. *Pediatric Annals, 13*, 525–536.

Bray, G. A., Sclafani, A., & Novin, D. (1982). Obesity-inducing hypothalamic knife cuts. Effects of lipolysis and blood insulin levels. *American Journal of Physiology, 243*, R445–R449.

Bray, G. A., & York, D. A. (1979). Hypothalamic and genetic obesity in experimental animals: An autonomic and endocrine hypothesis. *Physiological Reviews, 59*, 719–809.

Brobeck, J. R. (1946). Mechanism of the development of obesity in animals with hypothalamic lesions. *Physiological Reviews, 26*, 541–559.

Brooks, C. M., Lockwood, R. A., & Wiggins, M. L. (1946). A study of the effect of hypothalamic lesions on the eating habits of the albino rat. *American Journal of Physiology, 147*, 735–741.

Colpaert, F. E., & Wiepkema (1976). Ventromedial hypothalamus: Fear conditioning and passive avoidance in rats. *Physiology & Behavior, 16*, 91–95.

Corbit, J. D. (1965). Hyperphagic hyperreactivity to adulteration of drinking water with quinine HCl. *Journal of Comparative & Physiological Psychology, 60*, 123–124.

Corbit, J. D., & Stellar, E. (1964). Palatability, food intake, and obesity in normal and hyperphagic rats. *Journal of Comparative & Physiological Psychology, 58*, 63–67.

Cox, J. E., & Smith, G. P. (1986). Sham feeding in rats after ventromedial hypothalamic lesions and vagotomy. *Behavioral Neuroscience, 100*, 57–63.

Falk, J. L. (1961). Comments on Dr. Teitelbaum's paper. In M. R. Jones (Ed.), *Nebraska symposium on motivation* (pp. 65–68). Lincoln, NE: University of Nebraska Press.

Ferguson, N. B. L., & Keesey, R. E. (1975). Effect of a quinine-adulterated diet upon body maintenance in male rats with ventromedial hypothalamic lesions. *Journal of Comparative & Physiological Psychology, 89,* 478–488.

Finger, S., & Stein, D. G. (1982). *Brain damage and recovery: Research and clinical perspectives.* New York: Academic Press.

Franklin, K. B. J., & Herbert, L. J. (1974). Ventromedial syndrome: The rat's "finickiness" results from the obesity, not from the lesions. *Journal of Comparative & Physiological Psychology, 87,* 410–414.

Gale, S. K., & Sclafani, A. (1977). Comparison of overian and hypothalamic obesity syndromes in the female rat: Effects of diet palatability on food intake and body weight. *Journal of Comparative & Physiological Psychology, 91,* 381–392.

Gold, R. M. (1975). Anodal electrolytic brain lesions: How current and electrode metal influence lesion size and hyperphagiosity. *Physiology & Behavior, 14,* 625–632.

Gold, R. M., Kapatos, G., & Carey, R. J. (1973). A retractory wire knife for stereotaxic brain surgery made from a microliter syringe. *Physiology & Behavior, 10,* 814.

Gold, R. M., & Proulex, D. M. (1972). Bait-shyness acquisition is impaired by VMH lesions that produce obesity. *Journal of Comparative & Physiological Psychology, 79,* 201–209.

Gold, R. M., Sawchenko, P. E., DeLuca, C., Alexander, J., & Eng, R. (1980). Vagal mediation of hypothalamic obesity but not supermarket dietary obesity. *American Journal of Physiology, 238,* R447–R453.

Graff, H., & Stellar, E. (1962). Hyperphagia, obesity and finickiness. *Journal of Comparative & Physiological Psychology, 55,* 418–424.

Greenough, W. T., Fass, B., & DeVoogd, T. J. (1976). The influence of experience on recovery following brain damage in rodents: Hypotheses based on development research. In R. N. Walsh & W. T. Greenough (Eds.), *Environments as therapy for brain dysfunction* (pp. 10–50). New York: Plenum Press.

Greenwood, M. R. C., Quartermain, D., Johnson, P. R., Cruce, J. A. F., & Hirsch, J. (1974). Food motivated behavior in genetically obese and hypothalamic hyperphagic rats and mice. *Physiology & Behavior, 13,* 687–692.

Grossman, S. P. (1966). The VMH: A center for affective reactions, satiety, or both? *Physiology & Behavior, 1,* 1–10.

Grossman, S. P. (1972). Aggression, avoidance, and reactions to novel environments in female rats with ventromedial hypothalamic lesions. *Journal of Comparative & Physiological Psychology, 78,* 274–283.

Grossman, S. P. (1976). Neuroanatomy of food and water intake. In D. Novin, W. Wyrwicka, & G. A. Bray (Eds.), *Basic mechanisms and clinical implications* (pp. 51–59). New York: Raven Press.

Grossman, S. P. (1979). The biology of motivation. *Annual Reviews of Psychology, 30,* 209–242.

Grossman, S. P. (1984). Contemporary problems concerning our understanding of brain mechanisms that regulate food intake and body weight. In A. J. Stunkard & E. Stettar (Eds.), *Eating and its disorder* (pp. 5–13). New York: Raven Press.

Grossman, S. P., & Grossman, L. (1971). Food and water intake in rats with parasagittal knife cuts medial or lateral to the lateral hypothalamus. *Journal of Comparative & Physiological Psychology, 71,* 148–156.

Gunion, M. W., & Peters, R. H. (1979). Rats with hypothalamic knife cuts overeat an unpalatable diet. *Physiology & Behavior, 22,* 1037–1039.

Hamilton, C. L., & Brobeck, J. (1964). Hypothalamic hyperphagia in the monkey. *Journal of Comparative and Physiological Psychology, 57,* 271–278.

Harrell, L. E., & Remley, N. R. (1973). The immediate development of behavioral and biochemical changes following ventromedial hypothalamic lesions in rats. *Behavioral Biology, 9,* 49–63.

Harrell, L. E., & Balagura, S. (1974). The effects of dark and light on the functional recovery following lateral hypothalamic lesions. *Life Sciences, 15,* 2079–2088.

Hetherington, A. W., & Ranson, S. W. (1942). The relation of various hypothalamic lesions to adiposity in the rat. *Journal of Comparative Neurology, 76,* 475–499.

Hoebel, B. G. (1965). Hypothalamic lesions by electrocauterization: Disinhibition of feeding and self-stimulation. *Science, 149,* 452–453.

Hoebel, B. G. (1975). Brain reward and aversion systems in the control of feeding and sexual behavior. In J. K. Cole & T. B. Sonderegger (Eds.), *Nebraska symposium on motivation* (Vol. 22, pp. 49–112). Lincoln: University of Nebraska Press.

Hoebel, B. G., & Teitelbaum, P. (1966). Weight regulation in normal and hypothalamic hypophagic rats. *Journal of Comparative & Physiological Psychology, 61,* 189–193.

House, E. L., & Pansky, B. (1960). *Neuroanatomy.* New York: McGraw–Hill.

Hoyenga, K. B., & Hoyenga, K. T. (1982). Gender and energy balance: Sex differences in adaptation for feast and famine. *Physiology and Behavior, 28,* 545–563.

Inoue, S., & Bray, G. A. (1977). The effects of subdiaphragmatic vagotomy in rats with ventromedial hypothalamic obesity. *Endocrinology, 100,* 108–114.

Jacobs, H. L., & Sharma, K. N. (1969). Taste versus calories: Sensory and metabolic signals in the control of food intake. *Annals of New York Academy of Sciences, 157,* 1084–1125.

Kennedy, G. C. (1969). Interactions between feeding behavior and hormones during growth. *Annals of New York Academy of Sciences, 157,* 1049–1061.

Kent, M. A., & Peters, R. H. (1973). Effect of ventromedial hypothalamic lesions on hunger-motivated behavior in rats. *Journal of Comparative & Physiological Psychology, 83,* 92–97.

King, B. M. (1980). A re-examination of the ventromedial hypothalamic paradox. *Neuroscience & Behavioral Reviews, 4,* 151–160.

King, B. M., Alheid, G. F., & Grossman, S. P. (1977a). Factors influencing active avoidance behavior in rats with ventromedial hypothalamic lesions. *Physiology & Behavior, 18,* 901–913.

King, B. M., Carpenter, R. G., Stamoutsos, B. A., Frohman, L. A., & Grossman, S. P. (1977b). Hyperphagia and obesity following ventromedial hypothalamic lesions in rats with subdiaphragmatic vagotomy. *Physiology & Behavior, 20,* 643–651.

King, B. M., Carrington, C. D., & Grossman, S. P. (1978). Passive avoidance behavior in lean and obese rats with ventromedial hypothalamic lesions. *Physiology & Behavior, 20,* 57–65.

King, B. M., & Frohman, L. A. (1982). The role of vagally-mediated hyperinsulinemia in hypothalamic obesity. *Neuroscience & Biobehavioral Reviews, 6,* 205–214.

King, B. M., & Frohman, L. A. (1985). Nonirritative lesions of VMH: Effects on plasma insulin, obesity and hyperreactivity. *American Journal of Physiology, 248,* E669–E675.

King, B. M., & Frohman, L. A. (1986). Hypothalamic obesity: Comparison of radio-frequency and electrolytic lesions in male and female rats. *Brain Research Bulletin, 17,* 409–413.

King, B. M., & Gaston, M. G. (1973). The effects of pretraining on the bar-pressing performance of VMH-lesioned rats. *Physiology & Behavior, 11,* 161–166.

King, B. M., & Gaston, M. G. (1976a). Factors influencing the hunger and thirst motivated behavior of hypothalamic hyperphagic rats. *Physiology & Behavior, 16,* 33–41.

King, B. M., & Gaston, M. G. (1976b). Impaired free-operant avoidance behavior following ventromedial hypothalamic lesions in rats. *Physiology & Behavior, 16,* 719–726.

King, B. M., & Grossman, S. P. (1977). Response to glucoprivic and hydrational challenges by normal and hypothalamic hyperphagic rats. *Physiology & Behavior, 18,* 463–473.

King, B. M., & Grossman, S. P. (1978). Impaired and enhanced shuttle box avoidance behavior following ventromedial hypothalamic lesions in rats. *Physiology & Behavior, 20,* 51–56.

King, B. M., Phelps, G. R., & Frohman, L. A. (1980). Hypothalamic obesity in female rats in absence of vagally mediated hyperinsulinemia. *American Journal of Physiology, 239,* E437–E441.

Kraly, F. S., Carty, N. J., & Smith, G. P. (1978). Effect of pregastric food stimuli on meal size and intermeal interval in the rat. *Physiology & Behavior, 20,* 779–784.

Larkin, R. P. (1975). Effect of ventromedial hypothalamic procaine injections on feeding, lever pressing, and other behavior in rats. *Journal of Comparative & Physiological Psychology, 89,* 1100–1108.

LeMagnen, J. (1983). Body energy balance and food intake: A neuro-endocrine regulatory mechanism. *Physiological Review, 63,* 314–386.

Levine, S., & Soliday, V. M. H. (1960). The effects of hypothalamic lesions on conditioned avoidance learning. *Journal of Comparative & Physiological Psychology, 53,* 497–501.

Marks, H. E., & Miller, C. R. (1972). Development of hypothalamic obesity in the male golden hamster (Mesocricetus auratus) as a function of food preference. *Psychonomic Science, 27,* 263–265.

Marks, H. E., & Remley, N. R. (1972). The effects of type of lesion and percentage body weight loss on measures of motivated behavior in rats with hypothalamic lesions. *Behavioral Biology, 7,* 95–111.

Miller, N. E., Bailey, C. J., & Stevenson, J. A. F. (1950). Decreased "hunger" but increased food intake resulting from hypothalamic lesions. *Science, 112,* 256–259.

Mook, D. G., & Blass, E. M. (1968). Quinine-aversion thresholds and "finickiness" in hyperphagic rats. *Journal of Comparative & Physiological Psychology, 65,* 202–207.

Nance, D. M., Gorski, R. A., & Panksepp, J. (1976). Neural and hormonal determinants of sex differences in food intake and body weight. In D. Novin, W. Wyrwicka, & G. A. Gray (Eds.), *Hunger: Basic mechanisms and clinical implications* (pp. 257–271). New York: Raven Press.

Nisbett, R. E., Braver, A., Jusela, G., & Kezur, D. (1975). Age and sex differences in behaviors mediated by the ventromedial hypothalamus. *Journal of Comparative & Physiological Psychology, 88,* 736–746.

Panksepp, J. (1976). On the nature of feeding patterns-Primarily in rats. In D. Novin, W. Wyrwicka, & G. H. Bray (Eds.), *Hunger: Basic mechanisms and clinical implications* (pp. 257–271). New York: Raven Press.

Peters, R. H., & Gunion, M. W. (1980). Finickiness in VMH rats also results from the lesions, not just from obesity. *Physiological Psychology, 8,* 93–96.

Peters, R. H., & Reich, M. J. (1973). Effects of ventromedial hypothalamic lesions on conditioned sucrose aversions in rats. *Journal of Comparative & Physiological Psychology, 84,* 502–506.

Porter, J. H., & Allen, J. D. (1977). Food-motivated performance in rats with ventromedial hypothalamic lesions: Effects of body weight, deprivation, and preoperative training. *Behavioral Biology, 19,* 238–254.

Powley, T. L. (1977). The ventromedial hypothalamic syndrome, satiety, and a cephalic phase hypothesis. *Psychological Review, 84,* 89–126.

Powley, T. L., & Opsahl, C. A. (1976). Autonomic components of the hypothalamic feeding syndromes. In D. Novin, W. Wyrwicka, & G. A. Bray (Eds.), *Hunger: Basic mechanisms and clinical implications* (pp. 313–326). New York: Raven Press.

Powley, T. L., Opsahl, C. A., Cox, J. E., & Weingarten, H. P. (1980). The role of the hypothalamus in energy homeostasis. In P. J. Morgane & J. Panksepp (Eds.), *Handbook of the hypothalamus: Behavioral studies of the hypothalamus* (Vol. 3, Pt. A, pp. 211–298). New York: Marcel Dekker.

Reeves, A. G., & Plum, F. (1969). Hyperphagia, rage, and dementia accompanying a ventromedial hypothalamic neoplasm. *Archives of Neurology, 20,* 616–624.

Reynolds, R. W. (1965). An irritative hypothesis concerning the hypothalamic regulation of food intake. *Psychological Review, 72,* 105–116.

Rosenzweig, M. R. (1986). Animal models for effects of brain lesions and for rehabilitation. In P. Bach-y-Rita (Ed.), *Recovery of function: Theoretical considerations for brain injury rehabilitation* (pp. 127–172). Toronto: Hans Huber.

Sanders, M. K., Lakey, J. R., & Singh, D. (1973). Sex differences in hyperphagia and body weight gains following goldthioglucose-induced hypothalamic lesions in mice. *Physiological Psychology, 1,* 237–240.

Schallert, T. (1982). Adipsia produced by lateral hypothalamic lesions: Facilitation of recovery by preoperative restriction of water intake. *Journal of Comparative and Physiological Psychology, 92,* 720–741.

Sclafani, A. (1971). Neural pathways involved in the ventromedial hypothalamic lesion syndrome in the rat. *Journal of Comparative & Physiological Psychology, 77,* 70–96.

Sclafani, A. (1976). Appetite and hunger in experimental obesity syndrome. In D. Novin, W. Wyrwicka, & G. Bray (Eds.), *Hunger: Basic mechanisms and clinical implications* (pp. 281–295). New York: Raven Press.

Sclafani, A. (1977). Effects of presurgical weight reduction on the development of hypothalamic hyperphagia in rats. *Behavioral Biology, 21,* 412–417.

Sclafani, A., Aravich, P. F., & Landman, M. (1981). Vagotomy blocks hypothalamic hyperphagia in rats on a chow diet and sucrose solution, but not on a palatable mixed diet. *Journal of Comparative & Physiological Psychology, 95,* 720–734.

Sclafani, A., Aravich, P. F., & Schwartz, J. (1979). Hypothalamic hyperphagic rats overeat bitter sucrose octa acetate diets but not quinine diets. *Physiology & Behavior, 22,* 759–766.

Sclafani, A., Berner, C. N., & Maul, G. (1975). Multiple knife cuts between the medial and lateral hypothalamus in the rat: A reevaluation of hypothalamic feeding circuitry. *Journal of Comparative & Physiological Psychology, 88,* 210–217.

Sclafani, A., & Grossman, S. P. (1971). Reactivity of hyperphagic and normal rats to quinine and electric shock. *Journal of Comparative & Physiological Psychology, 74,* 157–166.

Sclafani, A., & Kirchgessner, A. (1986). The role of medial hypothalamus in the control of food intake: An update. In R. C. Ritter, S. Ritter, & C. D. Burnes (Eds.), *Feeding behavior neural and hormonal controls* (pp. 27–66). New York: Academic Press.

Sclafani, A., & Kluge, L. (1974). Food motivation and body weight levels in hypothalamic hyperphagic rats: a dual lipostatic model of hunger and appetite. *Journal of Comparative & Physiological Psychology, 86,* 28–46.

Singh, D. (1969). Comparison of hyperemotionality caused by lesions in the septal and ventromedial hypothalamic areas in the rat. *Psychonomic Science, 16,* 3–4.

Singh, D. (1970). Sex differences in obesity and good-directed activity in normal and hyperphagic rats. *Psychonomic Science, 21,* 306–308.

Singh, D. (1972). Preference for mode of obtaining reinforcement in rats with lesions in septal or ventromedial hypothalamic areas. *Journal of Comparative & Physiological Psychology, 80,* 259–268.

Singh, D. (1973a). Effects of preoperative training on food-motivated behavior of hypothalamic hyperphagic rats. *Journal of Comparative & Psychological Psychology, 84,* 47–52.

Singh, D. (1973b). Comparison of behavioral deficits caused by lesions in septal and ventromedial hypothalamic areas of female rats. *Journal of Comparative & Physiological Psychology, 84,* 370–379.

Singh, D. (1974). Role of preoperative experience on reaction to quinine taste in hypothalamic hyperphagic rats. *Journal of Comparative & Physiological Psychology, 86,* 671–678.

Singh, D. (1975). Experimental ablation. In D. Singh & D. D. Avery (Eds.), *Physiological techniques in behavioral research* (pp. 45–67). Monterey, CA: Brooks/Cole.

Singh, D., Lakey, J. R., & Sanders, M. K. (1974). Hunger motivation in goldthioglucose-treated and genetically obese female mice. *Journal of Comparative & Physiological Psychology, 86,* 890–897.

Singh, D., & Meyer, D. R. (1968). Eating and drinking by rats with lesions of the septum and the ventromedial hypothalamus. *Journal of Comparative & Physiological Psychology, 65,* 163–166.

Teitelbaum, P. (1955). Sensory control of hythalamic hyperphagia. *Journal of Comparative & Physiological Psychology, 48,* 158–163.

Teitelbaum, P. (1961). Disturbances in feeding and drinking after hypothalamic lesions. In M. R. Jones (Ed.), *Nebraska symposium on motivation* (pp. 39–55). Lincoln, NE: University of Nebraska.

Thomas, J. B., & Smith, D. A. (1975). VMH lesions facilitate bait-shyness in the rat. *Physiology & Behavior, 15,* 7–11.

Valenstein, E. S., Cox, V. C., & Kakolewski, J. (1969). Sex differences in hyperphagia and body weight following hypothalamic damage. *Annals of New York Academy of Sciences, 157,* 1030–1046.

Weingarten, H. P. (1982). Diet pulutability modulates sham feeding in VMH-lesion and normal rats: Implications for finickiness and evaluation of sham-feeding data. *Journal of Comparative & Physiological Psychology, 96,* 223–233.

Weingarten, H. P., Chang, P., & Jarvie, K. R. (1983). Reactivity of normal and VMH-lesion rats to quinine-adulterated foods: Negative evidence for negative finickiness. *Behavioral Neuroscience, 97,* 221–233.

Weingarten, H. P., Chang, P., & McDonald, T. J. (1985). Comparison of the metabolic and behavioral disturbances following paraventricular-and ventromedial-hypothalamic lesions. *Brain Research Bulletin, 14,* 551–559.

Weisman, R. N., & Hamilton, L. W. (1972). Two-way avoidance responding following VMH lesions: Effects of varying shock intensity. *Physiology & Behavior, 9,* 243–246.

Weisman, R. N., Hamilton, L. W., & Carlton, P. L. (1972). Increased conditioned gustatory aversion following VMH lesions in rats. *Physiology & Behavior, 9,* 801–804.

Wheatley, M. D. (1944). The hypothalamus and affective behavior in cats. *Archives of Neurology & Psychiatry, 52,* 296–316.

Wiepkema, P. R. (1968). Behavior changes in CBA mice as a result of one goldthioglucose injection. *Behaviour, 32,* 179–210.

Young, P. T., & Greene, J. T. (1953). Quantity of food ingested as a measure of relative acceptability. *Journal of Comparative & Physiological Psychology, 46,* 288–294.

5

Modulatory Effects of Environmental and Social Interactions on the Behavioral Expression of Amygdaloid Damage

Ernest D. Kemble
Division of Social Sciences
University of Minnesota, Morris

INTRODUCTION

Since the original description of the Kluver–Bucy syndrome (Kluver & Bucy, 1939), an enormous literature on the behavioral effects of amygdaloid lesions has accumulated (see e.g., Bandler, 1984; Ben–Ari, 1981; Eleftheriou, 1972; Fonberg, 1986; Kesner & DiMattia, 1987; Livingston & Hornykiewicz, 1978; Mogenson, 1987; Sarter & Markowitsch, 1985, for recent reviews). In view of growing evidence for recovery of function following damage to other CNS sites (e.g., Stein, Finger, & Hart, 1983; Stein, Rosen, & Butters, 1974; Walsh & Greenough, 1976) and substantial protective effects produced by environmental enrichment (e.g., Finger, 1978), the possibility that preoperative experience might alter the effects of later amygdaloid damage has received relatively little attention. This neglect is probably in reaction to a number of studies which yielded apparently contradictory results or only task-specific recovery effects. It now seems increasingly probable, however, that the simultaneous placement of extensive lesions common in these experiments and the restricted range of species and behaviors examined obscured recovery effects. Although the amygdala has been known to be anatomically and functionally heterogeneous for some time (e.g., Fernandez de Molina & Hunsperger, 1962; Goddard, 1964; Ursin & Kaada, 1957), more recent data indicate that it, and nearby structures, contain a number of discrete systems which seem to modulate behavior by mutually antagonistic interactions (e.g., Fonberg, 1986; Henke, 1980; Ursin, 1965a). Limited evidence further suggests that major behavioral predispositions are reflected in the balance between such interacting systems and that stimulation-induced shifts in balance produce a corresponding shift in behavior (Adamec, 1978; Adamec & Stark–Adamec, 1984). These data suggest the exciting possibility that the bias of some amygdaloid systems might be experientially, as well as physiologically, modifiable.

Further, it is also clear that the effects of simultaneous bilateral lesions are ameliorated by the placement of serial two-stage lesions (McIntyre & Stein, 1973; Stein, Rosen, Graziadei, Mishkin, & Brink, 1969) or by preoperative environmental enrichment (Kemble & Davies, 1981). This chapter will survey the major experimental approaches to recovery of function in the amygdala and suggest further research to delineate more clearly the functional plasticity of this structure. Such data may reveal procedures which will provide protective effects or facilitate recovery from amygdaloid damage.

AGE AT THE TIME OF LESIONS

Since the age at which damage is sustained is the most thoroughly studied and effective manipulation in demonstrating sparing of function at other CNS sites (e.g., Finger, 1978; Stein et al., 1974), it is not surprising that this technique has dominated studies of the amygdala as well. In an extensive series of studies, Kling and his coworkers (Dicks, Myers, & Kling, 1969; Green & Kling, 1966; Kling, 1965, 1966, 1972; Kling & Green, 1967), provided early data suggesting that amygdaloid lesions placed in infancy resulted in major sparing of the deficits seen following damage to adults. These investigators contrasted the effects of lesions placed in adults to those placed at various earlier stages of maturation. In rats, cats, and monkeys Kling (1962, 1965, 1966) found that lesions placed in infancy had no detectable effects on nursing, weaning, growth rates, and the time at which play and aggressive behavior appeared. Aphagia did not appear in cats unless they were at least 72 days old and, if anything, lesions placed in infancy slightly speeded development. Two subsequent studies have shown that extensive amygdaloid lesions placed in infant rats reversed the lesion-induced impairments in avoidance acquisition seen in adults (Eclancher & Karli, 1980; Molino, 1975) but failed to spare lesion effects on acquisition of a conditioned emotional response (Molino, 1975) or open field behavior (Eclancher et al., 1980). Both studies are thus consistent with earlier data in suggesting at least some protective effects of placing lesions in infancy.

The most extensive analyses of age-related sparing have been carried out on primates who have sustained total amygdalectomies. Following such lesions, adult primates show a striking "taming" effect toward humans (e.g., Aggleton & Passingham, 1981; Dicks et al., 1969; Kling, Dicks, & Gurowitz, 1968; Kluver & Bucy, 1939; Weiskrantz, 1956). When placed in social settings, these animals show a marked decrease in aggressive behavior (e.g., Kling & Cornell, 1971; Kling, Lancaster, & Benitone, 1969), unresponsiveness to solicitation of social contact by other members of their group (e.g., Kling et al., 1969) and frequently

(Dicks et al., 1969; Kling et al., 1968, 1969; Plotnik, 1968), but not always (Kling, 1974; Rosvold, Mirsky, & Pribram, 1954), a precipitous drop in dominance rank. In free-ranging troops, this also typically results in social isolation, frequent wounding by conspecifics and, ultimately, death (Dicks et al., 1969; Kling et al., 1969). When such lesions were placed in 2–3-year-old members of free-ranging monkey troops, however, a brief period of isolation was followed by a return to normal relationships with their mothers and other members of the troop (Dicks et al., 1969).

Subsequent experiments by Thompson and his coworkers (Thompson, 1981; Thompson, Bergland, & Towfighi, 1977; Thompson, Schwartzbaum, & Harlow, 1969; Thompson & Towfighi, 1976) seem to stand in direct contrast to Kling's findings. Thompson placed two-stage lesions at 1.8 and 2.5 months of age in rhesus monkeys and followed their development in an extensive 6-year longitudinal study. At the end of the 6-year period, these monkeys were compared with adult-amygdalectomized subjects. The infant-amygdalectomized monkeys showed no immediate effects of the lesions but between 5 and 8 months of age began to show hyperactivity, fear, and avoidance of conspecifics characteristic of adult-amygdalectomized monkeys (Thompson et al., 1969). These symptoms grew progressively more pronounced during periodic testing over the 6-year period (Thompson & Towfighi, 1976) and when they were compared with adult-amygdalectomized monkeys at 6 years of age (Thompson, 1981; Thompson et al., 1977) were indistinguishable. Further, when infant- and adult-amygdalectomized monkeys were confronted by a dominant 10-year-old female they showed similar and indistinguishable impairments in normal social behavior (e.g., staring directly at the dominant animal after being attacked and, thus, provoking further aggression) and were subjected to unremitting attack throughout the test (Thompson, 1981). Finally, both infant- and adult-amygdalectomized monkeys showed comparable deficits in both a delayed alternation and successive reversal problem (Thompson, 1981). Like adults (Weiskrantz, 1956), infant-amygdalectomized monkeys were also deficient in conditioned avoidance acquisition (Thompson, 1981).

The above data hardly provide persuasive evidence for strong protective effects of age per se. Although both Eclancher and Karli (1980) and Molino (1975) agree that lesions placed in infancy spare active avoidance acquisition in adulthood, these effects do not extend to other behavioral measures. Since avoidance acquisition may be altered by a broad range of variables, interpretation of these results is difficult. The contradictory findings of Kling and Thompson are also quite disturbing. Thompson's failure to observe sparing is made more striking because his lesions were placed serially at 1.8 and 2.5 months of age, a procedure which should have facilitated recovery (McIntyre & Stein, 1973; Stein et al., 1969). Since total ablations were employed by both Kling and Thompson, it is unlikely that lesion differences contributed to these differences. However, the two approaches did differ considerably in the conditions under which observations were carried out. Thompson's monkeys were laboratory-reared and tested in small, homogeneous groups. In contrast, the most striking evidence for recovery was obtained from monkeys that were members of large, free-ranging troops on Cayo Santiago (Dicks et al., 1969). The more varied environment and social relationships experienced by the free-ranging monkeys would seem to be a leading reason for the striking difference in the expression of lesion effects. If so, age might be expected to interact with other experiential variables in determining recovery effects.

AGE–EXPERIENCE
INTERACTIONS

More recent data have provided direct support for an environment–lesion interaction. Kling and Dunne (1976) studied a group of amygdalectomized and normal adult monkeys in both the laboratory and later in a spacious free-ranging environment with a larger social group. When observed in the laboratory, the amygdalectomized monkeys showed hyperorality, hypersexuality, tameness, reduced grooming and threat, and a loss of social status. In the field, the operates showed no hyperorality or hypersexuality, were intensely fearful, and became social isolates. This dramatic reversal of amygdaloid symptoms has also been demonstrated when amygdalectomized monkeys are released from individual housing into the total free-ranging environment of the jungle (Kling et al., 1969). It appears obvious then, that the symptoms which follow total amygdalectomy in primates depend critically on the social/environmental context of the observations and are highly responsive to such manipulations regardless of age.

A parallel series of experiments with rats suggests a similar conclusion. In these studies Eclancher and Karli (1979, 1980) observed rats that were either individually or group housed from the time of weaning and which sustained amygdaloid lesions in either infancy or adulthood. Since both the infant- and adult-lesioned groups contained rats in which the amygdaloid damage was quite extensive and others in which lesions were largely restricted to the corticomedial region, some degree of localization was also possible. Although both infant and adult lesions, regardless of lesion site, increased open field behavior, this effect was considerably less marked among rats raised in social isolation (Eclancher & Karli, 1979). They (Eclancher & Karli, 1980) also found that among infant-lesioned rats with corticomedial lesions avoidance behavior was impaired in group-housed rats but facilitated in those that were reared in social isolation. Thus, although the age at which amygdaloid damage occurs may produce some limited sparing, this effect interacts with both preoperative experience and lesion site.

Further data (Eclancher, Schmitt, & Karli, 1975), however, question whether "sparing" is an appropriate description of the effect in other than the most narrow sense. These investigators found that amygdaloid lesions placed in infancy, but not adulthood, greatly increased the incidence of muricide among their rats above control levels at adulthood. Subsequent research (Vergnes, 1981) revealed that the strong inhibition of mouse-killing induced by prior familiarization could be reversed in many of her rats by damage to the cor-ticomedial, but not lateral, amygdala in adults. Taken together, these studies suggest that the major effect of amygdaloid lesions placed in infancy is to prevent the normal social interactions between rat and mouse which would later inhibit muricide and to interfere with mechanisms which would normally lessen the animal's reactivity to the environment in a more general way (Eclancher & Karli, 1979; Vergnes, 1981). Thus, these data might be interpreted as providing little evidence for sparing of function but rather a long-standing disruption of social interactions and reactivity remarkably similar to those described by Thompson (1981). Apparent protective effects on avoidance learning in infant-lesioned animals, then, might be secondary to a more global disruption in emotional/social behavior. It should be remembered, however, that all of the primate data were derived from animals sustaining total amygdalectomies. In rats, prior housing conditions alter the effects of subsequent medial, but not lateral, amygdaloid damage. Although at present the apparent plasticity may be interpreted as a lesion-induced reduction in social responsiveness, the conclu-sion is based primarily on studies of muricide. Direct observations of conspecific social interactions following regional ablation are needed to explore this pos-sibility more fully.

ENVIRONMENTAL ENRICHMENT

Some years ago a former student and I (Kemble & Davies, 1981) conducted a series of experiments that approached the problem of protective effects from a somewhat different angle. Environmental enrichment substantially ameliorates the effects of cortical or hippocampal lesions whether enrichment occurs prior to surgical treatment or during the recovery period (Finger, 1978). This protective effect is found in both sexes and at various ages. Thus, it seemed to us that early experience might promote changes in the CNS which would, in a sense, "inocu-late" the subjects from the effects of later amygdaloid damage. Since limited prior data also suggested that the medial amygdaloid nucleus is sexually di-morphic in a number of its anatomical (Staudt & Dorner, 1976), physiological (e.g., Westley & Salaman, 1977) and behavioral characteristics (Kemble & Strand, 1979; Kling, 1974; Meany, Dodge, & Beatty, 1981; Rosvold et al., 1954), we also wished to see if lesion and environmental enrichment effects might be sex-dependent. In these experiments, male and female rats were either individually housed (impoverished environment) or group-housed in a spacious

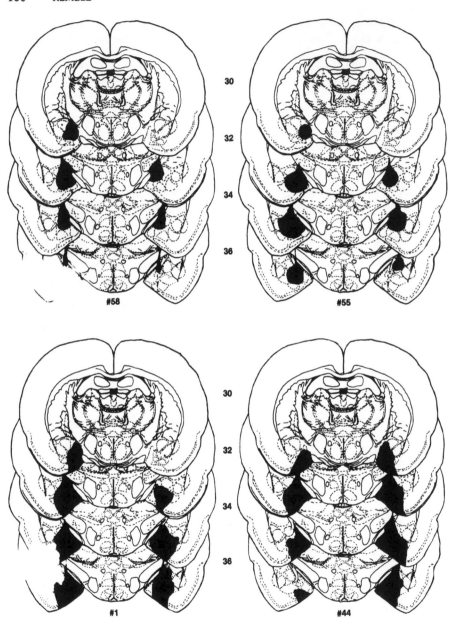

FIG. 5.1.   Representative large and small amygdaloid lesions of male (No. 58, No. 1) and female (No. 55, No. 44) rats reconstructed from the atlas of Konig and Klippel (1963). Plate numbers are indicated in the center column. Reprinted by permission of the Psychonomic Society Inc.

and complex enriched environment for 55–64 days after weaning. Half of the rats from each sex and housing condition then sustained amygdaloid lesions, which were centered in the corticomedial region. Representative small and larger lesions are reconstructed in Fig. 5.1. All rats were then individually housed for recovery and testing on a variety of consummatory measures, open field activity, insect predation and shuttlebox avoidance. Although the consummatory measures yielded a number of lesion effects and sex differences, there were no interactions between the sex of the subject, prior housing history, and lesion effects. The remaining tests yielded an interesting pattern of such interactions, however. A clear interaction between sex and prior enrichment was seen during the 3 days of open field testing. Although amygdaloid lesions had no consistent effect on the activity of males, regardless of previous housing, females with prior enrichment showed a more pronounced decline across days than did their impoverished female counterparts. Insect predation was observed for 2 consecutive days with all groups showing decreased kill latencies on the second day of testing. Amygdaloid lesions produced an overall increase in kill latencies but lesioned males with prior environmental enrichment killed more quickly on the first day than did their impoverished counterparts. No such first-day sparing effect was noted among females. Shuttlebox avoidance provided a particularly vivid, if somewhat more complex, demonstration of both sex and enrichment interactions. To facilitate description, the original figure depicting these results is reproduced in Fig. 5.2. It can be seen that females acquired this response more rapidly than males and that amygdaloid lesions generally facilitated acquisition. It can also be seen that the facilitatory effect of the lesion was much more marked in males than females and that prior enrichment produced an overall facilitation in acquisition in males but impairment in females. Finally, impoverished rats showed a greater lesion-induced facilitation in avoidance acquisition than did their enriched counterparts. This finding is in general agreement with the earlier report of Eclancher and Karli (1980). These results thus suggest that prior environmental enrichment can indeed alter the effects of later amygdaloid damage but that they do so in a task- and sex-dependent way. Prior enrichment seems to interact with the lesion to accelerate adaptation to an open field in females but not males, and to ameliorate the disruptive effects of the lesion on initial predatory attack and to facilitate avoidance acquisition in males only.

Protective effects of preoperative experience have also been demonstrated among adult animals. Although the retention of a panel-pressing avoidance response by monkeys (Weiskrantz, 1956) and a two-way shuttle avoidance response by cats (Horvath, 1963) is impaired by total (monkey) or basolateral (cat) amygdaloid lesions, no deficit is seen if extensive overtraining is carried out preoperatively in either cats (Brady, Schreiner, Geller, & Kling, 1954) or rats (Thatcher & Kimble, 1966). Unfortunately, it is not clear whether such overtraining protective effects are found among other preoperatively acquired behaviors.

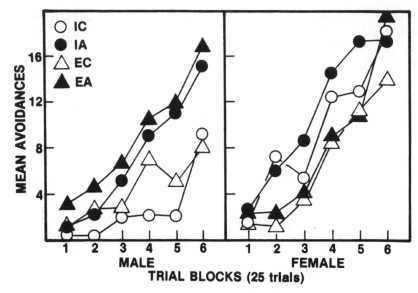

FIG. 5.2.   Mean avoidances for impoverished (I) and enriched (E) males follow-ing amygdaloid (A) or control (C) procedures (left panel) and their female counterparts (right panel). Scales are identical for both sexes. Reprinted by permission of the Psychonomic Society Inc.

To summarize, the above data clearly demonstrate at least some task-specific sparing of function via preoperative experience in both infants and adults. It also seems clear that this effect is modulated by the pattern of preoperative experi-ence, sex of the subject, and the site of amygdaloid damage. Clearly, however, our present data are far too limited to clarify the nature of these interactions. Since at least some sparing has been noted following both infant and adult lesions, systematic investigations of these variables at various ages should be of interest. Further, because the range of behavior examined in each of these experiments has been typically rather narrow, it is not clear how these sparing effects might relate, and possibly extend, to other major effects of amygdaloid damage. It is interesting to note, however, that Aggleton and Passingham (1981) failed to note deficits in serial discrimination reversals among monkeys unless their lesions were quite large and also produced taming effects. Given the robust protective effects of environmental enrichment at other CNS sites, it would seem of considerable interest to apply this technique to other amygdaloid lesion effects.

Finally, the sparing of retention deficits following preoperative overtraining clearly requires further investigation. We need to know if the sparing effect of overtraining on one task generalizes to related tasks and, if so, how widely and along which dimensions. Although the task-specificity noted by both Molino

(1975) and Eclancher and Karli (1979, 1980) suggests that such sparing might be rather restricted, this possibility remains to be investigated.

SERIAL LESIONS

In virtually all of the experiments described, bilateral lesions were placed during a single operation. A number of studies now show that the disruptive effects of such one-stage lesions at various cortical and limbic sites can be ameliorated or reversed if two unilateral lesions are placed with a 20–30-day interoperative interval (e.g., Stein et al., 1974, 1983). This serial lesion procedure eliminates impairments in discrimination learning, reversal, and delayed alternation which follow one-stage amygdaloid lesions and eliminates (Stein et al., 1969) or ameliorates (McIntyre & Stein, 1973) passive avoidance deficits. Such sparing effects are noted even after rather extensive amygdaloid lesions (Stein et al., 1969).

A major exception to this pattern of spared function, of course, is the long-term deficit noted by Thompson (1981) following serial lesions in monkeys. Since Stein's lesions were considerably less extensive than the total amygdalectomies performed by Thompson, it is possible that serial-lesion sparing occurs only if each lesion is subtotal and thus permits some functional reorganization within the amygdala during the interoperative interval. Obviously, it is also possible that species differences in the nature and/or time course of recovery processes were responsible for the contrasting results. In any case, serial lesion procedures seem to be quite effective in ameliorating the effects of subtotal amygdaloid lesions.

FUNCTIONAL LOCALIZATION

As mentioned previously, there is a dearth of careful localization data on amygdaloid recovery with virtually all information derived from subjects sustaining extensive or total ablation. Although disagreements about details of structure–function relationships continue (e.g., Grossman, Grossman, & Walsh, 1975; Ursin, 1965b), it has been clear for many years that the amygdala contains a number of anatomically distinct behavioral systems (e.g., Fonberg, 1986; Henke, 1980; Mogenson, 1987; Sarter & Markowitsch, 1985; Schoenfield & Hamilton, 1981; Siegel, 1984; Ursin, 1965a) some of which lie in close proximity. Thus, even regionally specific lesions (e.g., corticomedial amygdaloid) are likely to damage more than a single functional system and may, in turn, obscure recovery effects. Within this extensive literature are several studies revealing reciprocally antagonistic behavioral systems within the amygdala. Of particular interest, some effects of regional ablation or stimulation can be reversed by manipulations to other amygdaloid sites or closely related structures.

Extensive research by Fonberg (see Fonberg, 1972, 1986 for reviews) conducted primarily with dogs, reveals dorsomedial and basolateral amygdaloid systems which seem to reciprocally control appetitive and emotional/motivational behaviors. Dorsomedial lesions produce long-lasting hypophagia (Fonberg, 1968), impair appetitive conditioning (Fonberg, 1969) and produce behavioral changes variously described as apathy, indifference, sadness, and uncooperativeness (Fonberg, 1972). Basolateral lesions, in contrast, produce hyperphagia (Fonberg, 1971), and largely reverse dorsomedial impairments of appetitive conditioning (Fonberg, 1975) and emotionality (Fonberg, 1972). Though hypophagia probably results from damage outside the amygdala (Kemble, Studelska, & Schmidt, 1979; Schoenfeld & Hamilton, 1981), dorsomedial lesions result in loss of social rank in cats (Zagrodzka, Brudnias–Stepowska, & Fonberg, 1983) and have been strongly implicated in the mediation of fear in both rats (Werka, Skar, & Ursin, 1978) and rabbits (Kapp, Gallagher, Frysinger, & Applegate, 1981). Henke (1980) has also demonstrated mutually antagonistic medial-basolateral amygdaloid systems. Lesions within the medial amygdala or the ventral amygdalofugal pathway reduce restraint-produced gastric pathology while basolateral or stria terminalis lesions increase such pathology. He suggests that medial or ventral amygdalofugal lesions attenuate the effectiveness of noxious stimuli while basolateral or stria terminalis lesions interfere with such inhibitory effects.

Localized ablation or stimulation also reveals differential amygdaloid contributions to affective and predatory behavior in the cat. Early research demonstrated flight and defense zones within the amygdala (Kaada & Ursin, 1957), with basolateral lesions attenuating flight behavior (Ursin, 1965a) and impairing active avoidance acquisition (Ursin, 1965b), and corticomedial lesions impairing defensive behavior and passive avoidance. Selective reduction in flight and defensive attack behaviors have also been demonstrated following small lesions within the medial amygdala of feral rats (Kemble, Blanchard, Blanchard, & Takushi, 1984) suggesting that these opposing systems have some generality. Related research by Siegel (1984) also reveals opposing systems within the cat amygdala which modulate rat killing elicited by lateral hypothalamic stimulation. Basomedial amygdaloid stimulation slows attack (Egger & Flynn, 1963, 1967) while lesions temporarily abolish spontaneous attack (Zagrodzka & Fonberg, 1977). This effect is mediated by stria terminalis connections with the bed nucleus of the stria terminalis and medial hypothalamus and generally corresponds to the defensive system earlier described by Fernandez de Molina and Hunsperger (1962). In contrast, attack is speeded by stimulation of lateral or central nuclei. This facilitation is thought to be mediated by an indirect pathway to the lateral hypothalamus via the substantia innominata.

Despite major differences in species, procedures, and proposed anatomical localization, the data described herein suggest that some behaviors are modulated by anatomically dissociable and reciprocally interacting amygdaloid systems. Thus, the effect of localized manipulations might depend on quantitative disruptions in the balance between amygdaloid systems. If this interpretation is correct, then it should be possible to demonstrate a close relationship between behavioral and systems-balance changes and to manipulate such balance experimentally. An intriguing series of experiments by Adamec and coworkers (see, Adamec, 1978; Adamec & Stark–Adamec, 1984, for reviews) suggests just such a possibility. Adamec found that the rat-killing propensity of domestic cats was strongly related to their responsiveness to a novel environment or conspecific threat vocalizations and suggested that this broad behavioral propensity reflected quantitative variation along a developmentally stable aggressiveness–defensiveness dimension. Aggressive cats are more likely to kill rats spontaneously than defensive cats and react less fearfully to novel environments or threat vocalizations. These behavioral predispositions are closely related to the afterdischarge threshold (AD) in the basomedial amydala and ventral hippocampus. Aggressive cats have substantially higher AD thresholds in the amygdala and lower thresholds in the ventral hippocampus than defensive cats. Using a partial kindling technique (Goddard, McIntyre, & Leech, 1969), he found that reducing the amygdaloid AD threshold by repeated subthreshold stimulation, with no motor seizures, converted an aggressive cat to a more defensive one. As AD threshold decreased, the cats stopped killing rats and became generally more defensive. This change persisted for 4 months after the stimulation, did not depend on the occurrence of seizure activity in the amygdala and could be temporarily reversed by food deprivation. Aggressiveness–defensiveness seems to reflect the balance between an amygdaloventromedial hypothalamic (VMH) circuit and a second pathway connecting entorhinal cortex and dentate gyrus via the perforant pathway. Defensiveness is reflected in an increased propagation of activity from the amygdala to the VMH (increased limbic permeability) with a concomitant decrease in propagation of activity to the ventral hippocampus. If limbic permeability is blocked by repeated prior stimulation of the ventral hippocampus, lowering amygdaloid AD threshold does not increase defensiveness but actually increases aggressiveness. These experiments clearly demonstrate that aggressive–defensive propensities mirror differential propagation of activity in these two systems which can be altered by partial kindling and which do not depend on seizure activity per se. The fact that defensiveness can be temporarily reversed by food deprivation also suggests that this balance is experientially modifiable to some extent.

Adamec's data are important not only in elucidating reciprocal amygdaloid control mechanisms for aggression but also in suggesting some degree of experiential modifiability. If the previously described dorsomedial-basolateral and medial-lateral systems underlying appetitive conditioning, predation, flight–defense, and emotionality interact in similar ways, experiential modulation of amygdaloid function may prove to be more general than previously suspected.

Although little or no recovery seems to follow total amygdalectomy (Kling & Dunne, 1976; Thompson, 1981), prior experience may increase conduction efficiency within specific behavioral systems and, in turn, reduce the impact of partial destruction within the system. Alternatively, the extensive sparing noted after very large serial lesions (McIntyre & Stein, 1973; Stein et al., 1969) suggests that amygdaloid systems might undergo extensive reorganization extending to other systems under some conditions.

COMPARATIVE DATA

Finally, it must be recognized the available evidence for experiential modification of amygdaloid function is based on a pitifully narrow range of species. Although scattered reports clearly show that amygdaloid lesions disrupt one or more aspects of social behavior in a wide range of mammalian (e.g., Fonberg, 1986; Glendenning, 1972; Jonason & Enloe, 1971; Levinson, Reeves, & Buchanan, 1980) and even reptilian species (Keating, Kormann, & Horel, 1970; Tarr, 1977), systematic analysis has been restricted to monkeys, cats, and dogs. Even among primates, which have received most attention, virtually all data are derived from two genera and only one (i.e., large heterosexual groups) of several types of social structure (Stecklis & Kling, 1985). Even within this primate social system, there are marked species differences in the social consequences of total amygdalectomy (Kling & Cornell, 1971). A more broadly based comparative approach would be of the greatest value both in further clarifying amygdaloid function and in assessing experientially mediated recovery. It might be expected, for example, that prior experience would afford relatively greater protection from future amygdaloid damage among species whose social relationship and emotional responsiveness depend heavily on learning. Alternatively, such variables as developmental rate or ecological specializations (e.g., predation) might prove to be of primary importance. Whatever the outcome, comparative analyses could scarcely fail to increase understanding of amygdaloid function and recovery.

DISCUSSION

Perhaps the available data may be best characterized as providing some tantalizing clues about amygdaloid plasticity but, as yet, little knowledge of the parameters which maximize recovery. Though impairments following total amygdalectomy may be largely irreversible, it is equally clear that prior experience and the employment of serial lesions provide at least some protection from the effects of less massive damage. It remains to be determined what conditions will promote optimal recovery, the range and anatomical substrates of such effects, and their cross-species generality.

The moderate protective effects of standard laboratory environmental enrichment procedures (i.e., housing of small like-sex groups in a modestly complex cage) might be considerably enhanced by further increases in environmental complexity. Housing larger mixed-sex groups in a relatively spacious seminatural environment, for example, would increase environmental complexity and provide opportunities for expanded social interactions, burrowing, foraging for a more varied diet, and extensive exploration. If recovery from regional amygdaloid damage is partly mediated by prior experience, such changes should increase the degree and/or range of protective effects.

Since both environmental enrichment and the use of serial lesions independently produce some protective effects, another obvious strategy is to apply these techniques in combination. If the effects of these manipulations interact, it might be expected that serially lesioned subjects experiencing prior, and interoperative, environmental enrichment would show substantially greater, and perhaps more general, recovery than subjects experiencing either of these conditions alone. This approach should also be coupled with a broader range of behavioral tests. Since amygdaloid lesions markedly reduce reactions to frustration (Barta, Kemble, & Klinger, 1975; Henke & Maxwell, 1973), behavioral contrast (Henke, Allen, & Davison, 1972), and incentive shifts (Kemble & Beckman, 1969, 1970a; Schwartzbaum, 1960) and impair successive discrimination reversals (e.g., Aggleton & Passingham, 1981; Kemble & Beckman, 1970b; Thompson, 1981) these behaviors should be prime candidates for further study. Such investigations should also include a number of more ethologically oriented behavioral measures. Amygdaloid lesions strikingly alter flight and defensive attack (Kemble et al., 1984; Ursin, 1965a), conspecific social interactions (e.g., Glendenning, 1972; Jonason & Enloe, 1971; Kling, 1972) and predatory attack (e.g., Kemble & Davies, 1981; Zagrodzka & Fonberg, 1977) in a variety of species. Test batteries which include both types of measure would not only characterize the range of recovery effects more fully but would also help to clarify their adaptive significance.

As suggested previously, further localization data are needed and should provide valuable guidance for future research employing serial lesions and environmental manipulations. The correlated shifts in limbic permeability and defensiveness in cats (Adamec, 1978; Adamec et al., 1984) provide a promising model which should be thoroughly explored. The relationship of early experience, particularly the complexity and nature of social interactions with siblings and parents, to the emergence of aggressive–defensive behavior should receive careful scrutiny. Although Adamec's data suggest that these shifts reflect generalized propensities toward aggressiveness–defensiveness, a closer examination of the nature of the behavioral changes is needed. Since flight and defensive attack behavior are separately organized in both the cat (Ursin, 1965a) and rat (Kemble et al., 1984), it is important to know the relationship of these systems to limbic permeability. Observations should be extended to a wider range of social behaviors in cats (e.g., mating, maternal care) to explore more fully the social consequences of shifts in limbic permeability. Extension of this research to other species and a broader range of social behaviors is also needed. Although McIntyre (1978) found no inhibition of muricide in spontaneous mouse-killing rats with shifts in limbic permeability, the interpretation of this finding is not clear (e.g., Kemble, Flannelly, Salley, & Blanchard, 1985; O'Boyle, 1974). Some light might be shed on this question by more extensive use of feral or richly socialized species. Such animals show particularly striking changes in major behavioral propensities, such as flight, defensive attack, social grooming, following amygdaloid damage (e.g., Kling, 1972, 1986; Schreiner & Kling, 1956; Woods, 1956). These behaviors have been suggested as the most appropriate behavioral level ("natural fracture line") for the analysis of limbic function (Thomas, Hostetter, & Barker, 1968) and may be of particular value in behaviorally characterizing these systems. It would also be of great interest to know if other amygdaloid systems which seem to reciprocally interact (Fonberg, 1972, 1986; Henke, 1980; Siegel, 1984; Ursin, 1965a) also show shifts in their balance of conductivity and if such shifts are physiologically and experientially modifiable.

In view of increasing evidence for major species differences in the anatomical organization of the amygdala (e.g., Hopkins, 1975; Krettek & Price, 1977, 1978; Turner, 1981), species differences in the amygdaloid organization of such systems is to be expected. Nevertheless, much of the data discussed are consistent in pointing to the bed nucleus of the stria terminalis, substantia innominata, medial and lateral hypothalamus, and ventral hippocampus as nodal sites for converging amygdaloid interactions. The possibility that the activity of these sites can be modulated by reciprocally antagonistic amygdaloid systems which may be, in turn, capable of experientially mediated functional reorganization deserves careful consideration.

REFERENCES

Adamec, R. E. (1978). Normal and abnormal limbic system mechanisms of emotive biasing. In K. E. Livingston & O. Hornykiewicz (Eds.), Limbic mechanisms: The continuing evolution of the limbic system concept (pp. 405–455). New York: Plenum.

Adamec, R. E., & Stark–Adamec, C. (1984). The contribution of limbic connectivity to stable behavioral characteristics of aggressive and defensive cats. In R. Bandler (Ed.), Modulation of sensorimotor activity during alterations in behavioral states (pp. 325–339). New York: Alan Liss.

Aggleton, J. P., & Passingham, R. E. (1981). Syndrome produced by lesions of the amygdala in monkeys (Macaca mulatta). Journal of Comparative and Physiological Psychology, 95, 961–977.

Bandler, R. (Ed.). (1984). Sensorimotor activity during alterations in behavioral states. New York: Alan Liss.

Barta, S. G., Kemble, E. D., & Klinger, E. (1975). Abolition of cyclic activity changes following amygdaloid lesions. Bulletin of the Psychonomic Society, 5, 236–238.

Ben–Ari, Y. (Ed.). (1981). The amygdaloid complex. Amsterdam: Elsevier/North Holland.

Brady, J. V., Schreiner, L., Geller, I., & Kling, A. (1954). Subcortical mechanisms in emotional behavior: The effect of rhinencephalic injury upon the acquisition and retention of a conditioned avoidance response in cats. *Journal of Comparative and Physiological Psychology, 47,* 179–186.

Dicks, D., Myers, R. E., & Kling, A. (1969). Uncus and amygdala lesions: Effects on social behavior in the free-ranging rhesus monkey. *Science, 165,* 69–71.

Eclancher, F., & Karli, P. (1979). Effects of early amygdaloid lesions on the development of reactivity in the rat. *Physiology and Behavior, 22,* 1123–1134.

Eclancher, F., & Karli, P. (1980). Effects of infant and adult amygdaloid lesions upon acquisition of two-way active avoidance by the adult rat: Influence of rearing conditions. *Physiology and Behavior, 24,* 887–893.

Eclancher, F., Schmitt, P., & Karli, P. (1975). Effets de lesions precoces de l'amygdale sur le developpement de l'agressivite interspecifique du rat. *Physiology and Behavior, 14,* 277–283.

Egger, M. D., & Flynn, J. P. (1963). Effects of electrical stimulation of the amygdala on hypothalamically elicited attack behavior in cats. *Journal of Neurophysiology, 26,* 705–720.

Egger, M. D., & Flynn, J. P. (1967). Further studies on the effects of amygdaloid stimulation and ablation on hypothalamically elicited attack behavior in cat. In W. R. Adey & T. Takigan (Eds.), *Structures and function of the limbic system* (Vol. 27, pp. 165–182). *Progress in brain research,* Amsterdam: Elsevier.

Eleftheriou, B. E. (Ed.). (1972). *The neurobiology of the amygdala.* New York: Plenum.

Fernandez de Molina, A., & Hunsperger, R. W. (1962). Organization of the subcortical system governing defense and flight reactions in the cat. *Journal of Physiology* (London), *160,* 200–213.

Finger, S. (1978). Environmental attenuation of brain-lesion symptoms. In S. Finger (Ed.), *Recovery from brain damage: Research and theory* (pp. 297–329). New York: Plenum.

Fonberg, E. (1968). The instrumental alimentary-avoidance differentiation in dogs. *Acta Neurobiologica Experimentalis, 28,* 363–373.

Fonberg, E. (1969). Effects of small dorsomedial amygdala lesions on food intake and acquisition of instrumental alimentary reactions in dogs. *Physiology and Behavior, 4,* 739–743.

Fonberg, E. (1971). Hyperphagia produced by lateral amygdalar lesions in dogs. *Acta Neurobiologica Experimentalis, 31,* 19–32.

Fonberg, E. (1972). Control of emotional behavior through the hypothalamus and amygdaloid complex. In R. Porter & J. Knights (Eds.), *Physiology, emotion and psychosomatic illness* (pp. 131–161). Amsterdam: Elsevier/North Holland, Excerpta Medica.

Fonberg, E. (1975). Improvement produced by lateral amygdala lesions on the instrumental alimentary performance impaired by dorsomedial amygdala lesions in dogs. *Physiology and Behavior, 14,* 711–717.

Fonberg, E. (1986). Amygdala, emotions, motivation, and depressive states. In R. Plutchik, & K. Kellerman (Eds.), *Emotion: Theory, research, and experience* (pp. 301–331). New York: Academic Press.

Glendenning, K. K. (1972). Effects of septal and amygdaloid lesions on social behavior of the cat. *Journal of Comparative and Physiological Psychology, 80,* 199–207.

Goddard, G. V. (1964). Functions of the amygdala. *Psychological Bulletin, 62,* 89–109.

Goddard, G. V., McIntyre, D. C., & Leech, C. K. (1969). A permanent change in brain function resulting from daily electrical stimulation. *Experimental Neurology, 25,* 295–330.

Green, P. C., & Kling, A. (1966). Effects of amygdalectomy on affective behavior in juvenile and adult macaque monkeys. *American Psychological Association. Proceedings of the annual convention, 75,* 93–94.

Grossman, S. P., Grossman, L., & Walsh, L. (1975). Functional organization of the rat amygdala with respect to avoidance behavior. *Journal of Comparative and Physiological Psychology, 88,* 829–850.

Henke, P. G. (1980). The amygdala and restraint ulcers in rats. *Journal of Comparative and Physiological Psychology, 94,* 313–323.

Henke, P. G., Allen, J. D., & Davison, C. (1972). Effects of lesions in the amygdala on behavioral contrast. *Physiology and Behavior, 8,* 173–176.

Henke, P. G., & Maxwell, D. (1973). Lesions in the amygdala and the frustration effect. *Physiology and Behavior, 10,* 647–650.

Hopkins, D. A. (1975). Amygdalotegmental projections in the rat, cat and rhesus monkey. *Neuroscience Letters, 1,* 263–270.

Horvath, F. E. (1963). Effects of basolateral amygdalectomy on three types of avoidance behavior in cats. *Journal of Comparative and Physiological Psychology, 56,* 380–389.

Jonason, K. R., & Enloe, L. J. (1971). Alterations in social behavior following septal and amygdaloid lesions in the rat. *Journal of Comparative and Physiological Psychology, 75,* 286–301.

Kaada, B. R., & Ursin, H. (1957). Further localization of behavioral responses elicited from the amygdala in unanesthetized cats. *Acta Physiologica Scandinavica, 42,* 80–81.

Kapp, B. S., Gallagher, M., Frysinger, R. C., & Applegate, C. D. (1981). The amygdala, emotion and cardiovascular conditioning. In Y. Ben–Ari (Ed.), *The amygdaloid complex.* Amsterdam: Elsevier/North Holland, pp. 343–354.

Keating, G. E., Kormann, L. S., & Horel, J. A. (1970). The behavioral effects of stimulating and ablating the reptilian amygdala (*Caiman sklerops*). *Physiology and Behavior, 5,* 55–59.

Kemble, E. D., & Beckman, G. J. (1969). Escape latencies at three levels of electric shock in rats with amygdaloid lesions. *Psychonomic Science, 14,* 205–206.

Kemble, E. D., & Beckman, G. J. (1970a). Runway performance of rats following amygdaloid lesions. *Physiology and Behavior, 5,* 45–47.

Kemble, E. D., & Beckman, G. J. (1970b). Vicarious trial and error following amygdaloid lesions in rats. *Neuropsychologia, 8,* 161–169.

Kemble, E. D., Blanchard, D. C., Blanchard, R. J., & Takushi, R. (1984). Taming in wild rats following medial amygdaloid lesions. *Physiology and Behavior, 32,* 131–134.

Kemble, E. D., & Davies, V. A. (1981). Effects of prior environmental enrichment and amygdaloid lesions on consummatory behavior, activity, predation, and shuttlebox avoidance in male and female rats. *Physiological Psychology, 9,* 340–346.

Kemble, E. D., Flannelly, K. J., Salley, H., & Blanchard, R. J. (1985). Mouse killing, insect predation and conspecific attack by rats with differing prior aggressive experience. *Physiology and Behavior, 34,* 645–648.

Kemble, E. D., & Strand, M. (1979). A comparison of amygdaloid lesion effects in male and female rats. *Bulletin of the Psychonomic Society, 13,* 333–335.

Kemble, E. D., Studelska, D. R., & Schmidt, M. K. (1979). Effects of central amygdaloid nucleus lesions on ingestion, taste reactivity, exploration and taste aversion. *Physiology and Behavior, 22,* 789–793.

Kesner, R. P., & DiMattia, B. V. (1987). Neurobiology of an attribute model of memory. In A. N. Epstein & A. R. Morrison (Eds.), *Progress in psychobiology and physiological psychology* (Vol. 12, pp. 207–277). New York: Academic Press.

Kling, A. (1962). Amygdalectomy in the kitten. *Science, 137,* 429–430.

Kling, A. (1965). Behavioral and somatic development following lesions of the amygdala in the cat. *Journal of Psychiatric Research, 3,* 263–273.

Kling, A. (1966). Ontogenetic and phylogenetic studies on the amygdaloid nuclei. *Psychosomatic Medicine, 28,* 155–161.

Kling, A. (1972). Effects of amygdalectomy on social-affective behavior in non-human primates. In B. E. Eleftheriou (Ed.), *The neurobiology of the amygdala* (pp. 511–536). New York: Plenum.

Kling, A. (1974). Differential effects of amygdalectomy in male and female nonhuman primates. *Archives of Sexual Behavior, 3,* 129–134.

Kling, A. (1986). The anatomy of aggression and affiliation. In R. Plutchik & K. Kellerman (Eds.), *Emotion: Theory, research, and experience.* New York: Academic Press, pp. 237–264.

Kling, A., & Cornell, R. (1971). Amygdalectomy and social behavior in the caged stump-tailed macaque (*Macaca speciosa*). *Folia Primatologica, 14,* 190–208.

Kling, A., Dicks, D., & Gurowitz, E. M. (1968). Amygdalectomy and social behavior in a caged-group of vervets (C. aethiops). Proceedings of the Second International Congress of Primatology (Vol. 1, pp. 232–241). New York: Karger, Basel.

Kling, A., & Dunne, K. (1976). Social-environmental factors affecting behavior and plasma testosterone in normal and amygdala lesioned M. speciosa. Primates, 17, 23–42.

Kling, A., & Green, P. C. (1967). Effects of amygdalectomy in the maternally reared and maternally deprived neonatal and juvenile macaque. Nature, 213, 742–743.

Kling, A., Lancaster, J., & Benitone, J. (1969). Amygdalectomy in the free-ranging vervet (Cercopithecus aethiops), Journal of Psychiatric Research, 7, 3.

Kluver, H., & Bucy, P. C. (1939). Preliminary analysis of the functions of the temporal lobes in monkeys. Archives of Neurology and Psychiatry, 42, 979–1000.

Konig, J. F. R., & Klippel, R. (1963). The rat brain. Baltimore: Williams & Wilkins.

Krettek, J. E., & Price, J. L. (1977). Projections from the amygdaloid complex to the cerebral cortex and thalamus in the rat and cat. Journal of Comparative Neurology, 172, 687–722.

Krettek, J. E., & Price, J. L. (1978). Amygdaloid projections to subcortical structures within the basal forebrain and brainstem in the rat and cat. Journal of Comparative Neurology, 178, 225–234.

Levinson, D. M., Reeves, D. L., & Buchanan, D. R. (1980). Reduction in aggression and dominance status in guinea pigs following bilateral lesions in the basolateral amygdala or lateral septum. Physiology and Behavior, 25, 963–971.

Livingston, K. E., & Hornykiewicz, O. (Eds.). (1978). Limbic mechanisms: The continuing evolution of the limbic system concept. New York: Plenum.

McIntyre, D. C. (1978). Amygdala kindling and muricide in rats. Physiology and Behavior, 21, 49–56.

McIntyre, M., & Stein, D. G. (1973). Differential effects of one- vs two-stage amygdaloid lesions on activity, exploratory, and avoidance behavior in the albino rat. Behavioral Biology, 9, 451–465.

Meany, M. J., Dodge, A. M., & Beatty, W. W. (1981). Sex-dependent effects of amygdaloid lesions on the social play of prepuberal rats. Physiology and Behavior, 26, 467–472.

Mogenson, G. J. (1987). Limbic-motor integration. In A. N. Epstein & A. R. Morrison (Eds.), Progress in psychobiology and physiological psychology (Vol. 12, pp. 117–170). New York: Academic Press.

Molino, A. (1975). Sparing of function after infant lesions of selected limbic structures in the rat. Journal of Comparative and Physiological Psychology, 89, 868–881.

O'Boyle, M. (1974). Rats and mice together: The predatory nature of the rat's mouse-killing response. Psychological Bulletin, 81, 261–269.

Plotnik, R. (1968). Changes in social behavior of squirrel monkeys after anterior temporal lobectomy. Journal of Comparative and Physiological Psychology, 66, 369–377.

Rosvold, H. E., Mirsky, A. F., & Pribram, K. H. (1954). Influence of amygdalectomy on social behavior in monkeys. Journal of Comparative and Physiological Psychology, 47, 173–178.

Sarter, M., & Markowitsch, H. J. (1985). Involvement of the amygdala in learning and memory: A critical review, with emphasis on anatomical relations. Behavioral Neuroscience, 99, 342–380.

Schoenfeld, T. A., & Hamilton, L. W. (1981). Disruption of appetite but not hunger following small lesions of the amygdala of rats. Journal of Comparative and Physiological Psychology, 95, 565–587.

Schreiner, L., & Kling, A. (1956). Rhinencephalon and behavior. American Journal of Physiology, 184, 486–490.

Schwartzbaum, J. S. (1960). Changes in reinforcing properties of stimuli following ablation of the amygdaloid complex in monkeys. Journal of Comparative and Physiological Psychology, 74, 252–259.

Siegel, A. (1984). Anatomical and functional differentiation within the amygdala—behavioral state modulation. In R. Bandler (Ed.), *Modulation of sensorimotor activity during alterations in behavioral states* (pp. 299–323). New York: Alan Liss.

Staudt, J., & Dorner, G. (1976). Structural changes in the medial and central amygdala of the male rat following castration and androgen treatment. *Endokrinologie, 67,* 296–300.

Stecklis, H. D., & Kling, A. (1985). Neurobiology of affiliative behavior in nonhuman primates. In, M. Reite & T. Field (Eds.), *The psychobiology of attachment and separation* (pp. 93–134). New York: Academic Press.

Stein, D. G., Finger, S., & Hart, T. (1983). Brain damage and recovery: Problems and perspectives. *Behavioral and Neural Biology, 37,* 185–222.

Stein, D. G., Rosen, J. J., & Butters, N. (Eds.). (1974). *Plasticity and recovery of function in the central nervous system.* New York: Academic Press.

Stein, D. G., Rosen, J. J., Graziadei, J., Mishkin, M., & Brink, J. J. (1969). Recovery of function in the C.N.S. *Science, 166,* 528–530.

Tarr, R. S. (1977). Role of the amygdala in the intraspecies aggressive behavior of the iguanid lizard, *Sceloporus occidentalis. Physiology and Behavior, 18,* 1153–1158.

Thatcher, R. W., & Kimble, D. P. (1966). Effect of amygdaloid lesions on retention of an avoidance response in overtrained and non-overtrained rats. *Psychonomic Science, 6,* 9–10.

Thomas, G. T., Hostetter, G., & Barker, D. (1968). Behavioral functions of the limbic system. In E. Stellar & J. M. Sprague (Eds.), *Progress in physiological psychology* (Vol. 2, pp. 230–231). New York: Academic Press.

Thompson, C. I. (1981). Long-term behavioral development of rhesus monkeys after amygdalectomy in infancy. In Y. Ben–Ari (Ed.), *The amygdaloid complex* (pp. 259–270). Amsterdam: Elsevier/North Holland.

Thompson, C. I., Bergland, R. M., & Towfighi, J. T. (1977). Social and nonsocial behaviors of adult rhesus monkeys after amygdalectomy in infancy or adulthood. *Journal of Comparative and Physiological Psychology, 91,* 533–548.

Thompson, C. I., Schwartzbaum, J. S., & Harlow, H. S. (1969). Development of social fear after amygdalectomy in infant rhesus monkeys. *Physiology and Behavior, 4,* 249–254.

Thompson, C. I., & Towfighi, J. T. (1976). Social behavior of juvenile rhesus monkeys after amygdalectomy in infancy. *Physiology and Behavior, 17,* 831–836.

Turner, B. H. (1981). The cortical sequence and terminal distribution of sensory related afferents to the amygdaloid complex of the rat and monkey. In Y. Ben–Ari (Ed.), *The amygdaloid complex* (pp. 51–62). Amsterdam: Elsevier/North Holland.

Ursin, H. (1965a). The effect of amygdaloid lesions on flight and defense behavior in cats. *Experimental Neurology, 11,* 61–79.

Ursin, H. (1965b). Effect of amygdaloid lesions on avoidance behavior and visual discrimination in cats. *Experimental Neurology, 11,* 298–317.

Ursin, H., & Kaada, B. R. (1957). Functional localization within the amygdaloid complex in the cat. *Electroencephalography and Clinical Neurophysiology, 12,* 1–20.

Vergnes, M. (1981). Effect of prior familiarization with mice on elicitation of mouse-killing in rats: Role of the amygdala. In Y. Ben–Ari (Ed.), *The amygdaloid complex* (pp. 293–304). Amsterdam: Elsevier/North Holland.

Walsh, R. N., & Greenough, W. T. (Eds.). (1976). *Environments as therapy for brain dysfunction.* New York: Plenum.

Weiskrantz, L. (1956). Behavioral changes associated with ablation of the amygdaloid complex in monkeys. *Journal of Comparative and Physiological Psychology, 49,* 381–391.

Werka, T., Skar, J., & Ursin, H. (1978). Exploration and avoidance in rats with lesions in amygdala and piriform cortex. *Journal of Comparative and Physiological Psychology, 92,* 672–681.

Westley, B. R., & Salaman, D. F. (1977). Nuclear binding of the oestrogen receptor of neonatal rat brain after injection of oestrogens and androgens: Localization and sex differences. *Brain Research, 119,* 375–388.

Woods, J. W. (1956). Taming of the wild Norway rat by rhinencephalic lesions. *Nature, 197*, 869.

Zagrodzka, J., Brudnias–Stepowska, Z., & Fonberg, E. (1983). Impairment of social behavior in amygdalar cats. *Acta Neurobiologica Experimentalis, 43*, 63–77.

Zagrodzka, J., & Fonberg, E. (1977). Amygdalar area involved in predatory behavior in cats. *Acta Neurobiologica Experimentalis, 37*, 131–136.

6

An Odyssey in Behavioral Neuroscience: A Search for Common Principles Underlying Responses to Brain Damage

Peter J. Donovick
Richard G. Burright
Department of Psychology
State University of New York at Binghamton

INDIVIDUAL DIFFERENCES AND BRAIN INJURY

A hallmark of brain damage is decreased flexibility in capacities to adapt to changes in the environment. As such, "comparator processes," at many levels, appear to be particularly vulnerable to neural insult; in our view, such processes allow an individual to compare and alter plans of action vis-à-vis many ongoing demand contingencies of his or her internal and external milieus. The "final common path" (cf. Sherrington, 1941) of these comparator processes is represented in behavior. Indeed, the importance of such adaptive comparator processes in living organisms was, in part, eloquently recognized in the 19th century by C. Bernard's (1878) definition of a free and independent existence. Dysfunction(s) in such comparator processes may well underlie changes in emotionality which represent one of the earliest and most persistent symptoms of human neurological dysfunction (Livingston, Brooks, & Bond, 1985a, 1985b; Oddy, Coughlan, Tyerman, & Jenkins, 1985). Unfortunately, changes in emotionality often are highly disruptive to the interactions between the individual and his or her family, friends, and society in general (Brooks, 1984; Oddy, 1984).

We will discuss factors which influence changes in behavior associated with single-trauma brain injury as well as more clearly progressive damage to the central nervous system. For brain trauma produced at one time, we will review some aspects of the impact on behavior of closed-head injury in humans and septal lesions in rodents; for more clearly progressive damage, we will consider the behavioral consequences for aberrant hosts infected by *Toxocara canis* (the common round worm of dogs). Where available, we will discuss genetic and environmental events that influence the outcome from subsequent brain damage. First, however, we will discuss general methodological issues that have limited our understanding of the ongoing, gene–environment coactions which determine comparator-processing capabilities of individuals; processes which determine any individual's responses to, and ability to recover from, brain damage.

Sources and Consequences of Individuality

Individual differences are legion in psychology and the neurobehavioral sciences; yet they are poorly understood and rarely investigated directly. Furthermore, virtually all of our experimental designs and statistical techniques necessarily deal with the assessment of average differences among treatment conditions, and thus must view experimental error variance as extraneous to research questions specified by any given study; however, most extraneous variability is due to "individual differences" (i.e., differences which are readily observable both within as well as among subjects).

Our understanding of the origins of such marked variability in behavior demands insight into the ongoing, gene–environment coactions which occur at all levels of analysis and define the conscious and unconscious experiences of an individual; but it is unclear how these coactions are translated into the behavioral plasticity seen either among individuals, or within a given individual's performance over time (cf., Wilson, 1986), or how they influence the individual's reaction to brain damage (cf. Donovick, Burright, Fuller, & Branson, 1975). Virtually any attempt to put such chaos into order must assume consistent, identifiable, underlying principles which will serve to explain the exquisitely challenging diversity that can be readily observed within and among living organisms. The magnitude of the issue may be appreciated when it is noted that permuting only 13 items ("general principles"?) results in greater than 6 billion different outcomes ("individual differences"?); such logic helps define the almost infinite array of observed paths that any individual may take in "adaptively responding" to challenges, including neuropathological events, which arise in the ongoing commerce between one's internal milieu and the external environment (also see O'Kelly, 1963).

Any organism's genetic constitution, as John Fuller (e.g., 1979) likes to point out, provides an "invitation" to the environment; an invitation to channel the development of the individual through a subset of nearly limitless potential environmental possibilities. In some cases, the manifestation of such a spatiotemporal plan may be observed best as differences in longitudinal patterns of behavior. For example, Wilson (1986) noted that the longitudinal pattern of spurts and lags in the development of intellectual abilities is more similar in monozygotic than in dizygotic twins. Certainly, more longitudinal analyses of behavioral profile differences among individuals could help to illuminate important basic principles. Observed differences in response to brain injury of young and older organisms is undoubtedly related, in part, to this ongoing cumulative coaction of genetic and environmental factors.

Clearly the interplay between genetic consitution and the environment is anything but passive. The continual interaction between organism and environment demands active selection and development of plans and adjustment of response patterns in light of "feedback" from the internal and external environments. The experience of the individual in response to any fixed set of conditions can be quite different from one time to the next; it will depend on prior experiences, and whether external forces impose those conditions, or whether those conditions are "freely chosen"/"self-organized" by the individual (e.g., Kavanaugh, 1967). Not surprisingly then, it is difficult to identify factors responsible for the variability in responses to shared environmental conditions displayed by intact individuals, let alone those with brain injury. A large part of the difficulty in identifying critical underlying principles which serve to "explain" specific characteristics of individuals lies in the variability which exists in the very factor(s) under study; that is, the proportion of behavioral variability attributed to any directly manipulated factor(s) often is small relative to the total variance observed.

Minimally, any putative basic principle must afford marker(s) which are capable of at least differentiating pathological from "normal" conditions and how such individual characteristics influence the response to neuropathological processes. But finding useful and understandable behavioral or biological marker(s) for individuals who have, or are at risk for, CNS dysfunction will demand that we uncover basic principles. To overcome this "catch-22," programs of research concerned with identifying and improving markers to uncover truly basic principles will need to consider individual differences as critical source(s) of information, and not as extraneous to how the system works (also see Bullock, 1984).

Any potentially critical marker requires systematic investigation regarding its reliable and valid utility as a predictor and its etiological role in the context of basic principles. Furthermore, it should be clear that most, if not all, of even our "best" indicators cannot be expected to occur in pathological group(s) alone. Indeed, in dynamic, multiply-determined systems, average difference(s) among control and pathological groups frequently are "small." For instance, when considering polygenic inheritance, genetic factors which increase risk for neural/behavioral dysfunction typically are found to be: (1) recessive; (2) variable in their penetrance; and (3) variable in their expression (e.g., Goldin, Nurnberger, & Gershon, 1986). Thus, we currently have limited ability to predict, let alone explain, the outcome of brain injury at an individual level.

Improvements in our abilities to both define and prevent pathological susceptibility await better and more imaginative utilization of the critical sources of information contained in those "extraneous variables" some call "individual

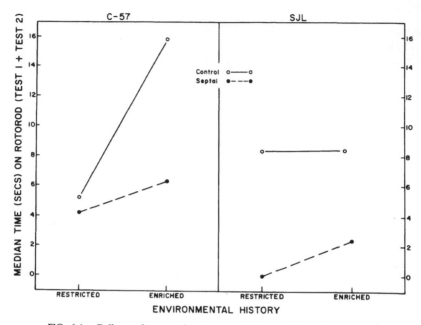

FIG. 6.1.   Differential impact of environmental history and brain damage in two strains of mice (Donovick et al., 1975).

differences" and others consider "nuisance variables." One thing is certain, the use of restricted behaviors, situations, and/or gene pools merely to reduce nuisance variability will continue to lead us to incomplete views of the intervening processes we hope to understand. For instance, most investigations of how presurgical manipulations influence response to brain lesions in animals have used rats. Conclusions based on such data are undoubtedly limited. Greater concern in the choice of subjects (Donovick & Horowitz, 1982) for experimental research would yield results of more general applicability. For instance, as seen in Fig. 6.1, the effect of septal lesions on rotorod ability of mice of two inbred strains was influenced by both their genotype and their presurgical rearing condition (Donovick, Burright, Fuller, & Branson, 1975). Thus any simple statement such as "septal lesions cause animals to . . . ," is inaccurate and misleading.

CLOSED-HEAD INJURY IN
HUMANS

Approximately 500,000 individuals in the United States suffer a new closed-head injury each year (Brooks, 1984; Frankowski, 1986; Levin, Benton, &

Grossman, 1982); the importance of understanding factors which contribute to the behavioral manifestations of brain injury is clear. Head injuries account for 70% of all the deaths from automobile injuries and a higher percentage of continuing disabilities that follow nonfatal accidents. Damage to the CNS following such accidents may be represented in focal contusions, shearing of fibers, or most likely both (Brooks, 1984; Levin et al., 1982). Additional injury may be secondary to changes in pressure within the skull. Such damage to the CNS is not necessarily obvious, even with remarkable new advances in relatively noninvasive technologies such as computer-assisted, and positron emission tomographic scans, as well as magnetic resonance imaging.

Several lines of evidence suggest that head injury does not occur randomly in the population, nor are its consequences a simple by-product of the resultant neurotrauma. Closed-head injury is more frequent in males than females; this difference is most dramatic between the ages of 18 and 25 (Frankowski, 1986; Levin et al., 1982), and is more frequent in individuals who are alcoholics than those who are not (e.g., Hillbom & Holm, 1986). Educational level of the individual also is related to the probability of closed-head injury (e.g., Brooks, 1984); that is, less educated individuals are more likely to be involved in accidents which produce sufficient CNS trauma to be noted in medical records.

Obviously, prospective studies of humans are infrequent but important. For instance, premorbid behavioral characteristics of the head-injured individual clearly impact his or her integration with family and society (e.g., Brooks, 1984; Brown, Chadwick, Shaffer, Rutter, & Traub, 1981; Chadwick, Rutter, Brown, Shaffer, & Traub, 1981; Oddy, 1984; Rutter, Chadwick, Shaffer, & Brown, 1980). Often, interpersonal difficulties attributed to brain injury appear to be "exaggerations" of behavior patterns expressed prior to the injury in a given individual. Difficulties in impulse control are often associated with individuals with antisocial tendencies. Such a person is at increased risk for closed-head injury; the disinhibition seen following injury is thus not a new pattern of behavior, even though it may become a more prominent characteristic of the individual. Recent data (Hillbom & Holm, 1986) suggest that a history of alcohol abuse may potentiate the neuropsychological manifestation of subsequent minor head injury. Unfortunately, a history of brain damage may, in turn, increase the risk for future head trauma and other neurological disorders (Mortimer & Pirozzolo, 1985). The role that exaggerated behavioral characteristics play in this increased propensity for brain injury is virtually unexplored.

From a familial, and more broadly societal perspective, the individual with CNS damage frequently is referred to as hyperemotional, irritable, or impatient; and such behavior often is ascribed to the individual's unawareness of environmental/social cues. In many cases, such resultant behavior can be viewed as a failure on the part of the individual to compare appropriately, in timely fashion, intended outcome(s) of the behavior and its subsequent effects.

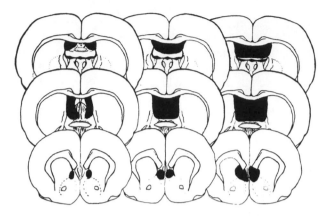

FIG. 6.2. Typical small, medium, and large septal lesions in rodents. (McDaniel et al., 1980).

BRAIN INJURY IN ANIMALS:
SEPTAL LESIONS

Changes in emotional reactivity following brain injury in humans should not be surprising in light of the extensive literature on the impact of brain damage in animals. As reviewed elsewhere (cf., Aslin, 1981; Donovick & Burright, 1982, 1984; Greenough, 1976; LeVere, 1980; Marshall, 1984; Meyer & Meyer, 1984; Stein, Finger, & Hart, 1983) both the pre- and postsurgical environmental history, genotype of the individual animal and the specific testing situation complexly coact to determine the behavioral (and physiological) manifestations of brain damage. Such coactions, occurring at all levels of analysis, begin even prior to conception and continue until death—and those cumulative coactions (experiences) determine our observations at any given point(s) in time.

In animals, selectively produced brain damage can result in behavioral changes which are strikingly parallel to those changes seen in humans following closed-head injury. Although we will discuss here the impact of lesions of the septal area of the forebrain (see Fig. 6.2) many other forms of neural dysfunction would serve as well. Interestingly, the first report (Ransom, 1895) of "the septal-rage syndrome" was described for a 24-year-old woman in whom a tumor in the anterior subcallosal region of the brain was found upon autopsy. Behavioral description suggested that she was extremely irritable and restless. Since that time, the septal-rage syndrome has been: (1) Shown to occur in a variety of species (cf. Donovick, Burright, & Bengelloun, 1979); (2) To persist for long periods following the production of the lesion (Krieckhaus, Simmons, Thomas, & Kenyon, 1964; Reynolds, 1965); and (3) Used as a model for certain human psychopathological processes (e.g., Gorenstein & Newman, 1980).

Shortly after surgery a variety of animals typically will exhibit an increase in emotionality and irritability in response to stimulation such as handling (Brady & Nauta, 1953) or placement of a probe on the back or near the snout (Engellenner, Goodlett, Burright, & Donovick, 1982). Level of emotionality has been assessed by measurements of biting and attempts to escape during handling (Slotnick & McMullen, 1972) and of vocalization, urination and defecation (Engellenner et al., 1982). However, hyperemotionality is not a necessary consequence of septal damage. Thus, the syndrome has been shown to be dependent on: (1) Location of lesion within the septal region (Harrison & Lyon, 1957; Schnurr, 1972; Turner, 1970); (2) The amount and distribution of handling during the postoperative period (Gotsick & Marshall, 1972; Turner, 1970); (3) Testing procedures employed (Max, Cohen, & Lieblich, 1974). In addition, several presurgical manipulations have been shown to alter the manifestation of postsurgical emotionality.

For instance, male rats castrated when they were 23–30 days old failed to exhibit hyperemotionality following septal lesions that were produced when they were adults (Lieblich, Gross, & Cohen, 1977; Phillips & Lieblich, 1972). Bengelloun, Nelson, Zent, and Beatty (1976) confirmed and extended these findings by showing that ovariectomy in juvenile female rats did *not* attenuate postsurgical emotionality. Furthermore, testosterone replacement following juvenile castration failed to reinstate the rage syndrome in male rats (Lieblich et al., 1977).

Furthermore, manipulating the animals presurgical environment has been shown to be effective in altering the manifestation of emotionality associated with damage to the septal region. We compared mice that had been reared under a relatively restricted condition with those that had prolonged experience in a socially and environmentally enriched condition (Engellenner et al., 1982). While there was evidence that these housing conditions altered emotionality in control mice, as can be seen in Fig. 6.3, the impact was much less than that seen for those animals that received septal lesions. In the brain-damaged group, the presurgical enrichment dramatically attenuated postsurgical emotional reactivity.

Changes in emotional reactivity following septal lesions must be viewed in the larger context of changes in responsiveness to a wide range of environmental stimuli. These septal lesions have been especially effective in changing reactions to stimuli that carry an obvious hedonic or affective component. For instance, immediately following surgery, rats that had received septal lesions or had undergone control operations, were returned to a recovery room and placed in individual wire-mesh cages where they were maintained in either continuous darkness or continuous light for 2 weeks (Zuromski, Donovick, & Burright, 1972). They were then transferred to environmental test chambers for a 2-week period in which they had a single lever through which the rat could control whether or not a light was on in its own chamber. The illumination condition

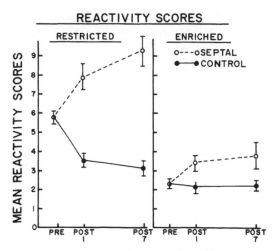

FIG. 6.3.   Impact of environmental history and septal lesions on emotionality (Engellenner et al., 1982).

remained constant until a bar press was made; thus the animal fully controlled both the amount of time spent in the light and how often the lighting condition was reversed. Fig. 6.4 shows that rats with septal lesions changed lighting conditions more frequently than controls; but, as illustrated in Fig. 6.5, septal animals spent less total time in the light than control rats. As these figures illustrate, there was a differential effect of the immediate pretesting housing condition on the brain-damaged and control animals. But can presurgical manipulations alter the environmental reactivity of animals with septal lesions?

One prominent example of a presurgical effect is found in the acceptance of preferred and nonpreferred tastants. Rats with septal lesions drink substantially more of a saccharin solution than controls, but almost totally reject unpalatable substances such as quinine (Beatty & Schwartzbaum, 1967, 1968; Carey, 1971; Donovick, Burright, & Gittleson, 1969; Donovick, Burright, & Zuromski, 1970). However, as shown in Table 6.1, social-environmental enrichment of animals from weaning until surgery (when they were young adults) markedly attenuated the overresponsiveness of animals with septal lesions to these tastants (Donovick, Burright, & Swidler, 1973).

Behavioral changes associated with the life history of brain-damaged and brain-intact organisms appear to depend on the specific nature of both the experience and the test conditions. For instance, when presurgical enrichment entailed only providing variety in available foodstuffs, dramatic and opposite effects were seen in rats which had undergone control or septal surgery (see Fig. 6.6; Donovick, Burright, & Bentsen, 1974). In this study presurgical mainte-

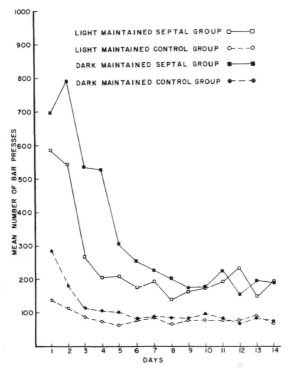

FIG. 6.4.   Impact of lighting history and septal lesions on bar pressing for change in lighting (Zuromski et al., 1972).

TABLE 6.1
Consummatory Behavior (ml/day)

Fluid Groups[1]	Water	0.1% NaSac	0.025% QHCL
ES	10.3	16.4	3.6
RS	12.2	19.3	0.5
EC	9.4	14.6	4.6
RC	10.4	14.8	4.7

[1]ES = enriched septal; RS = restricted septal; EC = enriched control; RC = restricted control.

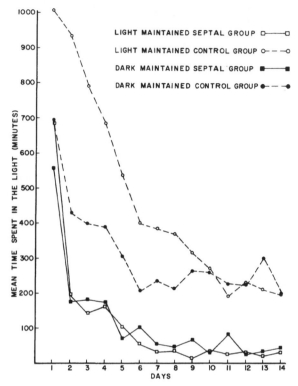

FIG. 6.5.   Influence of lighting history and septal lesions on time spent in the light (Zuromski et al., 1972).

nance conditions influenced a variety of behaviors including fluid consumption, exploration and learning.

Given such altered reactivity, interpreted in a framework of disrupted comparator processes, it is not surprising that septal lesions also can alter social reactivity, including agonistic behavior. However, increased and decreased intraspecific aggression, increased intraspecific defensive behavior, and increased nonaggressive social contact has been observed (cf. Albert, Walsh, Zalys, & Dyson, 1986; Donovick et al., 1979; Poplawsky & Johnson, 1973; Smith, Goodlett, Burright, Donovick, & Spear, 1983). Clearly, differences in the behavioral manifestations of septal lesions may be related to a variety of factors, such as the time since surgery and genotype of the lesioned animal (Gonsiorek, Donovick, Burright, & Fuller, 1974) as well as pre- and postsurgical experience (Goodlett, Engellenner, Burright, & Donovick, 1982).

As noted earlier, failure to modulate responding effectively in light of feed-

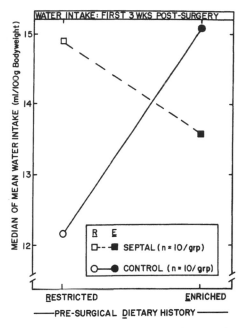

FIG. 6.6. The interaction between presurgical dietary history and septal lesions as manifested in water consumption (Donovick et al., 1974).

back from the environment often is correlated with closed-head injury in humans. Similarly, a failure to inhibit previously learned responses to otherwise highly salient cues frequently is observed following damage to the septal region in animals. For instance, rats and mice with septal lesions typically acquire a learned discrimination as readily as control animals. However, when reinforcement contingencies are changed—so that inhibition of a previously correct response is called for—rodents with septal damage have been shown to be deficient (cf. Donovick et al., 1979).

The evidence of perseverative behavior also suggests an important parallel between brain-injured rodents and brain-injured humans—a parallel which clearly has implications for rehabilitation efforts in humans with brain damage who often fail to transfer skills across tasks. For instance, while finding diminution of perseverative tendencies across repeated reversals within a single task, we failed to see generalization between tasks following septal lesions (Sikorszky, Donovick, Burright, & Chin, 1977). To improve rehabilitative strategies we need to understand better why and how brain damage reduces an individual's ability to compare and integrate internal and external environmental information in ways which allow adaptive behavior and how experience prior to damage may influence what "optimal" rehabilitative strategies might be for given individuals.

TOWARD RECOVERY OF FUNCTION

One relevant avenue of investigation has concentrated on the growing body of literature which suggests that the integrity of the norepinephrine system (NE) is important in the maintenance of *neural* plasticity of the brain (e.g., Kasamatsu & Shirokawa, 1985; Whishaw, Sutherland, Kolb, & Becker, 1986) in general, as well as pathways known to be influenced by experience, and thus assumed critical to preoperative effects (e.g., Dahl, Bailey, & Winson, 1983). Given that the NE system is dynamically influenced by the genotype of the organism (e.g., Donovick, Burright, Fanelli, & Engellenner, 1981), as well as long-term environmental conditions (Gray, 1982) and short-term stimulation (Aston–Jones & Bloom, 1981) the importance of its status prior to and following brain injury is clear. The implications of that literature, as we see them, for *behavioral* plasticity are outlined here (see also Finger & Almli, 1985; Marshall, 1984; Stein, Finger, & Hart, 1983).

Kasamatsu and Shirokawa (1985) noted that the early neuronal plasticity of the visual system, as represented in response to visual deprivation, is based upon the integrity of the NE system (but cf. Shinkman, Isley, & Rogers, 1985). The loss of adaptability that normally accompanies the developmental process can be restored by stimulation of the locus coeruleus (e.g., Kasamatsu, Watabe, Heggelund, & Scholler, 1985).

Several other lines of research also suggest the importance of this neural system in facilitating comparator processes involved in the dynamic interplay of the organism and its environment. For instance, rats treated neonatally with six-hydroxy-dopamine (to decrease NE) have lower cortical brain weights and apparently are less responsive to environmental enrichment than control animals (Brenner, Mirmiran, Uylings, & Van der Gugten, 1983). Similarly, thiamine deficiency, which also depletes brain NE, has been shown to impair acquisition of delayed, spatial-alternation tasks in rats (Mair, Anderson, Langlais, & McEntee, 1985).

These results, in conjunction with findings that suggest the frequent observation of enhanced recovery from neonatal lesions relative to those produced in adults are dependent on the integrity of the NE system (e.g., Sutherland, Kolb, Whishaw, & Becker, 1982), have major implications for how genotype and environment may coact to influence outcome from brain injury.

In keeping with findings such as these, the suggestion that the locus coeruleus plays a critical role in modulating vigilance to environmentally relevant stimuli, at times manifested in changes in emotional behavior (e.g., Aston–Jones, 1985;

Foote, Aston–Jones, & Bloom, 1983), is of interest. Since the locus coeruleus is the major source of brain norepinephrine, its diffuse efferent outflow affords the opportunity for these rather small nuclei to have a relatively synchronized effect throughout much of the neuraxis (e.g., Aston–Jones, 1985; Aston–Jones, Ennis, Pierbone, Nickell, & Shipley, 1986; Foote, Aston–Jones, & Bloom, 1983). In contrast to the diffuse pattern of efferent output from the *locus coeruleus*, its direct afferent innervation apparently is restricted primarily to the paragigantocellularis and prepositus hypoglossi nuclei in the dorsal medulla, with minor afferents from the paraventricular nucleus of the hypothalamus and intermediate gray regions of the spinal cord (Aston–Jones et al., 1986). Like the septal area (cf. Raisman, 1966; VanHoesen, Pandya, & Butters, 1972), this combination of afferents places the locus coeruleus in an ideal position for polymodal integration necessary for effective comparator processes which also may be critical in providing patterning of information for recovery from brain damage. Not surprisingly, levels of catecholamines found in an individual are a by-product of the coaction between the genetic constitution (Donovick, Burright et al., 1981) and the environmental history of that individual.

Given the apparent role of norepinephrine in behavioral plasticity, it is not surprising that a number of studies have suggested that manipulation of the system alters the recovery from direct brain damage. Both rats (Feeney, Gonzalez, & Law, 1982) and cats (Hovda & Feeney, 1984) treated with amphetamine following cortical brain lesions showed enhanced rates of recovery relative to control animals. Furthermore, early depletion of norepinephrine may retard recovery from cortical lesions in adult, environmentally restricted, rats (Whishaw et al., 1986). Such findings also are in keeping with those of Gage and coworkers, who have shown that reinnervation of brain regions depleted of noradrenergic fibers exhibit parallel recovery of behavioral capacity and sprouting of noradrenergic fibers (e.g., Kesslak & Gage, 1986). However, caution in interpretation of these findings is suggested by reports which have failed to find a relations between the behavioral dysfunction seen following brain damage and changes in catecholamine systems (e.g., Donovick, Burright et al., 1981). Unfortunately, often because of limitations in the experimental design and understanding of critical individual characteristics, our ability to predict the specific nature and/or degree of severity of outcome(s) from brain injury for an individual is limited.

PROGRESSIVE NEUROPATHOLOGY FROM TOXOCARIASIS

Thus far we have considered selected factors which ultimately impact the behavioral outcome(s) from brain damage that resulted from a traumatic event at one point in time. The impact of multiple-stage brain damage has been reviewed elsewhere (e.g., Donovick & Burright, 1984); but it is worth re-emphasizing that even a single, temporally well-defined event cannot be viewed as "static" with respect to its influence on the future course of the organism's behavioral plasticity and development. Nonetheless, we would like to discuss here the problem of how more continuous and progressive disease processes may affect the organism's behavior (also see Riese, 1960); to do this, our discussion will be limited to the behavior (and neuropathology) associated with the parasitic infection of mice with *T. canis,* the common round worm of dogs.

In abnormal hosts, such as humans or mice, the parasite's developmental cycle ends when second-stage larvae migrate to the brain (and other organs) where they can remain viable and active for long periods of time. Such infection causes extensive and continuing neuropathological and behavioral changes (cf. Donovick & Burright, 1987; Hay, Hutchison, & Aitken, 1983). Associated with the migration of *T. canis* larvae is extensive damage to large, myelinated fiber tracts in the brain. The progressive neuropathology would appear to be associated with mechanical disruption of the brain tissues through which the parasite moves, and probably also with neurotoxin(s) produced by the *T. canis* larvae. Mice infected with *T. canis* show alterations in a wide range of behaviors, including: reactivity to taste; exploration of the environment; and performance of learned tasks (cf., Donovick & Burright, 1987).

Somewhat to our surprise, in our original studies (Dolinsky et al., 1981; Donovick, Dolinsky et al., 1981), mice intubated with *T. canis* and simultaneously given lead as their sole source of fluid showed less of a change in behavior than those infected with the parasite alone (see Fig. 6.7). Despite the relatively smaller behavioral reaction(s) in the combined group, observable neuropathological changes were the same in those mice infected with *T. canis* alone and those infected with the parasite and administered lead (Summers, Cypess, Dolinsky, Burright, & Donovick, 1983).

To examine further the factors providing the organism with protection against *T. canis* we undertook two lines of research. In the first, at the time of birth of litters, dams and their pups were given either water or a 0.5% lead acetate solution as their sole source of fluid (Yuhl, Burright, Donovick, & Cypess, 1985). When the pups were approximately 40 days old, they were intubated with either the vehicle alone or with *T. canis.* At that time all mice were given water as their sole source of fluid. As can be seen in Table 6.2, the infected mice with no history of lead exposure were the least active of all groups before bedding was changed in their home cages; but the pattern and level of activity of the combined group was most similar to control mice. Obviously, these results complement the findings discussed previously, which suggest that the presurgical environment of the organism dramatically alters the response to brain damage.

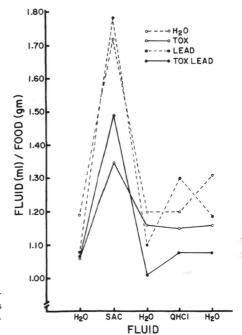

FIG. 6.7. Differential reactivity to tastants of mice exposed to lead, T. canis alone, or in combination (Donovick, Dolinsky, et al., 1981).

Our second approach has been based on the knowledge that humans, and other aberrant hosts, are most likely to experience repeated exposures to any parasite; thus, we recently examined the impact of single versus multiple exposures to T. canis (Draski, Summers, Cypess, Burright, & Donovick, 1987). Prior infection provided some protection for the mouse against subsequent exposures to T. canis; that is, pathology of peripheral organs and CNS, as well as the patterns of behavior exhibited by the mice were influenced by the infection

TABLE 6.2
Mean Activity Score (per minute)

Period Group	Bedding Change	
	Before	After
Control	33	32
Lead	26	40
Lead-T. Canis	25	26
T. Canis	21	30

regime. Earlier exposures may alter, among other things, the immunological competence of the organism to cope with subsequent exposures to the parasite. The potential for continual interactions between the nervous and immune systems, as reflected in behavior, has been discussed (e.g., Ader & Cohen, 1985).

Not surprisingly, the degree of reactivity to the environment, as reflected in responses of the immune system, is influenced by genetic factors (Raymond, Reyes, Tokuda, & Jones, 1986). Similarly, response to infection with T. canis is a by-product, in part, of the genotype of the host. While not explicitly investigated, we would expect to find a coactive relationship between geneotype, environmental history, and reactivity to infection with T. canis, as reflected in both the brain and the behavior of the host. Furthermore, it is interesting to note the parallel between the lessened effect(s) often observed when brain damage is produced in stages (cf. Donovick & Burright, 1984) and the "protection" afforded by successive exposure regimens.

PARTING SHOTS (TO THE HEAD)

To understand the relationship between brain injury and behavior it will be necessary to consider the unique attributes of the individual organism. As we look at the recent history of relevant disciplines we see several trends that influence our understanding. The concentration on molecular aspects of nervous system structure and function frequently overshadow behavioral analysis. Similarly, our examination of data—from motions in the petri dish to emotions in Times Square—commonly concentrates on descriptions of groups, with little apparent concern for how well such descriptions encompass the individual. And the choice of experimental model(s) rarely is based upon sound genetic (i.e., species or strain) rationale (cf. Donovick & Horowitz, 1982), let alone critical environmental or historical information. Furthermore, rarely do experiments examine cross-situation generalizations of behavioral patterns ascribed to brain damage (cf. Donovick, Burright et al., 1981). Thus it is not surprising that we understand so little about how the characteristics of the individual determine, in part, how he or she responds to neuropathological processes.

Obviously, the questions that we ask define the answers we receive. Thus, the very rapid expansion of our knowledge of molecular neuroscience has not been matched by an expanded understanding of brain-behavior relationships. In part, this state of affairs is attributable to the fact that ongoing, cumulative gene–environment coactions have not been central to our thinking; these dynamic coactions, at all levels of analysis, serve as the underpinning of the complex comparator processes associated with the continual unfolding of any individual's experience and behavior. As a consequence of such inattention to the bases for experiences as reflected in behavior, our models are not yet well suited to understanding, or even predicting, the neurobehavioral consequences of brain pathology for individuals, who as unique organisms with unique histories respond to brain injury in a fashion based upon their experiential history.

REFERENCES

Ader, R., & Cohen, N. (1985). CNS—immune system interactions: conditioning phenomena (with commentary). *Behavioral & Brain Sciences, 8*, 392–426.

Albert, D. J., Walsh, M. L., Zalys, C., & Dyson, E. (1986). Defensive aggression toward an experimenter: No differences between males and females following septal, medial accumbens, or medial hypothalamic lesions in rats. *Physiology & Behavior, 38*, 11–14.

Aslin, R. N. (1981). Experiential influences and sensitive periods in perceptual development: A unified model. In R. N. Aslin, J. R. Alberts, & M. R. Peterson (Eds.), *Development of perception: Psychobiological perspectives, Vol. 2, The Visual System* (pp. 45–93). New York: Academic Press.

Aston–Jones, G. (1985). Behavioral functions of Locus Coeruleus derived from cellular attributes. *Physiological Psychology, 13*, 118–126.

Aston–Jones, G., & Bloom, F. E. (1981). Norepinephrine-containing locus coeruleus neurons in behaving rats exhibit pronounced responses to non-noxious environmental stimuli. *Journal of Neuroscience, 1*, 887–900.

Aston–Jones, G., Ennis, M., Pierbone, V. A., Nickell, W. T., & Shipley, M. T. (1986). The brain nucleus locus coeruleus: Restricted afferent control of a broad efferent network. *Science, 234*, 734–737.

Beatty, W. W., & Schwartzbaum, J. S. (1967). Enhanced reactivity to quinine and saccharin following septal lesions in the rat. *Psychonomic Science, 8*, 483–484.

Beatty, W. W., & Schwartzbaum, J. S. (1968). Consummatory behavior for sucrose following septal lesions in the rat. *Journal of Comparative Physiological Psychology, 65*, 93–102.

Bengelloun, W. A., Nelson, D. J., Zent, H. M., & Beatty, W. W. (1976). Behavior of male and female rats with septal lesions: Influence of prior gonadectomy. *Physiology & Behavior, 16*, 317–330.

Bernard, C. (1878). *Leçons sur les phenomenes de la vie communs aux animaux et aux vegetaux*, Paris: Bailliere.

Brady, J. V., & Nauta, W. J. H. (1953). Subcortical mechanisms in emotional behavior: Affective changes following septal forebrain lesions in the albino rat. *Journal of Comparative and Physiological Psychology, 46*, 339–346.

Brenner, E., Mirmiran, M., Uylings, H. B. M., & Van der Gugten, J. (1983). Impaired growth of the cerebral cortex of rats treated neonatally with 6-hydroxydopamine under different environmental conditions. *Neuroscience Letters, 42*, 13–17.

Brooks, D. N. (1984). Head injury and the family. In N. Brooks (Ed.), *Closed head injury: Psychological, social, and family consequences*. Oxford, England: Oxford University Press, pp. 123–147.

Brown, G., Chadwick, O., Shaffer, D., Rutter, M., & Traub, M. (1981). A prospective study of children with head injuries: III. Psychiatric sequelae. *Psychological Medicine, 11*, 63–78.

Bullock, T. H. (1984). Comparative neuroscience holds promise for quiet revoluions. *Science, 225*, 473–478.

Carey, R. J. (1971). Quinine and sacharine preferences: Acquisition threshold determination in rats with septal ablation. *Journal of Comparative Physiological Psychology, 71*, 316–326.

Chadwick, O., Rutter, M., Brown, G., Shaffer, D., & Traub, M. (1981). A prospective study of children with head injuries: II. Cognitive sequelae. *Psychological Medicine, 11*, 49–61.

Dahl, D., Bailey, W. H., & Winson, J. (1983). Effect of norepinephrine depletion of hippocampus on neuronal transmission from perforant pathway through dentate gyrus. *Journal of Neurophysiology, 49*, 123–133.

Dolinsky, Z. S., Burright, R. G., Donovick, P. J., Glickman, L. T., Babish, J., Summers, B., &

Cypess, R. H. (1981). Behavioral effects of lead and *Toxocara canis* in mice. *Science, 213,* 1142–1144.

Donovick, P. J., & Burright, R. G. (1982). Genetic influences on responses to brain lesions. In I. Lieblich (Ed.), *The genetics of the brain* (pp. 178–205). Amsterdam: Elsevier Biomedical.

Donovick, P. J., & Burright, R. G. (1984). Roots to the future: Gene-environment coaction and individual vulnerability to neural insult. In C. R. Almli & S. Finger (Eds.), *Early brain damage* (Vol. 2, pp. 281–311). New York: Academic Press.

Donovick, P. J., & Burright, R. G. (1987). The consequences of parasitic infection for the behavior of the mammalian host. *Environmental Health Perspectives, 73,* 247–250.

Donovick, P. J., Burright, R. G., & Bengelloun, W. A. (1979). The septal region and behavior: An example of the importance of genetic and experiential factors in determining effects of brain damage. *Neuroscience & Biobehavioral Reviews, 4,* 83–96.

Donovick, P. J., Burright, R. G., & Bentsen, E. O. (1974). Presurgical dietary history differentially alters the behavior of control and septal lesioned rats. *Developmental Psychobiology, 8,* 13–25.

Donovick, P. J., Burright, R. G., Fanelli, R. J., & Engellenner, W. J. (1981). Septal lesions and avoidance behavior: Genetic, neurochemical and behavioral considerations. *Physiology & Behavior, 26,* 495–507.

Donovick, P. J., Burright, R. G., Fuller, J. L., & Branson, P. R. (1975). Septal lesions and behavior: Effects of presurgical raring and strain of mouse. *Journal of Comparative and Physiological Psychology, 89,* 859–867.

Donovick, P. J., Burright, R. G., & Gittleson, P. L. (1969). Body weight and food and water consumption in septal lesioned and operated control rats. *Psychological Reports, 25,* 303–310.

Donovick, P. J., Burright, R. G., & Swidler, M. A. (1973). Presurgical rearing environment alters exploration, fluid consumption, and learning of septal lesioned and control rats. *Physiology & Behavior, 11,* 543–553.

Donovick, P. J., Burright, R. G., & Zuromski, E. (1970). Localization of quinine aversion within the septum, habenula and interpedunucular nucleus. *Journal of Comparative and Physiological Psychology, 17,* 376–383.

Donovick, P. J., Dolinsky, Z. S., Perdue, V. P., Burright, R. G., Summers, B., & Cypess, R. H. (1981). *Toxocara canis* and lead alter consummatory behavior in mice. *Brain Research Bulletin, 7,* 317–323.

Donovick, P. J., & Horowitz, G. P. (1982). On the choice of subject populations for research in neurehavioral toxicology, *Journal of Toxicology & Environmental Health, 10,* 1–9.

Draski, L. J., Summers, B., Cypess, R. H., Burright, R. G., & Donovick, P. J. (1987). The impact of single versus repeated exposures of mice to *Toxocara canis. Physiology & Behavior, 40,* 301–306.

Engellenner, W. J., Goodlett, C. R., Burright, R. G., & Donovick, P. J. (1982). Environmental enrichment and restriction: Effect on reactivity, exploration and maze learning in mice with septal lesions. *Physiology & Behavior, 29,* 885–893.

Feeney, D. M., Gonzalez, A., & Law, W. A. (1982). Amphetamine, haloperidol, and experience intereact to affect rate of recovery after motor cortex injury. *Science, 217,* 855–857.

Finger, S., & Almli, C. R. (1985). Brain damage and neuroplasticity: Mechanisms of recovery or development? *Brain Research Review, 10,* 177–186.

Foote, S. L., Aston-Jones, G., & Bloom, F. E. (1983). The nucleus locus coeruleus: New evidence of anatomical and physiological specificity. *Physiological Reviews, 63,* 844–914.

Frankowski, R. F. (1986). Descriptive epidemiologic studies of head injury in the United States: 1974–1984. *Advances in Psychosomatic Medicine, 16,* 153–172.

Fuller, J. L. (1979). The taxonomy of psychophenes. In J. R. Royce & L. P. Mos (Eds.), *Theoretical advances in behavior genetics.* Netherlands: Sijthoff & Noordhoff, Ålphen aan den Rijn pp. 483–513.

Goldin, L. R., Nurnberger, J. I., Jr, & Gershon, E. S. (1986). Clinical methods in psychiatric genetics: II. The high risk approach. *Acta psychiatrica scandinavica, 74*, 119–128.

Gonsiorek, J. C., Donovick, P. J., Burright, R. G., & Fuller, J. L. (1974). Aggression in low and high brainweight mice following septal lesions. *Physiology & Behavior, 12*, 813–813.

Goodlett, C. R., Engellenner, W. J., Burright, R. G., & Donovick, P. J. (1982). Influence of environmental rearing history and postsurgical environment change on the septal rage syndrome in mice. *Physiology & Behavior, 28*, 1077–1081.

Gorenstein, E. E., & Newman, J. P. (1980). Disinhibitory psychopathology: A new perspective and a model for research. *Psychological Review, 87*, 301–315.

Gotsick, J. E., & Marshall, R. C. (1972). Time course of the septal rage syndrome. *Physiology & Behavior, 9*, 685–687.

Gray, J. A. (1982). *The neuropsychology of anxiety: An enquiry into the functions of the septo-hippocampal system.* New York: Oxford University Press.

Greenough, W. T. (1976). Enduring brain effects of differential experience and training. In M. R. Rosensweig & E. L. Bennett (Eds.), *Neural mechanisms of learning and memory.* Cambridge MA: MIT Press.

Harrison, J. M., & Lyon, M. (1957). The role of the septal nuclei and components of the fornix in the behaviour of the rat. *Journal of Comparative Neurology, 108*, 121–137.

Hay, J., Hutchison, W. M., & Aitken, P. P. (1983). The effect of *Toxocara canis* infection on the behaviour of mice. *Annals of Tropical Medicine and Parasitology, 77*, 543–544.

Hillbom, M., & Holm, L. (1986). Contribution of traumatic head injury to neuropsychological deficits in alcoholics. *Journal of Neurology Neurosurgery & Psychiatry, 49*, 1348–1353.

Hovda, D. A., & Feeney, D. M. (1984). Amphetamine with experience promotes recovery of locomotor function after unilateral frontal cortex injury in the cat. *Brain Research, 298*, 358–361.

Kasamatsu, T., & Shirokawa, T. (1985). Involvement of β-adrenoreceptors in the shift of ocular dominance after monocular deprivation. *Experimental Brain Research, 59*, 507–514.

Kasamatsu, T., Watabe, K., Heggelund, P., & Scholler, E. (1985). Plasticity in cat visual cortex restored by electrical stimulation of the locus coeruleus. *Neuroscience Research, 2*, 365–386.

Kavanaugh, J. L. (1967). Behavior of captive white-footed mice. *Science, 155*, 205–222.

Kesslak, J. P., & Gage III, F. H. (1986). Recovery of spatial alternation deficits following selective hippocampal destruction with kainic acid. *Behavioral Neuroscience, 100* (2), 280–283.

Krieckhaus, E. E., Simmons, H., Thomas, G., & Kenyon, J. (1964). Septal lesions enhance shock avoidance behavior in rats. *Experimental Neurology, 9*, 107–113.

LeVere, T. E. (1980). Recovery of function after brain damage: A theory of the behavioral deficit. *Physiological Psychology, 8*, 297–308.

Levin, H. S., Benton, A. L., & Grossman, R. G. (Eds.). (1982). *Neurobehavioral consequences of closed head injury.* New York: Oxford University Press.

Lieblich, I., Gross, R., & Cohen, E. (1977). Effects of testosterone replacement on the recovery from increased emotionality, produced by septal lesions in prepubertal castrated male rats. *Physiology & Behavior, 18*, 1159–1164.

Livingston, M. G., Brooks, D. N., & Bond, M. R. (1985a). Three months after severe head injury: Psychiatric and social impact on relatives. *Journal of Neurology, Neurosurgery, and Psychiatry, 48*, 870–875.

Livingston, M. G., Brooks, D. N., & Bond, M. R. (1985b). Patient outcome in the year following severe head injury and relatives' psychiatric and social functioning. *Journal of Neurology, Neurosurgery, and Psychiatry, 48*, 876–881.

Mair, R. G., Anderson, C. D., Langlais, P. J., & McEntee, W. J. (1985). Thiamine deficiency depletes cortical norepinephrine and impairs learning processes in the rat. *Brain Research, 360*, 273–284.

Marshall, J. F. (1984). Brain function: Neural adaptations and recovery from injury. *Annual Review of Psychology, 35,* 277–308.

Max, D. M., Cohen, E., & Lieblich, I. (1974). Effects of capture procedures on emotionality scores in rats with septal lesions. *Physiology & Behavior, 13,* 617–620.

McDaniel, J. R., Donovick, P. J., Burright, R. G., & Fanelli, R. J. (1980). Genetics, septal lesions, and avoidance behavior in mice. *Behavioral & Neural Biology, 28,* 285–299.

Meyer, D. R., & Meyer, P. M. (1984). Bases of recoveries from perinatal injuries to the cerebral cortex. In S. Finger & C. R. Almli (Eds.), *Early brain damage: Neurobiology and behavior* (Vol. 2, pp. 211–227). New York: Academic Press.

Mortimer, J. A., & Pirozzolo, F. J. (1985). Remote effects of head trauma. *Developmental Neuropsychology, 1*(3), 215–229.

Oddy, M. (1984). Head injury and social adjustment. In N. Brooks (Ed.), *Closed head injury: Psychological, social, and family consequences.* Oxford, England: Oxford University Press, pp. 108–122.

Oddy, M., Coughlan, T., Tyerman, A., & Jenkins, D. (1985). Social adjustment after closed head injury: A further follow-up seven years after injury. *Journal of Neurology, Neurosurgery, and Psychiatry, 48,* 564–568.

O'Kelly, L. I. (1963). The psychobiology of motivation. *Annual Review of Psychology, 14,* 57–92.

Phillips, A. G., & Lieblich, I. (1972). Developmental and hormonal aspects of hyperemotionality produced by septal lesions in male rats. *Physiology & Behavior, 9,* 237–242.

Poplawsky, A., & Johnson, D. A. (1973). Open-field social behavior of rats following lateral or medial septal lesions. *Physiology & Behavior, 11,* 845–854.

Raisman, G. (1966). The connections of the septum. *Brain, 89,* 317–348.

Ransom, W. B. (1895). On tumors of the corpus callosum with account of a case. *Brain, 18,* 531–550.

Raymond, L. N., Reyes, E., Tokuda, S., & Jones, B. C. (1986). Differential immune response in two handled inbred strains of mice. *Physiology & Behavior, 37,* 295–297.

Reynolds, R. (1965). Equivalence of radio-frequency and electrolytic lesions in producing septal rage. *Psychonomic Science, 2,* 35–36.

Riese, W. (1960). Dynamics in brain lesions. *Journal of Nervous and Mental Disease, 131,* 291–301.

Rutter, M., Chadwick, O., Shaffer, D., & Brown, G. (1980). A prospective study of children with head injuries: I. Design and methods. *Psychological Medicine, 10,* 633–645.

Schnurr, R. (1972). Localization of the septal rage syndrome in Long–Evans rats. *Journal of Comparative and Physiological Psychology, 81,* 291–296.

Sherrington, C. S. (1941). *Man on his nature.* New York: Macmillan.

Shinkman, P. G., Isley, M. R., & Rogers, D. C. (1985). Development of interocular relationships in visual cortex. In R. N. Aslin (Ed.), *Advances in Neural and Behavioral Development* (Vol. 1, pp. 187–269). Norwood, NJ: Ablex.

Sikorszky, R. D., Donovick, P. J., Burright, R. G., & Chin, T. (1977). Experiential effects of acquisition and reversal of discrimination tasks by albino rats with septal lesions. *Physiology & Behavior, 18,* 231–236.

Slotnick, B. M., & McMullen, M. F. (1972). Intraspecific fighting in albino mice with septal forebrain lesions. *Physiology & Behavior, 8,* 333–337.

Smith, G. J., Goodlett, C. R., Burright, R. G., Donovick, P. J., & Spear, N. E. (1983). The presence of home-cage stimuli attenuates spontaneous-alternation deficits in rats with septal lesions. *Physiological Psychology, 11,* 119–124.

Stein, D. G., Finger, S., & Hart, T. (1983). Brain damage and recovery: Problems and perspectives. *Behavioral and Neural Biology, 37,* 185–222.

Sutherland, R. J., Kolb, B., Whishaw, I. Q., & Becker, J. B. (1982). Cortical noradrenaline depletion eliminates sparing of spatial learning after neonatal frontal cortex damage in the rat. *Neuroscience Letters, 32,* 125–130.

Summers, B., Cypess, R. H., Dolinsky, Z. D., Burright, R. G., & Donovick, P. J. (1983). Neuropathological studies of experimental toxocariasis in lead exposed mice. *Brain Research Bulletin,* 10, 547–550.

Turner, B. H. (1970). Neural structures involved in the rage syndrome of the rat. *Journal of Comparative and Physiological Psychology,* 71, 103–113.

VanHoesen, G. W., Pandya, D. P., & Butters, N. (1972). Cortical afferents to the entorhinal cortex of the rhesus. *Science,* 175, 1471–1473.

Whishaw, I. Q., Sutherland, R. J., Kolb, B., & Becker, J. B. (1986). Effects of neonatal forebrain noradrenaline depletion on recovery from brain damage: performance on a spatial navigation task as a function of age of surgery and postsurgical housing. *Behavioral Neural Biology,* 46, 285–307.

Wilson, R. S. (1986). Continuity and change in cognitive ability profile. *Behavior Genetics,* 16, 45–60.

Yuhl, D. E., Burright, R. G., Donovick, P. J., & Cypess, R. H. (1985). Behavioral effects of early lead exposure and subsequent toxocariasis in mice. *Journal of Toxicology and Environmental Health,* 16, 315–321.

Zuromski, E. S., Donovick, P. J., & Burright, R. G. (1972). The effect of septal lesions on the albino rat's ability to regulate light. *Journal of Comparative and Physiological Psychology,* 78, 83–90.

7

Social Experience and Lesion-Induced Predation

David J. Albert
Department of Psychology
University of British Columbia

G. Lincoln Chew
Department of Psychology
Lethbridge University

Mike L. Walsh
Department of Kinesiology
Simon Fraser University

Mouse killing can be induced by lesions in various parts of the brain. An examination of the killing suggests that it is behaviorally similar to killing that occurs spontaneously or that is induced by food deprivation. An important feature of the killing is that it can be influenced by experience. Specifically, the simple procedure of exposing the rat to a mouse for a few hours preoperatively can prevent killing that would otherwise be induced by some lesions.

The focus of this chapter is on this interaction between preoperative experience and lesion-induced killing. However, to establish the context in which mouse killing occurs, we will begin by presenting evidence indicating that predatory behavior arises from a distinct motivational state and by describing observations suggesting that predation by a normal rat on a specific organism can be inhibited by prior social contact with that organism. We will then examine lesion-induced mouse killing in detail, first to establish that the mouse killing produced corresponds to the predatory behavior of normal animals, and then to present evidence indicating that preoperative social contact can prevent mouse killing induced by some lesions. Finally, we will discuss the role of preoperative experience in inhibiting lesion-induced predation in terms of both the normal role of social experience in inhibiting predatory behavior and the neurological substrate that mediates this function.

PREDATION AND EXPERIENCE

Predatory behavior arises from a distinct motivational state. This motive has a goal object, the prey. It is potentiated by hunger (Paul, 1972) and is elicited by stimuli such as the movement of small objects (Albert, Walsh, & Longley, 1985). The consummatory act of predatory killing is itself reinforcing (Van Hemel, 1972). This accounts for the otherwise paradoxical observation that rats continue to kill even when they are not allowed to consume the prey. Predatory killing is also influenced by reinforcement contingencies that may be superimposed upon the consummatory behavior. In common with other motivational states based on a positively reinforcing goal object, the addition of an aversive consequence (i.e., footshock) following the behavior will decrease or eliminate the predatory behavior (Baenninger, 1978). Conversely, if the consummatory act is followed by an additional reinforcement, it might be inferred that the behavior will be appropriately enhanced. Such a reinforcement does occur in the case of mouse killing, since the flesh of the mouse is highly palatable to the rat (Albert, Walsh, White, & Longley, 1984).

Predation is subject to an experiential influence that appears unique to this motive. It is inhibited by prior social contact with an otherwise potential prey object. Experiments examining the effect of nonkilling experience with a mouse on subsequent killing behavior appear to have emanated from Kuo's experiments demonstrating an inhibition of killing by cats reared with rats (Kuo, 1930). Denenberg, Paschke, and Zarrow (1968) and Myer (1969) reported analogous experiments using rats reared with mice. When tested for mouse killing in adulthood, these rats were far less likely to kill an unfamiliar mouse than were rats first exposed to a mouse at that time. Mouse killing induced by food deprivation is also suppressed by predeprivation exposure to a mouse (Paul, 1972). To demonstrate this, adult rats were cyclically food deprived (23 hr/day) for 7 days either with or without a mouse present. When tested for mouse killing on Day 6 with an unfamiliar mouse present, only 2 of 14 rats that cohabited with a mouse killed, compared with 12 of 16 animals that had never seen a mouse. Similar results were obtained with animals on a continuous food deprivation schedule. These findings demonstrate that the experience of cohabiting with a mouse is a powerful influence in preventing mouse killing that might occur spontaneously or that is induced by food deprivation.

MOUSE KILLING INDUCED BY BRAIN LESIONS

The ability of brain lesions to induce mouse killing has been known for many years. Lesions of the olfactory bulbs, medial accumbens, lateral septum, medial hypothalamus, or dorsal/median raphe can each induce mouse killing in rats that do not kill spontaneously (Fig. 7.1; Albert & Brayley, 1979; Albert, Nanji, & Chew, 1981; Grant, Coscina, Grossman, & Freedman, 1973; Karli, 1960; Karli, Vergnes, & Didiergeorges, 1969; Miczek & Grossman, 1972; Panksepp, 1971). The lesions induce killing in both male and female rats (for a review see Albert & Walsh, 1982b) and are effective when made in infancy as well as

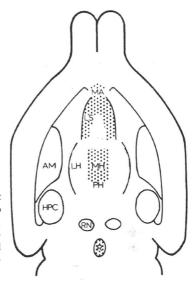

FIG. 7.1. A schematic horizontal section of the rat brain showing the locations where lesions appear to induce predatory behavior (stippled). AM-amygdala, HPC-hippocampus, LH-lateral hypothalamus, LS-lateral septum, MA-medial accumbens, MH-medial hypothalamus, PH-posterior hypothalamus, R-dorsal/median raphe nuclei, RN-red nucleus.

adulthood (Albert & Walsh, unpublished experiments; Eclancher & Karli, 1979).

Systemic injections of substances which deplete serotonin levels (para-chlorophenylalanine (PCPA); DiChiara, Camba, & Spano, 1971) or intracranial injections of a neurotoxin (5,7-dihydroxytryptophan; Marks, O'Brien, & Paxinos, 1977; Vergnes, Penot, Kempf, & Mack, 1977) which destroys serotonergic neurons in the raphe nuclei also induce mouse killing. It is usually argued that lesions of the raphe nuclei induce mouse killing by depleting brain serotonin.

Mouse killing can be induced by lesions of the medial amygdala (Vergnes, 1976). However, the induced killing manifests itself clearly only when the rats are food deprived before exposure to a mouse (Vergnes, 1976). In addition, a weak increase in mouse killing is induced by lesions of the bed nucleus of the stria terminalis (Albert & Brayley, 1979; for a more complete review of this literature, see Albert & Walsh, 1982b).

Recent experiments have examined the aggressive behavior of lesion-induced killers in a variety of situations in order to evaluate the extent to which the killing represents an enhancement of aggressive behavior in general. These experiments indicate that rats induced to kill by lesions are not necessarily aggressive toward an experimenter (Albert & Wong, 1978a, 1978b) and are actually deficient in testosterone-dependent intermale social aggression (Albert, Chew, Walsh, Ryan, & Lee, 1982; Albert, Dyson, Walsh, & Gorzalka, 1987; Albert & Walsh, 1982a; Olivier, 1977; Olivier, Olivier–Aardema, & Wiepkema, 1983).

A number of experiments suggest that lesions which induce mouse killing elicit the complete sequence of predatory behavior. These experiments demonstrate that in terms of latency to kill, pattern of attack, and tendency to eat following the kill, the behavior of rats with lateral septal, medial accumbens, or medial hypothalamic lesions or with depletion of brain serotonin (para-chlorophenylalanine injections) is similar to that of spontaneous killers, particularly spontaneous killers that are food deprived (Albert et al., 1981; Albert, Walsh, Ryan, & Siemens, 1982b; Albert, Walsh, Siemens, & Louie, 1986; Albert, Walsh, & White, 1985). Further, food-deprived spontaneous killers, as well as rats with lesions of the medial hypothalamus, medial accumbens, or lateral septum, all display an enhanced possessiveness of the prey following the kill (Albert, Walsh, & Longley, 1985; Albert, Walsh, & White, 1985; Panksepp, 1971).

These results suggest a substantial similarity in the predatory behavior of food-deprived rats that kill mice spontaneously and rats that are induced to kill by lesions of the lateral septum, medial accumbens, or medial hypothalamus, or by serotonin depletion (PCPA injections). However, the same cannot be said for rats induced to kill by olfactory bulb lesions. The killing induced by these lesions is clearly different from that of spontaneous killers in that it involves repeated biting at the prey and a long killing latency (Albert, Walsh, & White, 1985). As the killing induced by some lesions bears a close correspondence to that which occurs spontaneously, it is now reasonable to examine the extent to which the killing is subject to the same experiential inhibitory influences.

PREOPERATIVE EXPERIENCE

Exposure to the Prey

The mouse killing induced by lateral septal lesions is suppressed by preoperative exposure to a mouse. In rats reared with a mouse, the killing was completely eliminated (Table 7.1; Albert, Walsh, & White, 1984). However, the suppression of septal-lesion induced killing is not dependent on exposure to a mouse during rearing. Karli (1960) also failed to obtain mouse killing following septal lesions in male rats that preoperatively had lived with a mouse for 2 months as adults, and Penot and Vergnes (1976) obtained almost no killing with rats that had lived with a mouse for only a 24-hr period prior to a septal lesion.

In contrast, preoperative exposure to a mouse does not suppress mouse killing induced by medial hypothalamic or medial accumbens lesions. When rats were raised with mice from weaning to adulthood and then given lesions of the medial hypothalamus or medial accumbens, the proportion of animals that killed was not significantly different from that of lesioned animals that were not reared with mice (Table 7.1; Albert, Walsh, & White, 1984). Many killed within 10

TABLE 7.1
The Effect of Rearing Rats With Mice on the Induction of Mouse
Killing by Lesions in the Lateral Septum, the Medial Accumbens,
or the Medial Hypothalamus

Group	Proportion Killing	Kills within First 15 min
R-Lateral Septum	0/12	0/12
NR-Lateral Septum	8/12 *	5/12
R-Medial Accumbens	5/8 *	4/8
NR-Medial Accumbens	7/9 *	5/9
R-Medial Hypothalamus	5/10 *	4/10
NR-Medial Hypothalamus	6/10 *	2/10
R-Sham Lesion	1/13	1/13
NR-Sham Lesion	0/13	0/13

"R" indicates groups preoperatively reared with mice and "NR"
groups preoperatively reared without mice.
   * Significantly different from corresponding sham-lesioned control group, $p < .01$.
   Table modified from Albert, Walsh, & White, 1984.

to 15 min and most others did so within 24 hr. Appropriately, experiments in which rats were exposed to the mouse for a relatively short period (48 or 96 hr) have also found no suppression of the lesion-induced killing (Albert, 1979; Albert, Walsh, Ryan, Siemens, & White, 1983).

Preoperative exposure to a mouse also does not suppress the killing induced by olfactory bulb lesions. In the early experiments of Karli (1956, 1960), adult rats intermittently exposed to mice over several months were still induced to kill mice by olfactory bulb lesions.

The influence of prior exposure to a mouse on killing induced by electrolytic lesions of the dorsal/median raphe nuclei or serotonin depletion by para-chlorophenylalanine have not been subjected to a direct experimental analysis. However, mouse killing has been obtained with both procedures following preoperative exposure periods of 3 to 24 hours (Miczek, Altman, Appel, & Boggan, 1975; Paxinos, Burt, Atrens, & Jackson, 1977; Vergnes, Mack, & Kempf, 1973, 1974). In contrast, mouse killing induced by chemical lesions of the dorsal/median raphe nuclei is suppressed by preoperative exposure to a mouse (Marks et al., 1977; Vergnes et al., 1977). The exposure consisted of either three 1-hr periods, or a single period of 24 hr (however, see Applegate, 1980). The reason for the discrepancy between the chemical and electrolytic lesion experiments is not clear.

Mouse killing induced by amygdala lesions is not suppressed by preoperative exposure to a mouse. With amygdala lesions, the killing only occurs if the animals are food deprived for 72 hr prior to the mouse killing test (Vergnes, 1975, 1976).

The marked difference in the influence of preoperative experience on mouse killing induced by electrolytic lesions in various brain structures raises the question of whether mouse killing induced by septal lesions is in some way weak or unstable and, as a result, susceptible to attenuation by a social experience. Quantitative comparisons indicate that the frequency and latency of killing in rats with septal lesions is comparable with that of rats with medial accumbens or medial hypothalamic lesions (Albert, Chew et al., 1981; Albert, Walsh, White, & Longley, 1984; Albert, Walsh, Ryan & Siemens, 1982a). The amount of prey eaten following the kill is also similar for each of these lesions (Albert, Walsh, White, & Longley, 1984). In terms of these measures, there is no obvious reason for the greater susceptibility of the septal-lesion induced mouse killing to inhibition by preoperative exposure to a mouse. Unfortunately, extensive data on the strength and stability of the mouse killing induced by chemical lesions of the dorsal/median raphe nuclei are not available.

Gentling

To appreciate the specificity of the suppression of lesion-induced mouse killing (or food-deprivation induced mouse killing), it is useful to examine the ease and extent to which another variable can influence mouse killing behavior. Gentling is a type of experience that reduces postoperative aggressiveness toward the experimenter (defensiveness) in rats with septal or medial accumbens lesions. However, preoperative gentling does not attenuate mouse killing induced by electrolytic lesions of the lateral septum, medial accumbens, or medial hypothalamus, or by chemical lesions of the dorsal/median raphe nuclei (Albert, Walsh, Ryan, & Siemens, 1982a; Marks et al., 1977).

POSTOPERATIVE EXPERIENCE

Although the aim of this chapter is to examine the influence of preoperative experience on lesion-induced changes in mouse killing, it is also relevant to examine the effect of experience intervening between a lesion and a mouse killing test on the frequency of mouse killing.

Cohabitation With Rats

Cohabitation with other rats has been found to attenuate the mouse killing induced by olfactory bulb lesions (Didiergeorges & Karli, 1966). In contrast, the attenuation can be reversed by a period of isolation. Rats with septal lesions made in infancy and housed in groups are reported to kill in spite of the social housing (Eclancher & Karli, 1979).

Cohabitation With Mice

We have individually housed rats with medial accumbens lesions with a mouse by placing the mouse in a protective hardware cloth enclosure within the rat's living cage (Albert, Walsh, & White, unpublished observations). Over a 48-hr period, rats with lesions more or less continually bit at the feet and tail of the mouse as it climbed about its wire enclosure and then readily killed it when the protective hardware cloth was removed.

Spontaneous Decay

Mouse killing induced by septal lesions has been reported to attenuate spontaneously over a 2-week period postoperatively (Miczek & Grossman, 1972). This effect has not been found in a second study which made lesions in young rats (Eclancher & Karli, 1979).

SUPPRESSION OF MOUSE KILLING BY SOCIAL EXPERIENCE: FUNCTION AND SUBSTRATE

There must be both an experiential and a neurological basis for the suppression of lesion-induced mouse killing. And, it is reasonable to infer that the two levels of explanation will facilitate one another. Why there should be a suppression of lesion- or food deprivation-induced mouse killing as a result of social contact is not obvious. Presumably, the suppression serves some function in the life of the animal even if it outwardly seems paradoxical. Neurologically, the substrate subserving this function must be complex. It must involve neural systems mediating perception, learning, and predatory motivation.

The Psychology of the Influence of Experience

The evidence is clear that predatory behavior is dramatically suppressed by experience with a potential prey. Some of this influence can be accounted for in terms of the positive and negative consequences that follow the behavior. However, it is not particularly noteworthy that when footshock follows mouse killing, the probability of mouse killing declines. While the events within the nervous system responsible for this change in behavior are unknown, it is clear that the nervous system readily mediates this kind of behavior change in an infinite variety of situations.

The inhibition of predation simply as a result of social contact is, however, an unusual behavioral sequence. There is no aversive or appetitive stimulus operating according to the traditional conceptualizations of operant or classical conditioning. The decrease in predatory killing caused by exposing a mouse to a rat appears to be a special kind of learning peculiar to predatory motivation. In this instance, the brain appears to make a specific association between a perceptual experience and predatory motivation. The process can be looked upon as bearing some resemblance to imprinting. Imprinting also occurs as the result of a perceptual experience, and it has the obvious utility of providing an association between infant and parent which enhances the chances of survival of the young.

The unique characteristics of the learning that suppresses predation suggests that this learning has a special and important function in the life of a predatory species. The suppression might serve to decrease the probability that certain organisms would be treated as prey. The organisms most likely to benefit by this process would be the young of the predatory species itself. This is true in rats where the altricial nature of the pups render them easy targets for adult predation. It is reasonable to expect, then, this predation-inhibiting experience should occur in adulthood when pup killing is most likely. Furthermore, unlike classical imprinting, there would be no single sensitive period in which the predation-inhibiting experience would exert its effect.

In a recent series of experiments examining pup killing by mice, vom Saal (1984) has found that in male mice, copulation produces a short-term inhibition of pup killing lasting about 4 weeks. Assuming a comparable mechanism exists in the rat, it could inhibit killing while the pups are very small, but there would still need to be a mechanism for inhibiting killing in the several weeks following weaning when the pups are still vulnerable to predation. An inhibition resulting from social contact would be the kind of mechanism that could perpetuate the inhibition of pup killing.

To examine the applicability of this line of reasoning to rats, we have compared the behavior toward unfamiliar pups (2–10 days old) of eight randomly chosen male rats previously housed only with other males and seven randomly chosen alpha male rats previously housed for several months with an intact female and, intermittently, her pups. When left in an unfamiliar cage with an unfamiliar female and her pups for 5 days, only one of seven alpha males killed pups whereas six of eight males inexperienced with pups did so (Albert, Walsh, & Longley, unpublished observations). This experiment demonstrates that an inhibition of pup killing exists in alpha male rats that have sired pups and cohabited with them. Further experiments are required to evaluate the role of copulation and prior experience with pups in producing the inhibition.

Stimuli which mediate the inhibition of pup killing are presumably visual and olfactory, since these stimuli both seem to play a role in predation. Since the smell of a female is imparted to her pups, this may be a stimulus which serves to decrease the probability that the pups will be preyed upon by familiar adult conspecifics. An important point to note in this context is that for rats, the inhibition of killing as a result of social familiarity has only been demonstrated with mice, an organism morphologically similar to rat pups (however, see also Kuo, 1930, for the analogous effect between cats and rats). The substantive nature of this morphological similarity is illustrated by the tendency of some lactating females to retrieve mice just as they do rat pups (Albert, Walsh, Zalys, & Dyson, 1987).

Neurological Basis of the Suppression

Mouse killing induced by lesions of the septum, medial accumbens, medial hypothalamus, dorsal/median raphe, and chemical injections depleting serotonin levels appears to correspond closely to that of food-deprived rats. We have argued that this killing represents a release of predatory motivation by these lesions.

From this perspective, it is not surprising that preoperative exposure to a mouse inhibits killing induced by septal lesions in the same way it inhibits killing induced by food deprivation. Septal lesions appear to potentiate predatory behavior as does hunger. As well, the inhibition of predation by social contact represents a normal influence of social experience on predatory motivation. Attempting to describe how the suppression is mediated neurologically is bound to be frustrating because this is tantamount to trying to identify the structures involved in learning, and in addition, inferring the way in they interact with neural tissue modulating predation.

Vergnes and Karli (Vergnes, 1976; Karli, Vergnes, Eclancher, & Penot, 1977) and Adams (1979) have proposed mechanisms which might account for the influence of social contact on predatory behavior. Neither appears to encompass the full complexity of the process and, accordingly, the neurological explanations they suggest are incomplete. Vergnes and Karli have suggested that the amygdala is the structure which interfaces past social experience with predatory motivation. They argue that amygdala lesions do not induce aggressive behavior directly. Rather, lesions in the amygdala prevent prior social contact with a mouse from attenuating mouse killing induced by food deprivation. This effect appears to be mediated by the stria terminalis, since lesions of this structure produce the same effect as medial amygdala lesions (Vergnes, 1976).

In support of this line of reasoning, Vergnes (1976) has gone on to demonstrate that medial amygdala lesions can have the same effect in the case of mouse killing induced by septal lesions. In a group of rats with combined septal and amygdala lesions, 76% killed mice even though they had been exposed to mice preoperatively. Without the amygdala lesions, the septal lesions induced mouse killing in only 8% of rats previously exposed to a mouse for a 24-hr period. Once again it is argued that the medial amygdala exerts this effect by way of the stria terminalis, since lesions in the bed nucleus of the stria terminalis facilitate mouse killing while lesions in the ventral amygdalofugal pathway to the hypothalamus cause a temporary inhibition of mouse killing.

This argument has one interesting piece of evidence to support it. What this hypothesis does not explain is why the amygdala does not serve this same function for mouse killing induced by medial accumbens or medial hypothalamic lesions.

The hypothesis of Adams (1979) is that the medial hypothalamus is a structure which mediates the influence of past experience on aggressive behavior. Specifically, it is suggested that the medial hypothalamus serves to inhibit attack on familiar individuals. This hypothesis is consistent with the evidence, insofar as rats with medial hypothalamic lesions that have previous experience with mice should kill them since the medial hypothalamus which would normally inhibit aggression toward a familiar individual is no longer present. However, the hypothesis does not explain why a similar effect should be obtained with medial accumbens lesions or raphe lesions.

CONCLUSION

The suppression of lesion-induced mouse killing by preoperative social contact seems to be an anomaly arising from a normal process in which predation on infant conspecifics by adult predators is inhibited. There is nothing to prevent the same inhibitory process from occurring toward mice. In fact, it may well be that the morphological similarity between mice and rat pups contributes to the strength of the suppression following preoperative contact. As has been noted, the early work of Kuo (1930) first brought this phenomenon to the attention of psychologists. However, there may well be a large array of anecdotal experience from individuals who have kept different species together that would confirm that this is a common phenomenon.

The inhibition of predation as a consequence of social contact must be complex. In addition to neural systems controlling learning and motivation, it must involve activation of neural circuitry that brings the motivational and experiential representations together. There is nothing in either the experience or the motivation that inherently demands that these two processes should interact with one another.

Differences in the extent to which lesions disrupt the normal experiential inhibition of predation should reveal something about where the neural systems mediating the motivational and experiential influences on predation interact. The suggestion of Adams (1979) that the medial hypothalamus may be a site for this interaction was a reasonable inference. The suggestion that the medial amygdala is a part of the neural circuitry mediating the interaction can be integrated into this framework. The amygdala has neural connections through the stria terminalis by which it might interact with the medial hypothalamus in particular (Gloor, 1960). It seems reasonable to suppose that the medial accumbens and dorsal/median raphe nuclei may also be functionally associated with the medial hypothalamus in producing the inhibition of mouse killing as a result of social contact.

While a process mediating the inhibition of killing appears crucial to predatory species, there is no evidence that this is an important element in human behavior. Humans do kill to obtain food, but this behavior may well be mediated by operant conditioning rather than a distinct motivational system. The association of various aggressive behaviors in animals with different aggressive motives is made by considering the circumstances in which they occur and by the occurrence of species typical forms of behavior, such as the bite to the back of the neck. In the case of mouse killing, it is the existence of a pattern of attack different from that associated with other forms of aggression and the fact that the successful attack is followed by eating that leads to the identification of mouse killing as predatory behavior.

To associate aggressive behaviors seen in nonhuman mammals with human behavior, it has not been possible to depend on cross-species similarities in behavior or on the observation of a rigid species typical pattern of behavior in humans. Parallels between human and animal aggression have been most successfully drawn using evidence for parallel biological substrates modulating aggression (Albert & Walsh, 1984). For example, similar limbic structures appear to modulate defensive aggression in both nonhuman and human mammals. The evidence for this in humans comes from observed increases in defensive behavior following naturally occurring brain damage. For predation, the neural substrate in nonhuman mammals is becoming increasingly well understood. However, there is no evidence from humans sustaining damage to the homologous neural substrate to indicate that an increase or decrease in predation occurs comparable with what has been observed in nonhuman mammals.

ACKNOWLEDGMENT

Supported by a grant from the Natural Sciences and Engineering Research Council of Canada. The authors are indebted to Dr. R. Wong for comments and helpful discussions.

REFERENCES

Adams, D. B. (1979). Brain mechanisms for offense, defense, and submission. *Brain and Behavioral Sciences, 2,* 201–241.

Albert, D. J. (1979). Induction of mouse killing in nonkiller rats by temporary chemical lesions in the medial hypothalamus. *Physiological Psychology, 7,* 64–66.

Albert, D. J., & Brayley, K. N. (1979). Mouse killing and hyperreactivity following lesions of the medial hypothalamus, the lateral septum, the bed nucleus of the stria terminalis, or the region ventral to the anterior septum. *Physiology and Behavior, 23,* 439–443.

Albert, D. J., Chew, G. L., Dewey, K. J., Walsh, M. L., Lee, C. S. Y., & Ryan, J. (1981). Mouse and weanling rat killing by spontaneous mouse killing rats, and by rats with lesions of the lateral septum or the region ventral to the anterior septum: Similarities in killing latency and prey eating. *Physiology and Behavior, 27,* 791–795.

Albert, D. J., Chew, G. L., Walsh, M. L., Ryan, J., & Lee, C. S. Y. (1982). Lesions of the region ventral to the anterior septum increase mouse killing and reactivity but not social attack. *Behavioral and Neural Biology, 34,* 283–295.

Albert, D. J., Dyson, E. M., Walsh, M. L., & Gorzalka, B. B. (1987). Intermale social aggression in rats: Suppression by medial hypothalamic lesions independently of enhanced defensiveness or decreased testicular testosterone. *Physiology and Behavior, 39,* 693–698.

Albert, D. J., Nanji, N., & Chew, G. L. (1981). Structures posterior to the olfactory bulb which are responsible for the mouse killing and hyperreactivity following lesions of the olfactory bulb. *Physiology and Behavior, 26,* 395–399.

Albert, D. J., & Walsh, M. L. (1982a). Medial hypothalamic lesions in the rat enhance reactivity and mouse killing but not social aggression. *Physiology and Behavior, 28,* 791–795.

Albert, D. J., & Walsh, M. L. (1982b). The inhibitory modulation of agonistic behavior in the rat brain: A review. *Neuroscience and Biobehavioral Reviews, 6,* 125–143.

Albert, D. J., & Walsh, M. L. (1984). Neural systems and the inhibitory modulation of agonistic behavior: A comparison of mammalian species. *Neuroscience and Biobehavioral Reviews, 8,* 5–24.

Albert, D. J., Walsh, M. L., & Longley, W. (1985). Medial hypothalamic and medial accumbens lesions which induce mouse killing enhance biting and attacks on inanimate objects. *Physiology and Behavior, 35,* 523–527.

Albert, D. J., Walsh, M. L., Ryan, J., & Siemens, Y. (1982a). A comparison of the effect of preoperative gentling on the mouse killing and reactivity induced by lesion of the lateral septum, the medial accumbens nucleus, and the medial hypothalamus. *Physiology and Behavior, 28,* 1117–1120.

Albert, D. J., Walsh, M. L., Ryan, J., & Siemens, Y. (1982b). Mouse killing in rats: A comparison of spontaneous killers and rats with lesions of the medial hypothalamus or the medial accumbens nucleus. *Physiology and Behavior, 29,* 989–994.

Albert, D. J., Walsh, M. L., Ryan, J., Siemens, Y., & White, R. (1983). Mouse killing in rats induced by lesions of the medial hypothalamus or medial accumbens: Short-term preoperative exposure to a mouse does not suppress the killing. *Behavioral and Neural Biology, 38,* 113–119.

Albert, D. J., Walsh, M. L., Siemens, Y., & Louie, H. (1986). Spontaneous mouse killing rats: Gentling and food deprivation result in killing behavior almost identical to that of rats with medial hypothalamic lesions. *Physiology and Behavior, 36,* 1197–1199.

Albert, D. J., Walsh, M. L., & White, R. (1984). Rearing rats with mice prevents induction of mouse killing by lesions of the septum but not lesions of the medial hypothalamus or medial accumbens. *Physiology and Behavior, 32,* 143–145.

Albert, D. J., Walsh, M. L., & White, R. (1985). Mouse killing induced by para-chlorophenylalanine injections or septal lesions but not olfactory bulb lesions is similar to that of food-deprived spontaneous killers. *Behavioral Neuroscience, 99,* 546–554.

Albert, D. J., Walsh, M. L., White, R., & Longley, W. (1984). A comparison of prey eating by spontaneous mouse killing rats and rats with lateral septal, medial accumbens, or medial hypothalamic lesions. *Physiology and Behavior, 33,* 517–523.

Albert, D. J., Walsh, M. L., Zalys, C., & Dyson, E. M. (1987). Maternal aggression and intermale social aggression: A behavioral comparison. *Behavioural Processes, 14,* 267–276.

Albert, D. J., & Wong, R. C. K. (1978a). Hyperreactivity, muricide, and intraspecific aggression in the rat produced by infusion of local anesthetic into the lateral septum or surrounding areas. *Journal of Comparative & Physiological Psychology, 92,* 1062–1073.

Albert, D. J., & Wong, R. C. K. (1978b). Interanimal aggression and hyperreactivity following hypothalamic infusion of local anesthetic in the rat. *Physiology and Behavior, 20,* 755–761.

Applegate, C. D. (1980). 5,7-Dihydroxytryptamine-induced mouse killing and behavioral reversal with ventricular administration of serotonin in rats. *Behavioral and Neural Biology, 30,* 178–190.

Baenninger, R. (1978). Some aspects of predatory behavior. *Aggressive Behavior, 4,* 287–311.

Denenberg, V. H., Paschke, R. E., & Zarrow, M. X. (1968). Killing of mice by rats prevented by early interaction between the two species. *Psychonomic Science, 11,* 39–41.

DiChiara, G., Camba, R., & Spano, P. F. (1971). Evidence for inhibition by brain serotonin of mouse killing behaviour in rats. *Nature, 233,* 272–273.

Didiergeorges, F., & Karli, P. (1966). Stimulations "sociales" et inhibition de l'agressivité interspecifique chez le rat privé de ses afferences olfactives. *Comptes Rendus de Séances pour le Société de Biologie, 160,* 2445–2447.

Eclancher, F., & Karli, P. (1979). Septal damage in infant and adult rats: Effects on activity, emotionality, and muricide. *Aggressive Behavior, 5,* 389–415.

Gloor, P. (1960). Amygdala. In Field, J., Magoun, H. W., & Hall, V. E. (Eds.), *Handbook of physiology: Sect. 1. Neurophysiology: Vol. 2.* (pp. 1395–1420). Washington, DC: American Physiological Society.

Grant, L. D., Coscina, D. V., Grossman, S. P., & Freedman, D. X. (1973). Muricide after serotonin depleting lesions of midbrain raphe nuclei. *Pharmacology Biochemistry and Behavior, 1,* 77–80.

Karli, P. (1956). The Norway rat's killing response to the white mouse: An experimental analysis. *Behaviour, 10,* 81–103.

Karli, P. (1960). Effets de lesions experimentales du septum sur l'agressivité intespecifique ratsouris. *Comptes Rendus de Séances pour le Société de Biologie, 154,* 1079–1082.

Karli, P., Vergnes, M., & Didiergeorges, F. (1969). Rat–mouse interspecific aggressive behavior and its manipulation by brain ablation and by brain stimulation. In S. Garrattini & E. B. Sigg (Eds.), *Aggressive behavior.* New York: Wiley, pp. 47–55.

Karli, P., Vergnes, M., Eclancher, F., & Penot, C. (1977). Involvement of amygdala in inhibitory control over aggression in the rat: A synopsis. *Aggressive Behavior, 3,* 157–162.

Kuo, Z. Y. (1930). The genesis of the cat's response toward the rat. *Journal of Comparative Psychology, 11,* 1–35.

Marks, P. C., O'Brien, M., & Paxinos, G. (1977). 5-7-DHT-induced muricide: Inhibition as a result of preoperative exposure of rats to mice. *Brain Research, 135,* 383–388.

Miczek, K. A., Altman, J. L., Appel, J. B., & Boggan, W. O. (1975). Para-chlorophenylalanine, serotonin and killing behavior. *Pharmacology, Biochemistry, and Behavior, 3,* 355–361.

Miczek, K. A., & Grossman, S. P. (1972). Effects of septal lesions on inter- and intraspecies aggression in rats. *Journal of Comparative & Physiological Psychology, 79,* 37–45.

Myer, J. S. (1969). Early experience and the development of mouse killing by rats. *Journal of Comparative & Physiological Psychology, 67,* 46–49.

Olivier, B. (1977). The ventromedial hypothalamus and aggressive behavior in rats. *Aggressive Behavior, 3,* 47–56.

Olivier, B., Olivier–Aardema, R., & Weipkema, P. R. (1983). Effects of anterior hypothalamic and mammillary area lesions on territorial aggression in the male rat. *Behavioural Brain Research, 9,* 59–81.

Panksepp, J. (1971). Effects of hypothalamic lesions on mouse killing and shock-induced fighting in rats. *Physiology and Behavior, 6,* 311–316.

Paul, L. (1972). Predatory attack by rats: Its relationship to feeding and type of prey. *Journal of Comparative & Physiological Psychology, 78,* 69–76.

Paxinos, G., Burt, J., Atrens, D. M., & Jackson, D. M. (1977). 5-Hydroxytryptamine depletion with para-chlorophenylalanine: Effects on eating, drinking, irritability, muricide, and copulation. *Pharmacology, Biochemistry, and Behavior, 6,* 439–447.

Penot, C., & Vergnes, M. (1976). Declenchement de reactions d'agression interspecifique par lesion septale après lesion prealable de l'amygdale, chez le rat. *Physiology and Behavior, 17,* 445–450.

Van Hemel, P. E. (1972). Aggression as a reinforcer: Operant behavior in the mouse killing rat. *Journal of the Experimental Analysis of Behavior, 17,* 237–245.

Vergnes, M. (1975). Declenchement de reactions d'agression interspecifique aprés lesions amygdalienne chez le rat. *Physiology and Behavior, 14,* 271–276.

Vergnes, M. (1976). Control amygdalien de comportements d'agression chez le rat. *Physiology and Behavior, 17,* 439–444.

Vergnes, M., Mack, G., & Kempf, E. (1973). Lesions du raphe et reaction d'agression interspecifique rat-souris. Effets comportementaux et biochemiques. *Brain Research, 57,* 67–74.

Vergnes, M., Mack, G., & Kempf, E. (1974). Controle inhibiteur du comportement d'agression interspecifique du rat: System serotoninergique du raphe et afferences olfactives. *Brain Research, 70,* 481–491.

Vergnes, M., Penot, C., Kempf, E., & Mack, G. (1977). Lesions selective des neurones serotoninergiques du raphe par la 5,7-dihydroxytryptamine: Effets sur le comportement d'agression interspecifique du rat. *Brain Research, 133,* 167–171.

vom Saal, F. S. (1984). Proximate and ultimate causes of infanticide and parental behavior in male house mice. In G. Hausfater & S. B. Hrdy (Eds.), *Infanticide: Comparative and evolutionary perspectives.* New York: Aldine, pp. 401–426.

8

The Effects of Preoperative Experience Upon Postoperative Performance of Rats Following Lesions of the Hippocampal System

David S. Olton
Department of Psychology
Johns Hopkins University

Alicja L. Markowska
Department of Neurophysiology
Nencki Institute of Experimental Biology
Warsaw, Poland

INTRODUCTION

The hippocampus plays an important role in some types of memory processes. As might be expected, lesions of the hippocampal system (the hippocampus proper, its subfields, and its afferent and efferent connections) can produce substantial impairments in the performance of tasks that require these types of memory (reviews in Gray & McNaughton, 1983; O'Keefe & Nadel, 1978; Olton, Becker, & Handelmann, 1978). The magnitude of this impairment is influenced by many variables: the location and size of the lesion (Jarrard, 1980; Kesner, Crutcher, & Measom, 1986; Raffaele & Olton, 1988), the amount of information to be remembered and the length of time during which it is to be remembered (see review in Squire & Zola–Morgan, 1983), the specific task requirements (Markowska & Lukaszewska, 1981, 1982), and the amount of interference (Jarrard, 1975; Winocur, 1979) to name a few.

Another variable that may affect the performance of animals following lesions of the hippocampal system is the amount and type of preoperative training. To our knowledge, there has not yet been a systematic investigation of the many different ways in which preoperative training may affect postoperative performance. Nonetheless, a few experiments have compared the effects of different types of preoperative experience on the postoperative performance of rats with lesions of the hippocampal system; their results indicate that preoperative experience can affect postoperative performance. However, most of these studies were designed to test other ideas (specific theories of hippocampal function, the neurochemical and electrophysiological changes accompanying behavioral recovery, etc.). Thus, many experimental parameters differ among these experiments, making a systematic comparison very difficult, and producing a complicated pattern of results.

In order to review this literature, we have divided this chapter into four sections: (1) Some general principles that should guide any investigation of the effects of preoperative experience on postoperative performance are outlined in order to provide an organizational framework for the material that follows. (2) The results of four experiments are presented in detail to illustrate some of the effects and provide information that is necessary for the ensuing discussion. (3) Some variables that affect the direction and magnitude of preoperative experience on postoperative performance are discussed with illustrations from the available literature. (4) Some conclusions are suggested, along with directions for future research. Overall, we think that many important issues remain unresolved, and that careful systematic investigations will be necessary to identify and quantify the parameters responsible for the influence of preoperative experience on postoperative performance.[1]

THE POSSIBLE EFFECTS
OF PREOPERATIVE EXPERIENCE

The first question has to do with the type of transfer expected in a normal animal without any lesions. Obviously, information from one task can have a whole spectrum of effects on performance in another. *Positive transfer* is indicated by superior performance in the second task as a result of experience in the first one (compared with an animal that learned just the second task). Perfect positive transfer is reflected by immediate perfect performance on the second task. *Negative transfer* is indicated by inferior performance in the second task, showing that information obtained from the first task interfered with the acquisition of the subsequent task. At the extreme, the initial experience can completely block the acquisition of the second task (Maier, 1949). In between these extremes, of course, ranges a whole spectrum of possible outcomes.

---

[1]We have chosen not to present examples of the lesions used in these studies. Precise information about the characteristics of the lesions is unquestionably necessary for final resolution of the issues discussed in this chapter. However, many different kinds of lesions have been used, and the results reported may differ for each one. Thus, we have chosen the alternative of not presenting any lesions, rather than presenting them all, which would have markedly increased the length of this chapter. Clearly, a systematic study, within the same experimental design, is necessary to manipulate both the type of the lesion and the type of training before the interactions between lesions and transfer can be thoroughly described.

The type of information responsible for the transfer effects can vary widely. In some cases, it can be very specific, as in a discrimination reversal. In a very simple case, the rat is given a discrimination between two different stimuli, A and B. After learning this discrimination, the response/reinforcement contingencies are reversed so that now the opposite stimulus is correct.

Alternatively, the transfer effects may be due to very general types of information. Positive transfer is involved in the development of a learning set, where the rule is learned independently of any particular application of it. Negative transfer is found in examples of "functional fixedness" (Luchins, 1942) and in the experiments of Maier (1949), dealing with frustration. In both these instances, general information about stimulus/response/reinforcement contingencies in one situation influenced behavior in another situation.

At the most general, animals may learn many different types of behaviors that influence performance of a specific task. For example, when initially placed on a maze, rats are cautious and unwilling to venture freely around the maze. After experience, however, rats run rapidly on the maze without difficulty. When transferred to a new maze, the rat may show some tendency to explore the new environment, but does so rapidly, moving about the new maze quickly and efficiently. A similar result may occur in an operant bar press task. Once the animal learns that an experimental situation has a series of responses and reinforcements, and that reinforcement can be obtained from responses, the animal proceeds to emit many different responses, presumably in an attempt to determine the one that is correct.

Consequently, in order to analyze appropriately the effects of preoperative experience on postoperative performance of animals with hippocampal lesions, the tasks must be analyzed to determine whether positive or negative transfer is expected from a normal rat, and to identify the type of information that can produce the transfer. This latter point is particularly important because most descriptions of hippocampal function emphasize that it is not equally involved in all types of memory processes. For some types of information, rats with hippocampal lesions should show normal transfer, while for other types of information, these rats should show abnormal transfer (either improved or impaired).

There are two reasons why positive transfer from preoperative experience to postoperative performance might not take place. The first arises from a consideration of state dependent effects produced by drugs (Overton, 1985). When an animal is trained normally and then tested while drugged in the same task, the animal may perform poorly because of a failure to generalize from the nondrugged state to the drugged state. While a physical lesion is not identical to a drug, nonetheless, both are changes in the state of the central nervous system. If the change from a normal state to a lesioned state has properties similar to the change from a normal state to a drugged state, then a lesion might prevent transfer of preoperative experience to postoperative testing for the same reasons that a change from a normal state to a drugged state prevents transfer.

A second reason to expect no transfer of preoperative training has to do with the functional organization of the brain. A lesion analysis is complicated by the fact that parts of the brain not directly affected by the lesion may not function in the same way that they did prior to the lesion (Gregory, 1961; Webster, 1973; Weiskrantz, 1974). If such is the case, then transfer of preoperative training should be minimal because the lesioned brain processes information differently than the normal brain.

The fact that preoperative training can produce positive transfer to postoperative performance suggests that neither of these two views is entirely correct. To our knowledge, neither of them has been subjected to parametric tests to determine the extent to which either of these possible effects actually occur. However, the available data indicate that if these effects do occur as a result of lesions, they are not sufficient to block the transfer of preoperative experience to postoperative testing.

FOUR EXAMPLES OF
PREOPERATIVE EFFECTS

Radial Arm Maze: Working and Reference Memory

Preoperative training reduced the impairment that otherwise occurred during the postoperative acquisition of two types of spatial discriminations in a radial arm maze (Gage, 1985). Hippocampal lesions were made by electrolytic current. Destruction was maximal in the anterodorsal hippocampus. The largest lesions destroyed the entire dorsal hippocampus and adjacent fimbria. The smallest lesions damaged the dorsal hippocampus but left the fimbria intact. All lesions spared the posterior and ventral parts of the hippocampus, and produced minimal damage to the posterior portions to the septum and the fornix between septum and hippocampus.

The maze had 8 arms extending away from a central platform. No specific cues were placed on the arms, so the task emphasized spatial locations as the discriminative stimuli. A guillotine door was placed at the entrance to each arm. Each of three *baited arms* had food placed at the end of each of them. The other five *unbaited arms* did not have food on them.

At the beginning of each session, the rat was placed on the maze. All the guillotine doors around the central platform were raised, and the rat was allowed to choose an arm. When the rat returned to the central platform, the guillotine doors were lowered for 7 seconds. This confinement procedure prevented response strategies which can complicate the analysis of behavior in spatial mazes (Feeser & Raskin, 1987; Olton & Papas, 1979). One session was given each day.

For Task 1, one set of three arms was baited. For Task 2, a different set of three arms was baited; three of the previously unbaited arms were baited, and the three previously baited arms were unbaited. Thus, Task 1 assessed the acquisition of performance on the baited and unbaited arms, while Task 2 assessed a change in that discrimination that included a discrimination reversal for six arms (three baited changed to unbaited, and three unbaited changed to baited). A *working memory error* was a response to a baited arm that no longer had food (i.e., any response other than the first one to a baited arm). A *reference memory error* was any response to an unbaited arm.

In Task 1, lesioned rats with no preoperative training had a severe impairment in all three behavioral measures (trials to criterion, reference memory errors, working memory errors). Lesioned rats that did receive preoperative training had normal scores for the number of trials to criterion; although the number of reference memory errors and working memory errors was increased, the differences were not statistically significant (Table 8.1).

A similar pattern of results was seen in Task 2. Lesioned rats without preoperative training had a substantial impairment in all three behavioral measures (although the difference in working memory errors was not statistically significant). Lesioned rats given preoperative training on Task 1, however, had normal scores for the number of trials to criterion, and although the number of reference memory errors and working memory errors was greater than that of controls, the differences were not statistically significant.

Unfortunately, the statistical analysis of postoperative behavior considered only the difference between control rats and lesioned rats within each training condition (controls vs. lesioned rats with preoperative training, controls vs.

TABLE 8.1
Summary of Data From Gage (1985)

Behavioral Measure	Group	Task 1		Task 2	
		No Preoperative Training	Preoperative Training on Task 1	No Preoperative Training	Preoperative Training on Task 1
Trials to criterion	Control	12.8	11.1	10.8	15.2
	Lesion[a]	57.7[b]	12.3	29.3	16.9
Reference memory errors	Control	2.9	1.3	2.8	2.8
	Lesion	5.0	3.3	4.3	3.7
Working memory errors	Control	.2	.2	.1	.02
	Lesion	.9	.5	.3	.1

[a]The lesion, made by electrolytic current, produced extensive damage to the dorsal hippocampus.

[b]Three rats failed to reach criterion.

lesioned rats without preoperative training). Consequently, no statistics are available to determine whether or not the difference between control rats and lesioned rats in the two training conditions was significant. This statistical test requires a two-way analysis with group (control, lesioned) and type of training (preoperative training on Task 1, no preoperative training). However, some of the differences in performance were substantial. With no preoperative training, the scores of the lesioned rats were five times (Task 1) and three times (Task 2) greater than the scores of control rats for the number of trials to reach criterion, while with preoperative training, these scores were virtually identical to those of controls. With the appropriate analysis, these differences should be statistically significant. For reference memory errors and working memory errors, however, the expected result of this analysis is not clear. The ratio of errors for the two groups (scores of lesioned rats divided by the scores of control rats) was similar in all cases.

These data show that preoperative training can reduce the magnitude of the impairment that would otherwise occur in rats with lesions of the dorsal hippocampus. The positive transfer was not specific to the task that was learned preoperatively. Preoperative training reduced the deficit not only for Task 1, but also for Task 2, a reversal that occurred only postoperatively. Thus, positive transfer was seen in a task that was not trained preoperatively.

The magnitude of this effect needs to be verified, especially given the small differences in the number of working memory errors and reference memory errors, and the small size of the hippocampal lesions. The complete elimination of an impairment in a task that requires spatial working memory as a result of preoperative training would be surprising, given the reliability of this type of impairment following hippocampal lesions. Thus, the positive transfer seen in this experiment might not have occurred with more complete lesions, and probably did not restore normal behavior even with the incomplete lesions used here. Nonetheless, the results do demonstrate that preoperative training can have some effect on postoperative performance in the task that was trained preoperatively and in a new task that was given only postoperatively.

Radial Arm Maze: Cued, Noncued
Spatial Discriminations

Preoperative training in a noncued spatial discrimination had no effect on postoperative performance of this same discrimination, and impaired postoperative performance of a cued spatial discrimination (Winocur, 1982). The hippocampal lesions, made with electrolytic current, produced slight destruction of the most anterodorsal portions of hippocampus, and left the adjacent fimbria and the anterior fornix intact.

The maze was a radial arm maze with eight arms extending from a central choice point. It did not have guillotine doors around the center to confine the rats between choices and interrupt response tendencies. The maze was surrounded by a plywood wall, 2.2 m high and 25 cm beyond the closest arm. In the *cued task,* a metal plate painted with a different visual pattern was placed on top of each arm. The position of these plates on the arms remained the same throughout each test session, and was changed only at the end of the session. Consequently, both the cues and the spatial locations of the arms were relevant discriminative stimuli. In the *noncued task,* the plates were removed so they could not function as discriminative stimuli.

Each rat was given one test session each day. Rats given preoperative training were trained to a criterion of no more than one error in the first eight choices for 5 consecutive days. Postoperatively, each rat was tested for 10 days.

Preoperative Training and Postoperative Testing in the Same Task. In the noncued task, lesioned rats without preoperative training had more errors in the entire test session and fewer correct responses in the first eight choices (although the latter difference failed to reach statistical significance). Lesioned rats with preoperative training in the same task had an identical pattern of results. Thus, there was little if any transfer from preoperative training to postoperative testing (Table 8.2).

This interpretation is complicated by the fact that control rats did not show positive transfer of preoperative training; the performance of control rats with and without preoperative training was essentially the same during subsequent

TABLE 8.2
Summary of Data From Winocur (1982): Preoperative Training
and Postoperative Testing in the Same Task

Group	Mean Number of Correct Responses in First 8 Choices		Mean Errors in Test Session	
	No Preoperative Training	Preoperative Training	No Preoperative Training	Preoperative Training
	Noncued			
	(Exp. 1)	(Exp. 2)	(Exp. 1)	(Exp. 2)
Controls	7.0	7.2	1.9	2.1
Lesion[a]	5.8	6.0	8.2	6.8
	Cued			
Controls	7.0	7.0	2.1	2.2
Lesion[a]	6.8	6.8	3.4	3.1

[a]The lesion, made with electolytic current, produced slight damage to the dorsal hippocampus.

testing. Thus, the task might not have been optimal to detect positive transfer. Nonetheless, the postoperative performance of lesioned rats given preoperative training was the same as that of lesioned rats not given this training, showing that preoperative training was not sufficient to alleviate the impairment seen in postoperative acquisition.

Preoperative Training and Postoperative Testing in Different Tasks. Lesions produced negative transfer when rats were trained preoperatively in the noncued task and tested postoperatively in the cued task. This conclusion results from a series of comparisons (Table 8.3). First, control rats performed the same in the cued task with and without prior training in the noncued task. Second, lesioned rats performed the same in the noncued task with and without prior training in this same task. Third, lesioned rats were impaired in the performance of the cued task if they had been trained preoperatively in the noncued task (but not, as previously mentioned, if they had been trained in the cued task).

Winocur (1982, pp. 167–168) sees this negative transfer as resulting from a deficit in stimulus processing. The pattern of results suggests that lesioned rats have two impairments. The lack of positive transfer in the noncued–noncued experiment indicates a permanent impairment in the ability to process spatial information. The presence of negative transfer in the noncued–cued experiment indicates an impairment in changing strategies (from memory for spatial loca-

TABLE 8.3
Summary of Data From Winocur (1982): Preoperative Training
and Postoperative Testing in Same and Different Tasks

	Mean Number of Correct Responses in the First 8 Choices		Mean Number of Errors in the Test Session	
	Preoperative Training		Preoperative Training	
	Cued	Noncued	Cued	Noncued
Cued Postoperatively				
Controls	7.0	7.2	2.2	1.5
Lesion[a]	6.8	5.9	3.3	8.5
Noncued Postoperatively				
Controls	7.3	7.2	1.4	2.1
Lesion[a]	5.9	6.0	6.2	8.2

[a]The lesion, made with electrolytic current, produced slight damage to the dorsal hippocampus.

tions to memory for cued locations). Together, these ideas suggest that preoperative training produced postoperative transfer of the spatial strategy used
preoperatively, but not the ability to use specific types of spatial information.

Place Learning in a Morris Water Maze

Extensive preoperative training in a spatial discrimination in a Morris water maze
produced transient savings in rats given retrohippocampal lesions. The lesions
were made with radio frequency current through a series of electrodes placed
posterior to the hippocampus; they destroyed much of the entorhinal cortex while
sparing the presubiculum and parasubiculum, and most of the subiculum itself.

The circular pool was 1.3 m in diameter filled with water that was made
opaque by the addition of some milk. A platform, 8.3 cm in diameter, was
placed so that its top was 1 cm below the water. For each *training trial*, the rat
was placed into the water facing the wall of the tank at one of four different
starting locations located 90 degrees apart around the edge of the tank. The rat
swam until it found the hidden platform and escaped from the water by standing
on it. Each rat was given a total of 28 training trials during 5 successive days.
The last training trial was followed by a *transfer test* in which the platform was
removed from the pool and the rat was allowed to swim for 60 sec. Two measures
were taken of the tendency to go to the area in which the platform had been
located: the amount of time spent in each of the four quadrants of the pool
(training quadrant, opposite quadrant, adjacent left, adjacent right), and the
number of *annulus crossings*, where an annulus was defined as the diameter of the
platform located in the center of each quadrant.

Control rats showed a rapid decrease in latency to find the platform during
the first six trials, after which they remained near asymptotic performance. In
the transfer test, the control rats spent more time in the training quadrant and
crossed the annulus in that quadrant more often.

In contrast, rats with lesions showed an impairment throughout testing. At
the start of testing, the mean latency to find the platform was 100 sec (compared
with 38 sec for controls). At the end of testing, the mean latency was 11 sec
(compared with 4 sec for controls). In the transfer test, lesioned rats did not
spend more time in the training quadrant and did not cross the annulus in the
training quadrant more often than expected by chance.

Lesioned rats given preoperative training and then tested postoperatively
showed considerable savings, although not normal performance. During the
initial postoperative trials, the mean latency to find the platform was 57 sec
(compared with 38 sec for controls), and much less than the scores of lesioned
rats not given preoperative training (100 sec). During the final trials, the groups
given preoperative training performed the same as the groups without pre-

operative training, with mean latencies of 8 sec and 3 sec for the lesioned control rats, respectively (see footnote 1). Statistical tests indicated a three-way interaction among groups (control, lesion), training condition (preoperative training, no preoperative training), and trials (1–28). These data support the conclusion that the preoperative training produced significant savings at the beginning of postoperative testing, but not at the end.

The results from the transfer test were complicated because the two measures of performance gave different patterns of results. Lesioned rats given pre-operative training spent no more time in the training quadrant than expected by chance, a result similar to that of rats without preoperative training. In contrast, these rats did show a greater number of annulus crossings in the training quadrant, a result similar to that of controls and different from rats without pre-operative training.

These data demonstrate positive transfer from preoperative training to post-operative testing. However, the type of preoperative information affecting the performance of the rats during postoperative testing is difficult to identify. As pointed out by Schenk and Morris (1985, p. 20), escape latency is a poor measure of the capacity to localize the platform. Consequently, the significant savings in escape latency may have been due to the learning of general informa-tion about the appropriate strategy to use to find the platform, irrespective of its spatial location (swim a certain distance away from the wall of the pool and stop when a submerged object is met). The data from the transfer test are most appropriate to measure the ability of the rats to identify the location of the platform. Unfortunately, the two different measures (time in the training quad-rant, number of annulus crossings) gave different results. Thus, although the latency measure clearly indicates that preoperative training had some effect on postoperative performance, the data from the transfer test do not provide strong evidence that specific information about the location of the platform was re-tained postoperatively. Subsequent experiments suggested that in spite of pre-operative training and substantial postoperative testing, rats with entorhinal lesions never had a normal ability to locate the platform, data that support the predictions of the cognitive mapping theory of hippocampal function (O'Keefe & Nadel, 1978). Although preoperative training in spatial tasks may change postoperative behavior (Winocur, 1982), postoperative performance is certainly not normal (Schenk & Morris, 1985).

Discrimination on a Radial Arm Maze

A complicated pattern of results indicated some influence of preoperative training on postoperative performance for rats with lesions of the CA3 region of the hippocampus with kainic acid (Handelmann & Olton, 1981b). Rats with lesions of the anterior and posterior regions, or just the anterior region alone, showed positive transfer in terms of the number of trials to reach criterion. Rats receiving lesions of just the posterior regions, however, showed negative transfer. The reasons for these different results are not clear, and there were no a priori predictions of this outcome.

The rats were trained in a spatial discrimination on a radial arm maze with eight arms. At the beginning of each trial, one pellet of food was placed at the end of each arm. A confinement procedure was used to interrupt response strategies; each time the rat returned to the center platform, guillotine doors were lowered to confine the rat to the platform for 5 sec before the next response could be made. One trial was given each day. Preoperatively, each rat was given at least 10 trials and tested until reaching a criterion of seven correct responses in the first eight choices of each trial for 5 consecutive days. Postoperatively, each rat was given at least 20 trials; testing continued until the rat reached a criterion of seven correct responses in the first eight choices of each trial for 10 consecutive trials, or until a total of 50 trials had been given.

Bilateral injections of kainic acid were made with a microsyringe. Rats in the *anterior group* received injections at two anterior coordinates on each side, rats in the *posterior group* received injections at two posterior coordinates, and rats in the *combined group* received injections at both sets of coordinates.

Control rats showed rapid acquisition and almost perfect retention. Rats in the combined group without preoperative training failed to reach criterion within the limit of 50 trials, and showed virtually no improvement in performance above the level expected by chance during that time. In contrast, all rats in the combined group given preoperative training did reach criterion, taking a mean of 34 trials to do so. Rats in the anterior group showed similar savings from preoperative training, taking 1.4 trials to reach criterion after preoperative training, compared with 16.4 trials with no preoperative training. However, the opposite pattern of effects was seen for rats in the posterior group: 17 trials to criterion for rats without preoperative training and 31 trials to criterion for rats with preoperative training (Table 8.4).

The data for the combined group and the anterior group show significant positive savings as a result of preoperative training. Because the task involved working memory and the acquisition of a new list of spatial locations during each trial, preoperative training must have facilitated not only the retention of general behavioral strategies (such as run to the ends of the arms to get food), but also the ability to learn specific new information (don't return to arm 1 during this trial). The negative transfer for rats in the posterior group complicates the conclusions from this study. Although the anterior and posterior parts of the hippocampus may have some different neuroanatomical connections, none of these leads to obvious expectations for positive transfer resulting from lesions in one location, and negative transfer resulting from lesions in another. Until confirmed by other studies, this pattern of results must remain in question.

TABLE 8.4
Summary of Data From Handelmann and Olton
(1981)

Group	Postoperative Performance: Number of Trials to Criterion	
	No Preoperative Training	Preoperative Training
Control	4.2	1.0
Anterior[a]	16.4	1.4
Posterior[a]	16.8	31.2
Combined[a]	50[b]	34.2

[a] The lesions were made with kainic acid injected into CA₃.

[b] No rat reached criterion.

DISCUSSION

The major experiments that are relevant to this discussion are summarized in two tables that present the results from experiments testing rats in the same (Table 8.5) or different (Table 8.6) tasks preoperatively and postoperatively. In each table we have indicated the citation, the type of lesion, the task, and the results. Information from experiments using just one of these designs (only postoperative acquisition, or only postoperative testing after preoperative training) will be mentioned when the data are relevant, but this chapter is not designed to review all the behavioral effects of every type of hippocampal lesion. Rather, its primary purpose is to compare postoperative performance following different types of preoperative experiences, and for this analysis, a direct comparison of results within a single experimental procedure is most informative.

Location and Completeness of the Lesion

The amount of transfer from preoperative training to postoperative testing may depend on the location and the completeness of the lesion. We use the term "completeness" rather than "size" to emphasize the fact that a complete lesion is one that destroys all of a particular neural component, irrespective of the size of that component. If this component is small, a complete lesion is small.

The evidence reviewed here suggests that preoperative training may influence postoperative choice accuracy following partial lesions of any hippocampal component (pyramidal cells in the CA1 and CA3 cell layers, granule cells in the

TABLE 8.5
Summary of Experiments That Used the Same Behavioral Tests
for Preoperative Experience and Postoperative Testing

Study	Lesion	Test	Transfer Effect
Buerger (1970)	ventral hippocampus and pyriform cortex	auditory brightness discrimination (successive go no-go)	yes-positive
Gage (1985)	dorsal hippocampus	spatial discrimination 3 out of 8 arms in radial maze	yes-positive
Handelmann & Olton (1981b)	anterior CA$_3$	spatial discrimination in radial maze	yes-positive
	posterior CA$_3$		yes-negative
	combined CA$_3$		yes-positive
Jarrard (1978)	CA$_1$	spatial discrimination in radial maze	yes-positive
	fimbria		No
	complete hippocampus		No
	dorsal fornix		No
	alveus		yes-positive
Jarrard (1986; personal communication)	complete hippocampus	spatial discrimination 4 out of 8 arms in radial maze	yes-positive
Port et al. (1986)	dorsal hippocampus	trace conditioning	No
Schenk & Morris (1985)	retrohippocampal	place learning in water maze	yes-transient positive
Winocur (1982)	small, dorsal hippocampus	spatial discrimination in radial maze	little if any
	small, dorsal hippocampus	cued discrimination in radial maze	No
Winocur & Mills (1970)	small, dorsal hippocampus	black-white discrimination in a maze	yes-positive

Note: We have summarized the transfer effects for each experiment with one result. However, in some experiments the transfer varied, depending on the behavioral measurement.

dentate gyrus, the dorsal hippocampus). The effects of complete lesions are less clear. Complete lesions of the fimbria-fornix or entorhinal cortex blocked the effects of preoperative training on postoperative performance. Complete lesions of the hippocampus proper had mixed effects; transfer occurred after some lesions but not others. The variables responsible for these different results can not yet be identified with certainty, but may include the extent of damage to fibers of passage (Jarrard, 1986). Lesions made by aspiration, which destroyed cell bodies and fibers of passage, generally blocked transfer completely, while lesions made by neurotoxins had smaller effects (Jarrard, 1986).

TABLE 8.6
Summary of Experiments That Used Different Behavioral Tests
for Preoperative Experience and Postoperative Testing

Study	Lesion	Preoperative Test	Postoperative Test	Transfer Effect
Buerger (1970)	ventral hippocampus and pyriform cortex	auditory brightness discrimination (successive go-no go)	visual pattern discrimination (successive go-no go)	no
Gage (1985)	dorsal hippocampus	spatial discrimination 3 out of 8 arms in radial maze	spatial discrimination different 3 arms out of 8 in radial maze	yes-positive
Winocur (1982)	small dorsal hippocampus	spatial discrimination in radial maze	cued discrimination in radial maze	yes-negative
	small dorsal hippocampus	cued discrimination in radial maze	spatial discrimination in radial maze	no
Winocur & Mills (1970)	small dorsal hippocampus	black-white simultaneous discrimination	visual pattern discrimination	yes-negative
Winocur & Salzen (1968)	small dorsal hippocampus	visual simultaneous two-choice discrimination	reversal of 1 discriminative stimulus	no

Input/Output Pathways.   Following destruction of the fimbria-fornix, one of the major extrinsic connections of the hippocampus, rats with and without preoperative training had a marked impairment of choice accuracy in a radial eight-arm maze. Immediately after surgery and at the end of postoperative testing, choice accuracy was at chance levels (Becker, Walker, & Olton, 1980; Olton, Becker, & Handelmann, 1979; Walker & Olton, 1979). Rats with fimbria-fornix lesions had many working memory errors for the 8 baited arms in a radial 17-arm maze, but they relearned very quickly to eliminate reference memory errors to the unbaited arms (Olton & Papas, 1979). Preoperatively trained rats with fimbria-fornix and entorhinal cortex lesions had a general impairment in working memory in both spatial and cue tasks (Jarrard, Okaichi, Steward, & Goldschmidt, 1984). Furthermore, rats with entorhinal cortex lesions were always impaired in their search for the hidden platform in the Morris water maze in spite of extensive preoperative training (Schenk & Morris, 1985). Rats with fimbria-fornix lesions and preoperative training had impaired performance and no signs of recovery of function (Olton & Feustle, 1981). Bilateral lesions of the septum, postcomissural fornix, and entorhinal cortex all caused severe impairments in spatial tasks that required working memory (Becker et al., 1980; Jarrard, 1978, 1980; Rawlins & Olton, 1982; Schenk & Morris, 1985). Bilateral lesions of fimbria-fornix also produced changes in memory for the time of reinforcement in spite of extensive preoperative training (Meck, Church, & Olton, 1984; Olton, Meck, & Church, 1987). Thus, complete lesions of hippocampal input/output pathways and closely related structures produced an impairment of postoperative performance whether or not preoperative training was given, and the rats showed no signs of recovery of function, even when tested for a long time.

CA3 Pyramidal Cells. On the other hand, preoperative experience influenced postoperative performance to some extent following incomplete lesions of the hippocampus itself or its subdivisions, but the ability to perform tasks that are sensitive to hippocampal lesions was still impaired. CA3 lesions produced an impairment in discrete trial rewarded alternation, and the magnitude of this impairment was affected by the amount of preoperative training (Fowler & Olton, 1984; Handelmann, Olton, O'Donohue, Beinfeld, Jacobowitz, & Cummins, 1983). Rats without preoperative training had an enduring impairment with no signs of recovery of function, similar to the impairment found after bilateral destruction of the extrinsic connections of the hippocampus. Rats with preoperative training also had a severe impairment of choice accuracy at the start of postoperative testing. With continued testing, however, the magnitude of the impairment decreased, and after 30 days, choice accuracy was normal.

Results from experiments not directly comparing the effects of preoperative training on postoperative performance in tasks sensitive to hippocampal lesions are also consistent with this view. Rats not given preoperative training prior to a CA3 lesion had impaired performance in the place discrimination in the Morris water maze (Sutherland, Wishaw. & Kolb, 1983). Rats given preoperative training prior to a CA3 lesion did not have impaired performance in postoperative performance in a radial maze task with baited and unbaited arms (Jarrard, 1983). Thus, rats with preoperative training had a smaller impairment following CA3 lesions than rats without this training.

Dentate Gyrus, CA1 Pyramidal Cells, and Subiculum. After dentate lesions, rats without preoperative training were impaired in the place discrimination in the water maze (Sutherland et al., 1983). However, rats given preoperative training on a spatial discrimination in a radial arm maze performed this discrimination with minimal problems after lesions of the dentate gyrus (Jarrard, Okaichi, Steward, & Goldschmidt, 1984). A similar pattern of results occurred following lesions of the CA1 pyramidal cells. Rats without preoperative training had impaired performance in a spatial discrimination on a radial arm maze, but rats with preoperative training did not (Jarrard, 1978). Rats trained pre-operatively in a radial arm maze performed poorly after subicular lesions, even after 50 trials (Jarrard, 1983).

The lesions of the hippocampal subfields were made with neurotoxins: ibotenic acid, kainic acid, or colchicine. Although these toxins can produce selective damage when used in optimal conditions, the anatomical organization of the hippocampus makes the surgery very difficult. The comparisons described all assume that the lesions were discrete and comparable in the different studies. However, careful histological analysis has indicated that these neurotoxins can injure other cell groups, and this unintended damage may be responsible for the behavioral changes (Jarrard, 1983).

Dorsal Hippocampus. Evaluation of the results following lesions of the dorsal hippocampus is difficult because variations in the size of the lesion can be crucial. Lesions that involve only the dorsal hippocampus proper, sparing the lateral fimbria, also spare the ventral and posterior hippocampus and the extrinsic connections of these hippocampal areas. These lesions may be considered incomplete lesions of the hippocampal system. Lesions that spread laterally into the fimbria may be equivalent to a complete fimbria-fornix transection. The behavioral effects of complete fimbria-fornix lesions are much more severe than those of partial hippocampal lesions, so that a slight variation in the lateral extent of the lesion can have a profound effect on behavior.

Rats without preoperative training were impaired in the performance of a spatial discrimination on a radial arm maze (Gage, 1985; Winocur, 1982), results similar to those found after partial lesions of the hippocampus or after lesions of the extrinsic connections of the hippocampus. Gage (1985) reported that preoperative training reduced the impairment of rats with dorsal hippocampal lesions when they were tested with three baited arms in a radial eight-arm maze. On the other hand, Jarrard (1983), reported different results. Even though he used a task similar to that of Gage (1985), rats given preoperative training prior to dorsal hippocampal lesions had severely impaired performance on both baited and unbaited arms during postoperative testing. These discrepant findings may be due to differences in the extent of the dorsal hippocampal lesions. In Jarrard (1983), the lesions included bilateral damage to the fimbria. In Gage (1985), only the largest lesions invaded the adjacent fimbria; the smallest lesions left the fimbria intact. Other factors may also have contributed to these discrepant results. For example, Gage (1985) used guillotine doors to confine the rats to the central platform after each choice while Jarrard (1983) did not. Confinement interrupts response tendencies and may reduce the tendency to make errors, especially on unbaited arms (compare Jarrard & Elmes, 1982; Olton & Papas, 1979). Differences in the amount of damage to neocortical tissue may also be relevant.

Preoperative training did not affect the performance of rabbits after dorsal hippocampal lesions that included fimbria, subiculum, and dorsal fornix. The rabbits were given a classically conditioned trace discrimination using closure of the nictitating membrane as the response. The onset latency of the conditioned response was altered during both acquisition and retention (Port, Romano, Steinmetz, Mikhail, & Patterson, 1986).

THE SPECIFICITY OF THE TRANSFER

Preoperative training includes many different types of experience, and relatively few experiments have tried to identify the types of preoperative information that influence postoperative performance. The following review indicates that general information about the training procedures clearly showed positive transfer, more specific information from the preoperative discrimination had less consistent effects.

Although not explicitly mentioned in most of the experiments, the general sensory-motor skills learned during preoperative training inevitably showed strong positive transfer to postoperative performance. For example, a naïve rat, when first placed on a maze, is very hesitant to move, rarely runs out arms, and cautiously explores before eating. In contrast, a rat that has had experience on a maze moves quickly around it, searches the places that might contain food, and eats food that it does find. Rats with preoperative training, when placed on the maze postoperatively, behaved like trained rats and not like naïve rats. This positive transfer was reliable and robust, and indicates that some aspects of preoperative training clearly transfer to postoperative performance.

A general cognitive strategy learned preoperatively also showed positive transfer. As reviewed earlier (Winocur, 1982, p. 156), rats trained preoperatively in a noncued spatial discrimination in a radial arm maze had impaired performance in a cued spatial discrimination postoperatively, while rats without this preoperative training (or with preoperative training in the same cued discrimination) did not. Winocur (1982) interprets this pattern of performance as follows. Preoperatively, the rats had learned to use a spatial strategy, and then had difficulty switching to a nonspatial strategy postoperatively. Because the lesioned rats had difficulty with the spatial discrimination, but not the cued discrimination, continued reliance on the spatial strategy learned in the cued procedure produced negative transfer in the noncued procedure.

More specific information may or may not show transfer, depending on the size of the lesion. In general, preoperative training had little effect on postoperative choice accuracy after complete lesions. Following complete lesions of the fimbria-fornix, rats with preoperative training still performed near the levels expected by chance in several different discriminations (Olton & Feustle, 1981). Likewise, the asymptotic performance of rats with entorhinal lesions in a place discrimination in the Morris water maze was no better following preoperative training than during postoperative acquisition (Schenk & Morris, 1985). As reviewed elsewhere, preoperative training prior to lesions of hippocampal subcomponents (pyramidal cells, granule cells, dorsal hippocampus) did often lead to positive transfer to postoperative choice accuracy.

Cats with ventral hippocampal lesions trained preoperatively in a successive go/no-go auditory-brightness discrimination task failed to show any transfer when tested postoperatively in a different go/no-go visual discrimination (Buerger, 1970).

These results suggest that in partly lesioned rats the protective effects of preoperative training are highly specific for the task learned preoperatively. However, other evidence (Gage, 1985, pp. 6–9), argues against specificity of the protective effect. As reviewed previously, rats were trained to retrieve food pellets from three baited arms in an eight-arm maze. Preoperatively trained rats were unimpaired in the retention test. Furthermore, preoperatively trained lesioned rats were unimpaired in the subsequent reversal of the discrimination with a different set of baited arms, even though they had not had specific preoperative experience in this task. In rats without preoperative training, lesions produced anterograde amnesia; the rats were severely impaired in acquisition of both spatial tasks. These results indicate a preservation of the ability to process specific spatial information.

Another explanation of this general effect might also be appropriate. Lesioned rats may show positive transfer from preoperative training only when they can use stimuli similar to those used in preoperative training. Rats with hippocampal lesions are very sensitive to interference. When preoperative training and postoperative testing are carried out with the same procedure and the same types of stimuli, the interference of previously acquired information with postoperative learning should be diminished more in situations than when new stimuli are introduced.

This idea can be tested in other experiments using different discriminations. For example, demonstration of positive transfer from a preoperatively trained delayed visual discrimination (i.e., delayed object nonmatching-to-sample) to a different postoperatively tested delayed visual discrimination (i.e., delayed color nonmatching-to-sample) would be a serious challenge to the idea that the protective effect of preoperative experience is limited to tasks with similar discriminative stimuli. Several reports concerned with the effects of hippocampal lesions on performance of spatial working/reference memory components of a preoperatively acquired task indicate that in spite of preoperative training, rats with hippocampal lesions have impaired performance even when postoperatively tested in the same task.

The transfer of preoperative training to postoperative testing is only one example of many different types of transfer. Thus, the effects of the lesions in the experimental designs using preoperative training and postoperative testing might reflect a more general function of the hippocampus in all types of transfer. Winocur has made this point in a series of experiments suggesting that hippocampal lesions may produce a failure to integrate relevant sensory information (Winocur & Salzen, 1968) and respond effectively to changes in experimental situations (Winocur & Mills, 1970).

Neural Mechanisms

The neural mechanisms mediating the effects of preoperative training on postoperative performance have not yet been identified, and this endeavor requires considerable effort. Consider the possibilities following CA3 lesions, for example. Entorhinal cells have two sets of projections to the CA1 pyramidal cells. The first is through successive synapses in the dentate gyrus and the CA3 pyramidal cells (Anderson, Bland, & Dudar, 1973; Swanson & Cowan, 1977; Swanson, Wyss, & Cowan, 1978), the second is direct to the CA1 pyramidal cells (Steward & Scoville, 1976). Destruction of CA3 cells leaves the direct pathway intact, and it might mediate the effects of preoperative training. Alternatively, the effects of preoperative training might be mediated by the surviving CA3 cells, which can sprout and produce collaterals (Fowler & Olton, 1984; Handelmann & Olton, 1981b; Handelmann et al., 1983). Electrophysiological changes in the CA1 cells in response to stimulation of the dentate gyrus indicate that any remaining CA3 cells do establish strong functional connections (Fowler & Olton, 1984). The only way to distinguish between these two alternatives (and others) is to produce a second lesion in the pathway thought to mediate the effects of preoperative training and see if these effects still remain. If the remaining CA3 cells mediate the effect, a subsequent lesion of the remaining CA3 cells or their afferents from the dentate gyrus should abolish this effect. If direct connections from the entorhinal cortex to the CA1 cells are responsible, then cutting these connections should abolish this effect. If neither of these pathways is involved and the effects of preoperative training are not mediated by the hippocampal system, these effects should remain following both lesions.

Neurochemical changes after CA3 damage may also mediate the effects of preoperative training (Handelmann et al., 1983). Behavioral testing that accelerated behavioral recovery produced three neurochemical changes. (1) It prevented the decline of the biosynthetic enzyme, choline acetyltransferase activity (ChAT), suggesting that septohippocampal projections were activated. (2) It increased concentrations of glutamic acid decarboxylase (GAD), the biosynthetic enzyme to GABA, which is used as a neurotransmitter in the inhibitory influence of GABA-ergic fibers. (3) It increased the concentration of cholecystokinin (CCK), which is in several intrinsic neurons and may help to modulate the activity of each of the major hippocampal cells groups. Training also produced an increased release of endorphin (Izquierdo et al., 1981). Hippocampal pyramidal neurons are generally excited by opioid peptides, by inhibiting adjacent inhibitory interneurons (Nicoll, 1982; Zieglgänsberger, French, Siggins, & Bloom, 1979). Moreover, the opioids may also modulate transmitter effects at a postsynaptic level (Izquierdo et al., 1980; Izquierdo et al., 1981). All of these changes might modulate the activity of surviving neurons in the hippocampus and influence behavioral performance.

CONCLUSIONS

A number of variables might be expected to influence the extent to which preoperative experience has an effect on postoperative performance. These include the following: the type of information that is learned preoperatively, the amount of training that takes place preoperatively, the amount of time between preoperative training and the surgery, and the magnitude of the lesion. The studies reviewed here generally were not designed as a parametric examination of these (and other variables) that might affect the interaction of preoperative experience and postoperative performance. Consequently, drawing firm conclusions about the quantitative effects of these variables is not possible now. However, some general points may be made.

First, preoperative training does affect postoperative performance in some circumstances. This transfer generally occurred with relatively small lesions. In several cases, the transfer involved not only specific stimulus/response/reinforcement contingencies that were the same preoperatively and postoperatively (reference memory), but also the ability to process new information that changed from trial to trial (working memory).

So many differences exist among the studies that firm conclusions about the variables affecting the magnitude of transfer from preoperative training to postoperative testing can not be made. Nonetheless, we would like to make the following suggestions. Greater transfer from preoperative training to postoperative testing will occur with the following: more extensive rather than less extensive preoperative training; reference memory rather than working memory; smaller lesions rather than larger lesions.

The mechanisms involved in the transfer of preoperative training to postoperative testing clearly need further investigation. Analysis is necessary at both the psychological level and the neural level. Psychologically, preoperative training may result in transfer because specific information is stored preoperatively and then retrieved postoperatively, general rules are learned preoperatively so that the information obtained postoperatively can be processed more effectively, and stimulation of psychological mechanisms may activate further psychological development.

At a neural level, much remains to be specified. For example, a fundamental question concerns whether positive effects of preoperative training are caused by changes in the structures in which lesions are made (assuming that they are partial lesions), or whether these effects are mediated by entirely independent neural mechanisms, ones that are not directly altered by the lesion. Training in normal animals can produce a variety of changes in neurochemical, neuroanatomical, and electrophysiological functioning. These types of changes have just begun to be examined in detail in the normal brain, and they may also affect functioning of the damaged brain.

ACKNOWLEDGMENTS

The authors thank L. Jarrard and G. Winocur for many helpful comments on a previous draft, and D. Harris for typing the manuscripts.

REFERENCES

Anderson, P., Bland, B. H., & Dudar, J. D. (1973). Organization of the hippocampal output. *Experimental Brain Research, 17,* 152–168.

Becker, J. T., Walker, J. A., & Olton, D. S. (1980). Neuroanatomical bases of spatial memory. *Brain Research, 200,* 307, 320.

Buerger, A. A. (1970). Effects of preoperative training on relearning a successful discrimination by cats with hippocampal lesions. *Journal of Comparative and Physiological Psychology, 72,* 462–466.

Feeser, H. R., & Raskin, L. A. (in press). The effects of neonatal dopamine depletion on spatial ability during ontogeny. *Behavioral Neuroscience, 101,* 812–818.

Fowler, K. R., & Olton, D. S. (1984). Recovery of function following injections of kainic acid: Behavioral, electrophysiological and neuroanatomical correlates. *Brain Research, 321,* 21–32.

Gage, P. D. (1985). Performance of hippocampectomized rats in a reference/working-memory task: Effects of preoperative versus postoperative training. *Physiological Psychology, 13,* 235–242.

Gray, J. A., & McNaughton, N. (1983). Comparison between the behavioural effects of septal and hippocampal lesions: A review. *Neuroscience & Biobehavioral Reviews, 7,* 119–188.

Gregory, R. L. (1961). The brain as an engineering problem. In W. H. Thorpe & O. L. Zangwill (Eds.), *Current problems in animal behavior* (pp. 307–330). Cambridge, England: Cambridge University Press.

Handelmann, G. E., & Olton, D. S. (1981a). Recovery of function following neurotoxic damage to the hippocampus: Importance of recovery interval and task experience. *Behavioral Neural Biology, 33,* 453–464.

Handelmann, G. E., & Olton, D. S. (1981b). Spatial memory following damage to hippocampal CA3 pyramidal cells with kainic acid: Impairment and recovery with preoperative training. *Brain Research, 217,* 41–58.

Handelmann, G. E., Olton, D. S., O'Donohue, T. L., Beinfeld, M. C., Jacobowitz, D. M., & Cummins, C. J. (1983). Effects of time and experience on hippocampal neurochemistry after damage to the CA3 subfield. *Pharmacology Biochemistry & Behavior, 18,* 551–561.

Izquierdo, I., Dias, R. D., Souza, D. O., Carrasco, M. A., Elisabetsky, E., & Perry, M. L. (1980). The role of opioid peptides in memory and learning. *Behavioral Brain Research, 1,* 451–468.

Izquierdo, I., Perry, M. L., Dias, R. D., Souza, D. O., Elisabetsky, E., Carrasco, M. A., Orsingher, D. A., & Netto, C. A. (1981). Endogenous opioids memory modulation, and state dependency. In J. L. Martiner, R. A. Jensen, R. B. Messing, H. Rigter, & J. L. McGaugh (Eds.), *Behavioral biology—An international series* (pp. 270–286). New York: Academic Press.

Jarrard, L. E. (1975). Role of interference in retention by rats with hippocampal lesions. *Journal of Comparative and Physiological Psychology*, 89, 400–408.

Jarrard, L. E. (1978). Selective hippocampal lesions: Differential effects on performance by rats of a spatial task with preoperative vs postoperative training. *Journal of Comparative and Physiological Psychology*, 92, 1119–1127.

Jarrard, L. E. (1980). Selective hippocampal lesions and behavior. *Physiological Psychology*, 8, 198–206.

Jarrard, L. E. (1983). Selective hippocampal lesions and behavior: Effects of kainic acid lesions on performance of place and cue tasks. *Behavioral Neuroscience*, 97, 873–889.

Jarrard, L. E. (1986). Selective hippocampal lesions and behavior: Implications for current research and theorizing. In R. L. Isaacson & K. H. Pribram (Eds.), *The hippocampus* (Vol. 4, pp. 93–126). New York: Plenum Press.

Jarrard, L. E., & Elmes, D. G. (1982). Role of retroactive interference in the spatial memory of normal rats and rats with hippocampal lesions. *Journal of Comparative and Physiological Psychology*, 96, 699–711.

Jarrard, L. E., Okaichi, H., Steward, O., & Goldschmidt, R. B. (1984). On the role of hippocampal connections in the performance of place and cue tasks: Comparisons with damage to hippocampus. *Behavioral Neuroscience*, 98, 946–954.

Kesner, R. P., Crutcher, K. A., & Measom, M. O. (1986). Medial septal and nucleus basalis magnocellularis lesions produce order memory deficits in rats which mimic symptomatology of Alzheimer's Disease. *Neurobiology of Aging*, 7, 287–295.

Luchins, A. S. (1942). Mechanization in problem-solving: The effects of Einstellung. *Psychological Monographs*, 1942, 54(Whole No. 248). Described in H. Gleitman, (1987), *Basic psychology* (p. 227). New York: W. W. Norton.

Maier, N. R. F. (1949). *Frustration: The study of behavior without a goal.* Ann Arbor: University of Michigan Press.

Markowska, A., & Lukaszewska, I. (1981). Response to stimulus change following observation or exploration by the rat: Differential effects of hippocampal damage. *Acta Neurobiologie Experimentalis*, 41, 323–336.

Markowska, A., & Lukaszewska, I. (1982). Response to stimulus change following observation or exploration by the rat: A confirmation of differential effects of hippocampal damages. *Acta Neurobiologie Experimentalis*, 42, 433–437.

Meck, W. H., Church, R. M., & Olton, D. S. (1984). Hippocampus, time, and memory. *Behavioral Neuroscience*, 98, 3–22.

Nicoll, R. A. (1982). Responses of central neurons to opiates and opioid peptides. In E. Coste & M. Trabucchi (Eds.), *Regulatory peptides: From molecular biology to function* (pp. 337–346). New York: Raven Press.

O'Keefe, J., & Nadel, L. (1978). *The hippocampus as a cognitive map.* Oxford, England: Oxford University Press.

Olton, D. S., Becker, J. T., & Handelmann, G. E. (1979). Hippocampus, space, and memory. *Behavioral and Brain Sciences*, 2, 352–359.

Olton, D. S., & Feustle, W. (1981). Hippocampal function required for nonspatial working memory. *Experimental Brain Research*, 41, 380–389.

Olton, D. S., Meck, W. H., & Church, R. M. (1987). Separation of hippocampal and amygdaloid involvement in temporal memory dysfunctions. *Brain Research*, 404, 180–188.

Olton, D. S., & Papas, B. C. (1979). Spatial memory and hippocampal function. *Neuropsychologia*, 17, 669–682.

Overton, D. A. (1985). Contextual stimulus effects of drugs and internal states. In P. D. Balsam & A. Tomie (Eds.), *Context and learning* (pp. 357–384). Hillsdale, NJ: Lawrence Erlbaum Associates.

Port, R. L., Romano, A. G., Steinmetz, J. E., Mikhail, A. A., & Patterson, M. M. (1986). Retention and acquisition of classical trace conditioned responses by rabbits with hippocampal lesions. *Behavioral Neuroscience, 100,* 745–752.

Raffaelle, K., & Olton, D. S. (1988). Hippocampal and amygdaloid involvement in working memory for nonspatial stimuli. *Behavioral Neuroscience, 102,* 349–355.

Rawlins, J. N. P., & Olton, D. S. (1982). The septo-hippocampal system and cognitive mapping. *Behavioral Brain Research, 5,* 331–358.

Schenk, F., & Morris, R. G. M. (1985). Dissociation between components of spatial memory in rats after recovery from the effects of retrohippocampal lesions. *Experimental Brain Research, 58,* 11–28.

Squire, L. R., & Zola–Morgan, S. (1983). The neurology of memory: The case for correspondence between the findings for human and nonhuman primate. In J. A. Deutsch (Ed.), *The physiological basis of memory* (pp. 199–268). New York: Academic Press.

Steward, O., & Scoville, S. A. (1976). Cells of origin of entorhinal cortical afferents to the hippocampus and fascia dentat of the rat. *Journal of Comparative Neurology, 169,* 347–370.

Swanson, L. W., & Cowan, W. M. (1977). An autoradiographic study of the organization of the efferent connections of the hippocampal formation in the rat. *Journal of Comparative Neurology, 172,* 49–84.

Swanson, L. W., Wyss, J. M., & Cowan, W. M. (1978). An autoradiographic study of the organization of intrahippocampal association pathways in the rat. *Journal of Comparative Neurology, 181,* 681–715.

Sutherland, R. J., Wishaw, I. Q., & Kolb, B. (1983). A behavioural analysis of spatial localization following electrolytic, kainate- or colchicine-induced damage to the hippocampal formation in the rat. *Behavioural Brain Research, 7,* 133–153.

Walker, J., & Olton, D. S. (1979). Spatial memory deficit following fimbria-fornix lesions: Independent of time for stimulus processing. *Physiology and Behavior, 23,* 11–15.

Webster, W. G. (1973). Assumptions, conceptualizations, and the search for the functions of the brain. *Physiological Psychology, 1*(4), 346–350.

Weiskrantz, L. (1974). Brain research and parallel processing. *Physiological Psychology, 2*(1), 53–54.

Winocur, G. (1979). The effects of interference on discrimination learning and recall by rats with hippocampal lesions. *Physiology and Behavior, 22,* 339–345.

Winocur, G. (1982). Radial-arm-maze behavior by rats with dorsal hippocampal lesions: Effects of cuing. *Journal of Comparative and Physiological Psychology, 96,* 155–169.

Winocur, G., & Mills, J. A. (1970). Transfer between related and unrelated problems following hippocampal lesions in rats. *Journal of Comparative and Physiological Psychology, 73,* 162–169.

Winocur, G., & Saizen, E. A. (1968). Hippocampal lesions and transfer behavior in the rat. *Journal of Comparative and Physiological Psychology, 65,* 303–310.

Zieglgänsberger, W., French, E. D., Siggins, G. R., & Bloom, F. E. (1979). Opioid peptides may excite hippocampal pyramidal neurons by inhibiting adjacent inhibitory interneurons. *Science, 205,* 415–417.

9

Preoperative Training Provides No Protection Against Lesion-Induced Decrements in Explicit Processes

E. E. Krieckhaus
Department of Psychology
University of Massachusetts, Amherst

INTRODUCTION

In general, localized cortical brain damage in humans has little effect on old memories but if it does, most of the loss usually fills in over a few years (Squire, 1987). This is an observation in line with Lashley's famous notion of the distributed nature of memory (Lashley, 1950). One of the most well-investigated behavioral deficits following fairly localized cortical lesions in man is that of a relatively pure, so-called "anterograde amnesia," characterized by the inability to learn anything new following neural insult except for implicit, procedural tasks (Squire, 1987). Although lesions in several locations are reported to produce varying degrees of this symptomatology, the densely amnestic patient, such as H. M., presumably has fairly circumscribed bilateral lesions in the medial temporal lobe critically involving hippocampal gyrus and perhaps amygdala (Mishkin & Petri, 1984).

This relatively pure anterograde amnesia, where neural connections established prior to the lesion are largely preserved, might be seen as a prime example of the topic of this volume: preoperative learning protecting an organism from otherwise deleterious effects of brain damage, the so-called "protection" effect. However, if we think not of the information already stored, but rather of the function of the hippocampus, which is to store or consolidate new explicit associations, then the amnestic patient shows no preoperative protection. Whereas H. M. remembers almost everything prior to the lesion, including his extensive preoperative experience with, for example, learning word associations, these general experiences are of no help postoperatively when he must explicitly learn some new set of word associations. This interpretation of the human amnestic syndrome is commensurate with Olton's claim in this volume of little protection in animals following complete hippocampal lesions. Like H. M., rats show no loss in their memory of the general circumstances surrounding the learning of, for example, the radial arm maze where they must learn to remember which arm they have just visited. Yet for all of the rats' preoperative experience on this task they, like H. M., are not protected in their ability to make any such new explicit associations postoperatively.

Here we examine possible protection effects in mammals with lesions of the mammillothalamic system (MTS), the chief subcortical structure projected to by hippocampus. The MTS consists of: (a) the neurons of the mammillary bodies (MBs) that occupy the posterior hypothalamus, (b) their axons comprising the mammillothalamic tract (MTT), and (c) their site of termination, the anterior thalamic nuclei (ATN). The examination will center around two well-established but previously unconnected observations.

The first observation is that animals with MTS lesions show profound decrements in two apparently quite different tasks. One is an appetitively motivated delayed alternation task that requires holding episodic information as a trace in "representational" memory, and the other is an "unnatural" shock avoidance task. It is apparently unnatural for an animal to be shocked in an enclosed box and not have his action provide for his escape. However, the two-way or shuttle avoidance task is only semiunnatural in that at least the response itself (i.e., running) is natural, whereas the lever-press task is totally unnatural in that the response of reaching out to press a lever to avoid shock to one's feet is apparently quite unnatural (Bolles, 1972; Krieckhaus, 1966).

The second fact forms the basis of this chapter. Whereas cats who are taught this unnatural lever-press avoidance task are apparently not at all protected by preoperative training, rats taught the more natural two-way avoidance task, which is as difficult for them as the lever-press task is for cat, are well protected by preoperative learning. To explain this lack of a protection effect on the totally unnatural lever-press avoidance task in cats following MTS lesions, I will suggest that MTS mediates explicit or intentional processes that are necessary for integrated action in real time.

This claim seems to depend on the validity of two general conditions, one functional, the other structural: first, that the function of MTS is cognitive, not regulatory or emotional; second, that MTS is strongly influenced by multimodal highly abstracted sensory inputs and has powerful effects on both the voluntary and involuntary motor systems. Because neither of these conditions are generally well known, a brief excursion into the structure and function of the MTS is presented in the following two "Empirical" sections. Unless referenced explicitly, documentation for anatomical claims can be found in Brooks (1986) and Nauta and Feirtag (1986) and documentation for functional claims can be found in Squire (1987) and Squire and Cohen (1984).

EMPIRICAL: STRUCTURE

Let us begin our discussion of the mammalian forebrain by considering a very comprehensive, uniquely mammalian "sensory system" made up of the large posterior part of the thalamus and its reciprocally connected, extensive sensory isocortex, including both primary and association areas. This comprehensive sensory system not only contains the neuronal connections and synaptic conductances embodying stored information, but also dramatically alters the form of the representation of incoming sensory information.

This later function is vividly portrayed in the visual system: After information reaches the primary visual cortex, V1, where it is represented retinotopically as features, the inward flow splits into two prominent forebrain systems each quite different in both architecture and function (Ungerleider, 1985). The dorsal system extracts spatial information about the location of objects and their probable trajectories whereas the ventral portion recognizes objects. Using hierarchical cascades of cortical-cortical connections, the ventral system synthesizes from the feature array progressively more abstract patterns as the information travels through the sequential components of the extrastriate cortex, finally arriving at the inferior temporal cortex. The receptive fields of single neurons in this system progress from so-called simple and complex units in the several layers of V1 that respond to simple features such as lines of differing orientation, to units in the inferior temporal cortex that respond selectively to abstract patterns, categories, or concepts such as hands or faces. These abstract patterns are independent of retinal size of the adequate stimulus (Rolls, 1985). In sheep, some units even respond differentially to the faces of different members of the sheep's immediate group (Kendrick & Baldwin, 1987), true "grandmother" cells.

This categorical or pattern information abstracted by this mammalian sensory system is then available to be focused into the primary reverberating forebrain loop of higher mammals and especially man. This archi cortical loop, Papez circuit, consists of four nodes: the hippocampal gyrus (focus node) projects massively via the fornix to MBs (base node) which equally impressively project, via MTT, to ATN (thalamic node). The ATN has reciprocal connections with the cingulate cortex (cortical node), which in turn is diffusely connected with the hippocampal gyrus, thus closing Papez circuit. Hippocampus also projects directly to ATN. Apparently this four-node reverberating architecture, first described by Papez (1937) for the archi system, is characteristic of both parts of the limbic forebrain, paleo, and archi systems. It is instantiated in the paleo system by the projections from amygdala (focus) to the ventral medial nucleus of the hypothalamus (VMH) (base) to the dorsomedial thalamic nucleus (DM) (thalamus) to the prefrontal cortex (cortex) and back to amygdala. As in the archi loop, the focus node also projects directly to the thalamic node. This

mammalian, four-node, loop architecture, characterized by funneling of progressively more highly abstracted and categorized information to each of the two
limbic, thalamic nuclei, ATN and DM, reaches its phylogenetic culmination in
the massive MTS of man. Both fornix and MTT contain roughly as many
myelinated fibers as the optic nerve in man (Krieckhaus, 1966).

Based on this four-node forebrain architecture and other known connections
(Brooks, 1986; Nauta & Feirtag, 1986), the following model of MTS physiology
is proposed. The hippocampus that receives the abstracted information from the
ventral sensory system projects massively to the MBs. The MBs, which have
strong reciprocal connections with the midbrain via the mammillotegmental
tract and the mammillary peduncle, have their primary effect on the cingulate
cortex, both anterior and posterior parts, through ATN which includes both the
anteroventral thalamic nucleus (AV) and anteromedial thalamic nucleus (AM).
Cingulate cortex, the cortical node of the archi loop, appears to be responsible
for organizing complex mammalian behavioral patterns (MacLean, 1986). This
motoric effect is mediated through extensive indirect connections to the mammalian pyramidal, or "voluntary," motor system, whose axons completely bypass
the entire hindbrain motor system and terminate directly on the alpha motor
neurons. In particular posterior cingulate, largely driven by AV, affects this
voluntary system indirectly through the posterior parietal cortex, area 7, whereas anterior cingulate, driven largely by AM, affects the voluntary system through
prefrontal cortex. Cingulate also effects the more primitive midbrain via direct
connections to the motor systems of the superior colliculus and the limbic
midbrain area of Nauta. Thus the MTS, both directly and through its cortical
node, cingulate cortex, can exert a powerful simultaneous effect on both the
involuntary (midbrain), and voluntary (pyramidal) motor systems.

EMPIRICAL: FUNCTION

Many secondary sources on MTS function for the last 50 years or so implicate
MTS primarily in memory and autonomic, regulatory functions (e.g., American
Psychiatric Association, 1987; Carlson, 1986; Glass & Holyoak, 1986). Both
implications are probably unwarranted.

The case against autonomic regulatory behavior seems clear. Careful localization of function using electrophysiological stimulation of many sites in the
posterior hypothalamus, ventral subthalamus, and rostral midbrain that mediates such autonomic effects as heart rate, respiration, blood pressure, and
arousal, showed conclusively that the critical areas for eliciting these effects lie
dorsal, caudal, and somewhat lateral to MBs. No effects were found within MBs
themselves (Risse, 1972). This lack of involvement of MTS in typical hypothalamic regulatory behavior is supported by the lack of any reliable changes in such
behavior following lesions of MTS. Similarly, no deficits in a variety of typical

higher level hypothalamic regulatory tasks such as regulation of water, nutrients, and sex are found following MTS lesions (Krieckhaus, 1966). Thus the MBs, the most posterior part of what is traditionally identified as "hypothalamus," which grow progressively larger within mammalia and reach their culmination in man, seem to have lost their typical hypothalamic functions.

The second popular function attributed to MTS is that of playing a role in memory consolidation in a manner similar to that of hippocampus. When based simply on the fact that MTS is the chief subcortical projection of hippocampus, attribution of this function has always been frustrated by the general lack of noticeable behavioral deficits in man (Squire, 1987), or animal (Krieckhaus, 1966) following lesions of fornix, which connects hippocampus to MTS.

More importantly, there is little support in the animal literature for this notion that the function of hippocampus is similar to that of MTS (Krieckhaus, 1966). In rats and cats, effects of hippocampal lesions on most tasks involving avoidance of pain are directly opposite those of MTS lesions. On the semiunnatural two-way avoidance task it has been shown repeatedly that animals with hippocampal lesions show improvement, whereas animals with MTS lesions show decrements (Gray, 1982). Further, on natural fear-motivated tasks such as one-way avoidance or passive avoidance, hippocampal lesions have adverse effects, whereas MTS lesions have no effect (Gray, 1982). This double dissociation of behavioral function also appears in the electrophysiology of ATN. Units in ATN activated by electrical stimulation of hippocampus are often inhibited by concomitant MB stimulation (Krieckhaus & Krieckhaus, 1969). Thus, if we assume, perhaps erroneously, that the general function of these archi limbic structures has not changed appreciably in phylogeny, we would expect in humans, as in animals, that lesions of MTS would show quite different effects than lesions of medial temporal lobe critically involving hippocampal gyrus.

This idea that MTS, like hippocampus, is involved in consolidation of memory springs primarily from the extensive and complicated literature on the nature of the Korsakoff psychosis with its anatomical substrate, usually considered to be MTS. However, most investigators now agree that the symptoms of the Korsakoff patient and those of amnestic patients with lesions of hippocampus, though both limited to explicit processes, are fundamentally different (Squire, 1987; Squire & Cohen, 1984). For instance the extensive temporally graded retrograde amnesia, the very common and often florid confabulation, and the shallow processing, all typical of Korsakoff psychosis are rarely seen in the amnestic patient.

Now let us consider the similarities in the behavior of the two clinical populations, amnestic and Korsakoff. Although there are many experimental conditions that are claimed to discriminate between those tasks that these patients can and cannot perform postoperatively, those that seem to best discriminate are "repetition priming" tasks such as lexical decision, word identification, and word stem or fragment completion (Schacter, 1987). When the instructions to the subject in the test phase of, for instance, a paired-associate memory experiment, are to produce explicitly the word that was paired with the target word during training (recall paradigm) or even to say "yes" or "no" as to whether he has seen the word before (recognition paradigm), amnestic and Korsakoff patients do very poorly. However, if the test instructions are only implicit, "just say whatever comes to mind," the patients can produce the previously associated word as well as controls (Schacter, 1987; Sherry & Schacter, 1987; Shimamura, 1986). This functional independence of explicit and implicit processes is also shown by their stochastic independence in normal subjects (Tulving, 1985). Thus in spite of the several important differences in the two populations of patients with lesions of the archi loop, the fact that only explicit processes are affected in both groups suggests that the function of the archi loop or Papez circuit is largely a cognitive one and not an emotional one, as suggested by Papez (1937).

In an evaluation of the nature of the deficit in Korsakoff patients, where lesions could be reasonably accurately localized to the MTS, I concluded some years ago that "the behavioral deficits . . . are often those of . . . inability to order memories along a time continuum" (Krieckhaus, 1962). This interpretation of the Korsakoff psychosis as a deficit in time ordering and integration, forcefully argued as early as 1942 by Rapaport (1971), and later by Talland (1965), and extensively documented in terms of recent animal and human experiments by Squire and Cohen (1984), postulates a single, general, primary cognitive deficit in explicitly processing information, which in turn accounts for the apparent deficit in explicit consolidation of information. Indeed if Korsakoff patients are given enough extra time in viewing test stimuli so that their immediate recall is similar to that of controls then their rate of forgetting is also similar (Huppert & Piercy, 1978).

From our own older work on experimental animals, most of it summarized more than 20 years ago (Krieckhaus, 1966), the behavioral effects of MTT lesions appeared limited to unnatural avoidance tasks, with one exception reported later. For instance cats preoperatively trained in the very unnatural lever-press avoidance task following MTT lesions could not relearn even after twice the number of trials required for original learning (Krieckhaus & Lorenz, 1968). This severe decrement in the totally unnatural lever-press avoidance task is in marked contrast to the absence of any effect in the quite natural one-way avoidance task as well as in many other simple fear-motivated tasks, such as conditioned emotional response (CER) and passive avoidance. The semiunnatural two-way avoidance task was quite significantly but often only mildly impaired following MTT lesions in cats. Finally, there were no decrements in a wide variety of difficult appetitively motivated tasks, including those involving consolidation of information into long-term storage (LTS).

Returning to the exception just noted, it has been reported recently by Thomas and Gash (1985) that in rats, lesions of MTT severely interfere with relearning a sequence of appetitively motivated delayed matching problems with delays of about 10 sec. This ability to integrate temporally ordered episodes as discussed by Thomas (1984) is identified by him as "representational" memory. Each problem, tested in a standard two-choice situation, consists of an information trial designating one or the other condition as critical. Then after the 10 sec. delay the rat must choose the condition opposite the one that was critical on the information trial. Because there are many such two-part problems in a daily session that differ only in which condition was critical in the immediately preceding information trial, it is assumed the rat cannot use LTS but must explicitly rehearse or keep in mind a representation of what occurred on the immediately preceding trial, while systematically suppressing information from all previous trials.

In a somewhat different appetitively motivated, delayed, reversal task we also found significant decrements following MTT lesions with a delay of 30 sec (Krieckhaus & Randall, 1968). It now appears that there are probably little or no lesion effects with delays of less than 5 sec, whereas deficits are found routinely with delays of greater than 30 sec (Beracochea & Jaffard, 1987). Similar effects on representational memory have been found by several investigators in a variety of delayed tasks in monkeys with archi lesions (Mishkin & Petri, 1984; Zola-Morgan & Squire, 1985).

This temporal extent of 5–30 sec seen in several animal species with archi forebrain lesions is similar to the temporal extent of short-term memory (STM) in normal humans who are prevented from rehearsing and thus from maintaining a representation, by using tasks such as the Brown-Peterson distractor task (Peterson & Peterson, 1959). Further, there is good evidence in both amnestic and Korsakoff patients that, although typical STM tasks such as digit span are not affected by the archi lesions (Squire, 1987), tasks requiring the holding of episodic, representational information beyond 5–30 sec are severely affected. This effect is seen in both the Konorski "same-different" task using, for instance, tones of different pitches (Prisco, 1963) and in the remembrance of the eccentricity of ellipses (Sidman, Stoddard, & Mohr, 1968).

Thus presumably the mechanism that allows mammals to temporally integrate their instrumental response with the subsequent non-occurrence of pain in an unnatural avoidance paradigm is the same mechanism that provides for both the temporal integration of the representational memories necessary to solve the appetitively motivated delayed alternation tasks in normal animals, and the ability to maintain, through rehearsal, the representations of, for instance, words, tones, and ellipses in normal humans. The explicit, intentional aspect of these representational processes is indicated by the finding that the loss of explicit processing is usually found to occur in conjunction with inability to extend memory representationally beyond the 5–30 sec cutoff of STM in patients with archi lesions. That these explicit process in humans are manipulated through verbal instructions and monitored by verbal report does not imply that explicit processes are themselves inherently linguistic.

To account for these several types of concomitant decrements in unnatural avoidance behavior, delayed matching, and explicit processing, I propose, using the functional data outlined in this section, that the archi forebrain system, Papez circuit, mediates intricately timed reverberating neural processes necessary to integrate disparate episodes over wide ranges of time and content. As we have seen in the "Empirical: Structure" section, the archi loop could not be better equipped for these functions with its highly abstracted multi-modal sensory input and its widespread motor effects on both the voluntary sensory-motor cortex and the involuntary mesencephalon via both MTS and cingulate cortex. This reverberating circuit basically serves two distinct but intimately related functions. One, mediated by hippocampus, is to consolidate systematically such information into pertinent isocortical and subcortical association areas specialized for information storage. The other, mediated by MTS, is that of mediating deliberate decisions in difficult or unnatural situations requiring explicit integration of episodes in real time.

PREOPERATIVE PROTECTION

As we have seen, well-substantiated behavioral effects of MTT transection in animals appear to be limited to decrements in tasks involving representational memory or unnatural avoidance. The actual learning of these avoidance tasks and the effects of MTT lesions on their acquisition and retention is not completely straightforward, largely because the acquisition scores for intact animals are not at all normally distributed, but rather fall into three distinct groups.

Figure 9.1 is a frequency histogram depicting the performance of a large number of normal unlesioned rats and cats on the two-way avoidance task. For details of training see Krieckhaus (1966). On the basis of this distribution each animal may be located in one of 12 different levels of performance based on the number of times the animal avoided the shock in 120 trials. Poor performance (few avoidances in 120 trials) is to the left on the horizontal axis in the figure and good performance is to the right. It is clear that the performance of most rats is poor and largely distributed into two distinct groups, a "bad" group, and a "mid" group. A few animals (<10%) fell into a possible third, "good" group. The generality of these three learning groups is indicated by a similar trimodal distribution in this task for many varieties of avian species, which, interestingly, have no MTS (Krieckhaus, 1988). In marked contrast to the performance scores of rats that are bimodal and poor, the cat's performance on this two-way task resembles that seen on most natural learning tasks. All fell into the good group, with a reasonably normal distribution and a mean of 10–15 trials.

Similarly, Figure 9.2 shows the distribution of performance scores on the totally unnatural lever-press avoidance task for rat, cat, and also squirrel monkey. Notice that similar to the rat in the two-way task, the cat's performance on the lever-press task, is also not normally distributed, its scores being distributed roughly equally among all three learning groups. Thus, the lever-

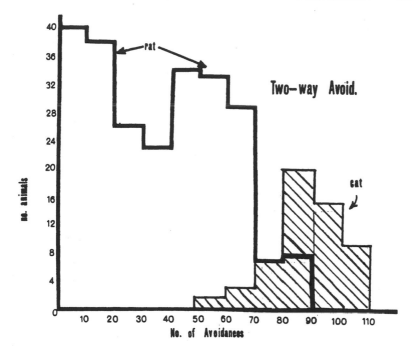

FIG. 9.1.   A frequency histogram of number of animals in each of the 10 performance groups based on the number of avoidances in 120 trials on the two-way
avoidance task for the rat and cat. Poor performance is to the left and good to the
right. The performance of the rats is distributed in two distinct groups, a "bad"
group, and a "mid" group. For the cat, the animals are roughly normally distributed in yet a third group, the "good" group.

press task for cat is apparently only slightly easier than the two-way task for rat.
This strong species-by-task interaction in acquisition of unnatural avoidance
behavior is dramatically seen by comparing rat with squirrel monkey in learning
lever-press avoidance. All rats are in the bad group whereas all monkeys are in
the good group.

   Although, as we have just seen, normal cats trained in the two-way task are
largely all in the good group with few (<10%) in the mid group, Thomas, Fry,
Fry, Slotnick, and Krieckhaus (1963) showed that cats initially acquiring this
task following MTT lesions are distributed extremely bimodally with roughly
two-thirds still in the good group but the remaining one-third mostly in the bad
group. Similarly, postoperative relearning of the two-way task following MTT
lesions (although significantly and often markedly reduced in some cats, particularly when evaluated under extinction conditions) showed considerable savings
in most cats (Krieckhaus, 1964). Although it is always difficult to find a single
behavioral measure by which to compare retention deficits with acquisition

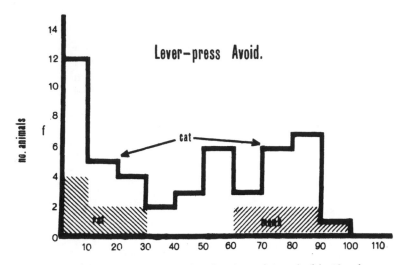

FIG. 9.2.   A frequency histogram of number of animals in each of the 10 performance groups based on the number of avoidances in 120 trials on the lever-press avoidance task for the three species of rat, cat, and monkey.

deficits (a condition necessary to measure the degree of preoperative protection) there certainly does not appear to be much of a protection effect on this two-way avoidance task in cats, because neither acquisition nor retention is that severely affected. This lack of preoperative protection in the two-way task is in marked contrast to the cat's retention of the totally unnatural lever-press task, which is completely eliminated following MTT transection. This severe impairment in cat's retention of the lever-press task would presumably also hold for the acquisition of this totally unnatural avoidance task following MTT lesions. Thus we will suppose that during acquisition, unlike the roughly one-third distribution of the intact cats in each of the three learning groups, the cats with MTT lesions would all be in the bad group and would not learn at all.

Contrary to this lack of a protection effect seen in cats on the lever-press task, there appears to be a large protection effect in the rats in the retention of the semiunnatural two-way avoidance task which is roughly as difficult as the lever-press task is for cats. Because most of the rats that were ultimately lesioned had to reach our learning criteria of 17 out of 20 successful avoidances for each of 3 successive days (usually over the course of several days to a week or so) by and large such successful learners would have to have been in the mid group in order to be lesioned. (The number of shocks each rat received preoperatively is shown in column 7 of Table 9.1.). But as we have seen, analysis of the initial acquisition of the two-way task following MTT lesions in rats reveals that status in the mid group is not attained without an intact MTT; at least 90% of the rats with MTT lesions initially acquiring the two-way task were in the bad group, indicating that the MTT is necessary for initial acquisition. Yet we can see from column 9 of Table 9.1 that integrity of MTS is only marginally related to retention: At least half of the MTT lesioned rats (presumably in the mid group initially, and thus presumably requiring an intact MTT for initial acquisition) did not show retention deficits following MTT lesions any larger than those of controls. Furthermore, the remaining half of the rats by and large showed only

TABLE 9.1

Postoperative Retention of Two-Way Avoidance Behavior in the Rat
as a Function of % MTT Lesion, Shock Level, Preoperative Training Level,
Number of Preoperative Shocks, and Lesion Size

Rat No.	Exp. No.	% MTT Left	Lesion Right	Shock Level	Preop. Level	Shocks Preop.	Lesion Size	Postop. Shocks
70	2	100	0	0.75	19	59	1.02	43
17	1	100	100	1	19	109	0.79	37
3	2	100	100	0.75	20	48	1.63	32
649	3	80	80	0.75	17	50	1.39	31
79	2	100	100	0.75	18	75	2	27
652	3	100	50	0.75	20	18	1.44	26
648	3	100	100	0.75	17	10	1.65	25
623	3	100	100	0.75	17	66	1.26	23
509	3	100	60	1.5	18	80	1.13	20
588	5	100	100	0.75	18	132	0.73	17
14	2	100	100	0.75	18	56	2.08	16
655	5	100	100	0.75	18	121	1.51	13
18	1	95	90	0.5	18	103	0.86	12
646	3	100	100	0.75	17	84	1.34	10
635	3	100	90	0.75	18	27	1.07	10
601	3	100	90	0.75	17	64	1.07	8
416	3	100	100	1	17	73	1.85	7
643	3	100	90	0.75	18	27	1.07	6
25	2	100	100	0.75	19	73	1.16	6
650	3	100	100	0.75	18	44	0.89	5
522	3	100	100	1.5	20	66	1.24	5
642	3	100	100	0.75	18	68	1.25	4
579	3	100	90	0.5	20	50	1.28	4
690	3	100	100	0.75	19	52	1.11	4
607	3	100	50	0.75	19	37	1.14	3
496	3	100	100	1.5	19	100	0.84	2
460	3	100	100	1	20	144	1.63	2
21	2	100	80	0.75	18	62	0.87	2
493	3	100	60	1.5	20	136	1.05	0
421	3	100	100	1	20	76	1.34	0
606	3	100	90	0.75	19	52	1.07	0
Means:								
Lesioned				0.86	18.5	70	1.25	13
Controls				0.80	18.3	76	1.14	4

small deficits. Even the largest deficit, 43 shocks, is still no worse than original learning for most rats. The contrast of this mild retention deficit to the large acquisition deficit indicates a very strong protection effect in rats in the semiunnatural two-way avoidance task.

The following is a summary of the results on protection afforded by preoperative training on unnatural avoidance behavior. Although cat and rat are similar in their initial acquisition of the lever-press and two-way avoidance tasks respectively (being distributed roughly equally in the three learning groups), and are similarly affected by MTT lesions made prior to acquisition (moving most all of the animals into the bad learning group), the two species are markedly different in retention of their respective tasks following MTT lesions. The rat shows only a slight decrement, good savings and thus a large protection effect, whereas the cat shows a large decrement, negative savings and thus no protection effect. It appears then that, unlike the totally unnatural lever-press avoidance response that cannot be executed at all without an intact MTS in rat or cat, the semiunnatural two-way avoidance task, in rat requires an intact MTS for initial acquisition but does not require the MTS once the rat has learned this task.

CONCLUSION

That the rat, in the semiunnatural two-way avoidance task, which is certainly as challenging for him as the lever-press task is for the cat, shows considerable protection from his preoperative learning is presumably attributable to his explicitly solving this semiunnatural problem preoperatively by a representational integration of the relevant episodes. In this way the explicit, attention demanding task is cast as an implicit, automatic sequence of natural responses chained together into a habit or script, the neural traces of which are presumably stored in the remaining forebrain, the association cortex, paleo loop, and/or basal ganglia. For instance, during initial learning a rat with an intact MTS, in just a few key trials, might explicitly decide, for instance, to turn 180 degrees to the right (or left) after entering the safe side of the shuttle-box, and then at CS presentation just move forward out of the now "bad" place designated as the place in which a turn had just been executed. Such initial explicit integration presumably requires the MTS because the rat shows virtually no learning of this two-way task without an intact MTS. Yet once this explicitly learned automatization has occurred, the world is now really much simpler for the rat and the services of MTS are no longer needed.

On the other hand, for the cat in the totally unnatural lever-press task where it must reach out and press something so that its feet will not be shocked, there is apparently no safe place to identify and there is no reasonable relationship between its instrumental response and the eventual non-occurrence of the pain.

No matter how many times the cat successfully executes the lever-press response to avoid pain preoperatively, the task probably remains unnatural, requiring constant, explicit, focused attention and thus cannot be integrated and relegated to the subattentional, automatic processes mediated by the rest of the forebrain. But there are other possibilities; the task could be integrated and thus explicitly stored but not retrieved, or perhaps it is stored and retrieved but not utilized by the rest of the nervous system because the chief output of the archi loop, MTS, is cut. Both of these alternatives are unlikely because the rat with MTT lesions had no such trouble in either retrieval or expression of the equally difficult, semiunnatural two-way avoidance task. However such possibilities are commensurate with the consistent finding that moderate doses of amphetamine can markedly improve performance following MTS lesions in cats and rats (Krieckhaus & Lorenz, 1968).

In conclusion, I suggest that because this integrative function of MTS apparently cannot be relegated to the other forebrain structures, successful execution of explicit episodic behavior such as delayed matching and totally unnatural lever-press avoidance shows no preoperative protection. Thus, we find that the two observations identified at the beginning of the chapter, that MTT lesions affect two different kinds of tasks, unnatural and representational, and that there is a lack of a protection effect on the unnatural lever-press task in cat, are not only intimately related, but, taken together, give strong support to this idea that MTS mediates the explicit representational processes necessary for deliberate, integrated living. This notion certainly makes sense of the observation that what is most us as humans is thoughtful concern for long term goals and a greatly enlarged MTS.

REFERENCES

American Psychiatric Association. (1987). *Diagnostic and statistical manual of mental disorders* (3rd ed.). Washington, DC.: Author.

Beracochea, D. J., & Jaffard, R. (1987). Impairments of spontaneous alternation behavior in sequential test procedures following mammillary body lesions in mice: Evidence for time-dependent interference-related memory deficits. *Behavioral Neuroscience, 101*(2), 187–197.

Bolles, R. C. (1972). The avoidance learning problem. In G. E. Bower (Ed.), *The psychology of learning and motivation, Vol. 6.* New York: Academic Press.

Brooks, V. B. (1986). *The neural basis of motor control.* New York: Oxford University Press.

Carlson, N. R. (1986). *Physiology of behavior* (3rd ed.). Boston: Allyn & Bacon.

Glass, A. L., & Holyoak, J. K. (1986). *Cognition* (2nd ed.). New York: Random House.

Gray, J. A. (1982). *The neuropsychology of anxiety: An enquiry into the functions of the septo-hippocampal system.* New York: Oxford University Press.

Huppert, F. A., & Piercy, M. (1978). Dissociation between learning and remembering in organic amnesia. *Nature, 275,* 317–318.

Kendrick, K. M., & Baldwin, B. A. (1987). Cells in temporal cortex of conscious sheep can respond preferentially to the sight of faces. *Science, 236,* 448–450.

Krieckhaus, E. E. (1962). *Behavioral changes in cats following lesions of the mammillothalamic tracts.* Unpublished doctoral dissertation, University of Illinois.

Krieckhaus, E. E. (1964). Decrements in avoidance behavior following mammillothalamic tractotomy in cats. *Journal of Neurophysiology, 27,* 753–767.

Krieckhaus, E. E. (1966). The mammillary bodies: Their function and anatomical connections. *Acta. Biol. Exper. (Warsaw), 27,* 319–337.

Krieckhaus, E. E. (1988). *The mammillothalamic system and avoidance of pain—comparative, psychological and neuroanatomical considerations.* Unpublished manuscript.

Krieckhaus, E. E., & Krieckhaus, S. (1969). *Effect of electrical stimulation on the mammillary bodies on autonomic and regulatory functions in the acutely prepared cat.* Unpublished manuscript.

Krieckhaus, E. E., & Lorenz, R. (1968). Retention and relearning of lever-press avoidance following mammillothalamic tractotomy. *Physiology and Behavior, 3,* 433–438.

Krieckhaus, E. E., & Randall, D. (1968). Lesions of mammillothalamic tract in rat produce no decrements in recent memory. *Brain, 91,* 369–378.

Lashley, K. S. (1950). In search of the engram. *Symp. Soc. Exp. Biol., 4,* 454–482.

MacLean, P. D. (1986). Culminating developments in the evolution of the limbic system: The thalamocingulate division. In B. K. Doane & K. E. Livingston (Eds.), *The limbic system: Functional organization and clinical disorders.* New York: Raven Press.

Mishkin, M., & Petri, H. L. (1984). Memories and habits: Some implications for the analysis of learning and retention. In L. R. Squire & N. Butters (Eds.), *Neuropsychology of memory.* New York: Guilford Press.

Nauta, W. J. H., & Feirtag, M. (1986). *Fundamental neuroanatomy.* New York: W. H. Freeman.

Papez, J. W. (1937). A proposed mechanism of emotion. *Archives of Neurology and Psychiatry (Chicago), 38,* 725–743.

Peterson, L. R., & Peterson, M. J. (1959). Short-term retention of individual verbal items. *Journal of Experimental Psychology, 58,* 193–198.

Prisco, I. (1963). *Short term memory in cerebral damage.* Unpublished doctoral dissertation, McGill University, Montreal.

Rapaport, D. (1971). *Emotions and memory* (5th ed.). New York: International University Press.

Risse, G. (1972). *Effects of electrical stimulation of the mammillary bodies on autonomic and regulatory functions in the anesthetized cat.* Unpublished master's thesis, University of Massachusetts, Amherst.

Rolls, E. T. (1985). Neuronal activity in the relation to the recognition of stimuli in the primate. In C. Chagas, R. Gattass, & C. Gross (Eds.), *Pattern recognition mechanisms.* New York: Springer-Verlag.

Schacter, D. L. (1987). Implicit memory: History and current status. *Journal of Experimental Psychology: Learning, Memory, and Cognition, 13,* 501–518.

Sherry, D. F., & Schacter, D. L. (1987). The evolution of multiple memory systems. *Psychological Review, 94,* 439–454.

Shimamura, A. P. (1986). Priming effects in amnesia: Evidence for a dissociable memory function. *Quarterly Journal of Experimental Psychology, 38A,* 619–644.

Sidman, M., Stoddard, L. T., & Mohr, J. P. (1968). Some additional quantitative observations of immediate memory in a patient with bilateral hippocampal lesions. *Neuropsychologia, 6,* 245–254.

Squire, L. R. (1987). *Memory and brain.* New York: Oxford University Press.

Squire, L. R., & Cohen, N. (1984). Human memory and amnesia. In G. Lynch, J. L. McGaugh, & N. M. Weinberger (Eds.), *Neurobiology of learning and memory.* New York: Guilford Press.

Talland, G. A. (1965). *Deranged memory.* New York: Academic Press.

Thomas, G. T. (1984). Memory: Time binding in organisms. In L. R. Squire & N. Butters (Eds.), *Neuropsychology of memory.* New York: Guilford Press.

Thomas, G. T., & Gash, D. M. (1985). Mammillothalamic tracts and representational memory. *Behavioral Neuroscience*, 99, 621–630.

Thomas, G. T., Fry, W. J., Fry, F. J., Slotnick, B. M., & Krieckhaus, E. E. (1963). Behavioral effects of mammillothalamic tractotomy in cats. *Journal of Neurophysiology*, 26, 857–876.

Tulving, E. (1985). How many memory systems are there? *American Psychology*, 40, 385–398.

Ungerleider, L. G. (1985). The corticocortical pathways for object recognition and spatial perception. In C. Chagas, R. Gattass, & C. Gross (Eds.), *Pattern recognition mechanisms*. New York: Springer-Verlag.

Zola-Morgan, S., & Squire, L. R. (1985). Medial temporal lesions in monkeys impair memory on a variety of tasks sensitive to human amnesia. *Behavioral Neuroscience*, 99, (1), 22–34.

10

Sparing, Loss, and Recovery of Function in the Telencephalon Ablated Teleost Fish

J. Bruce Overmier
Department of Psychology
University of Minnesota, Minneapolis

INTRODUCTION

When the diagnosis of "severe stroke," "brain damaged," or "brain tumor" is applied to a loved one, we are emotionally crushed. This is because, in contrast to diseases, no "cure" is at hand, and we see the effects persisting endlessly into the future. This despair is most marked when we believe the damage to be in the cerebral hemispheres to which we attribute most higher associative and cognitive functions. But is the future so bleak as is assumed? Oftentimes we in fact do see recovery of some functions. Or, with slow-growing tumors—those that Hughlings Jackson (1873) described as of "low momentum"—behavioral consequences can be very modest. How does recovery occur, or, at least, when can we expect it to occur. Why does slowly developing destruction have lesser effects? Are there prior or postdamage experiences that can modulate the rates of recovery? These important questions are being addressed in retrospective clinical studies with human patients and more directly with a variety of animal models. Each animal model is selected because of some special neuroanatomical, neurophysiological, or functional behavioral advantage or opportunity that it affords. Although the fish brain shares the same gross anatomical divisions as all vertebrates, it has some special features (see Hollis & Overmier, 1978; Laming, 1981), and some work on the problem of sparing and recovery of function is going forward using the teleost or "bony" fish as the model.

Why the Teleost Fish?

The telencephalon of the teleost fish is of special interest because it differs ontogenetically and anatomically from that of all other vertebrates. In most vertebrates, the development of the forebrain from the anterior portion of the neural tube is accomplished through evagination and an outpouching of the *lateral* walls followed by an inversion of the dorsal lateral wall resulting in paired hemispheres *each* with a central ventrical. In contrast, expansion in teleosts is accomplished by eversion and the *dorsal* parts bulge and bend outward resulting in two solid hemispheres separated by one median ventricle. This likely results in an inversion of anatomical relationships within the teleost telencephalon relative to that seen in other vertebrates. The importance of this is that the functional anatomy is at best uncertain and identification of homologous sub-structures a matter of vigorous controversy (Aronson 1981; Nieuwenhuys, 1967; Northcutt & Bradford, 1980; Scalia & Ebbesson, 1971; Schnitzlein, 1968). Accompanying these ontological differences is a reorganization of the vasculature supplying the brain.

The unique anatomy of the teleost telencephalon has resulted in it receiving relatively little attention in comparative-evolutionary studies of structure and function because, I suppose, it stands "outside" the main sequences. Additionally because fish are sometimes—incorrectly (Hodos & Campbell, 1969)—thought of as "lower species," the amount of neurobehavioral research on fish in general and teleosts in particular is relatively limited.

On the other hand, one could well argue that this very uniqueness of the alternative set of structural relationships found in the teleost telencephalon ought to make it of very special interest for both functional and physiological-behavioral research. Are the behavioral capacities of these fish different in kind from those of other vertebrates? Are the effects of CNS insults to the teleost telencephalon different? Are the adaptive and recuperative capacities of the fish following such insults different in kind from other vertebrates?

The first question has been subject to research by some psychologists (e.g., Bitterman, 1975) with the finding that there may well be some differences in basic learning processes. With respect to the second question, scientists are still trying to get a detailed picture of the effects of telencephalic lesions upon teleost behavior (see Davis & Kassel, 1983; Overmier & Hollis, 1983). To date, the bulk of that work has used gross ablations of the telencephalon as the primary manipulation although other techniques are now becoming the methods of choice (viz. Laming, 1981a). Nonetheless, even relying on the data from gross ablations, analytical efforts have been made to answer whether the effects of telencephalic ablations in teleosts are functionally analogous to "similar" ablations in other vertebrate classes, and the answer for at least some tasks is "yes" (Flood, Overmier, & Savage, 1976; Hollis & Overmier, 1978). The third question on the adaptive and recuperative capacities and how these may be optimized are the focus of the present chapter, but to anticipate, teleost behavior seems surprisingly "impervious" to telencephalic ablations yet for those deficits known, preoperative experiences result in little amelioration of the deficit.

A Bit of History

The first experiments on the functions of the teleost telencephalon date back at least 150 years (Desmoulins, 1825) but with only intermittent additional efforts until well into this century. Little, if anything, was learned from 19th-century studies except that fish could survive the radical surgery of complete telencephalonectomy.

The questions of whether a particular lesion or ablation produces a behavioral deficit and whether there is recovery of function are deceptively simplistic. The former is deceptive in that a given failure to observe a deficit in a particular set of circumstances or task does not allow the inference that there is none (you cannot prove the null hypothesis), only that you have failed to detect one. This is well illustrated by reference to the literature on the consequences of telencephalon ablation in the teleost fish.

The early experiments on telencephalic functions (perhaps better labeled "forebrain" or "prosencephalon" because the ablations also removed the olfactory bulbs and possibly diencephalic structures beyond the cerebral hemispheres) reported that the fish were essentially normal following the ablations (Desmoulins, 1825, Meader, 1939). The fish swam normally, ate normally, and showed no major behavioral disruptions except for a loss of initiative and variability (e.g., Janzen, 1933). There was of course the obvious loss of olfaction, and this loss was given prominence. This "rhinencephallic" view of the teleost telencephalon has persisted (incorrectly) into relatively recent times (e.g., Prosser & Brown, 1961). However, it is true that olfaction is integral in not yet understood ways to several aspects of normal behavior in various species (e.g., aggression); thus some later detected disruptions of such behaviors attributed to lost telencephalic functions may in fact be due to lost olfaction (see Colyer & Jenkins, 1976; Kleerekoper, 1969; Koyama, Satou, Oka, & Ueda, 1984; Kyle & Peter, 1982). Beyond olfaction, there is as yet no other demonstrated permanent sensory loss, although there is a very brief (a few hours) disruption in color vision which appears to be merely postsurgical trauma from exposure of the optic tectum (Bernstein, 1961a, 1961b, 1962, 1970). Representative brains are shown in Fig. 10.1.

It seemed unlikely that the early reports could be correct in that total ablation of the fish's cerebral hemispheres—hemispheres thought so important in other vertebrates—could be without significant effect in fish. As interest in the functional analysis of the teleost telencephalon began to grow by midcentury, two functional domains were focused upon: (a) reproductive behaviors (including territoriality, defense, nesting, mating, parenting), and (b) associative

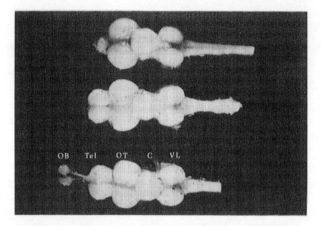

FIG. 10.1. From top of figure to bottom are shown representative telencephalon ablation, a bulbectomized/sham operation, and normal goldfish brain. Key: OB = olfactory bulbs; Tel = telencephalon; OT = optic tectum; C = cerebellum; VL = vagal lobes.

learning (classical conditioning and appetitive- and avoidance-based instrumental behaviors). The goal was to find and identify deficits. Scant attention was paid to recovery of function—much less special manipulations that might promote sparing and/or recovery.

DEFICITS AND RECOVERY OF FUNCTION

To study recovery of function, its modulating factors, and mechanisms, one must identify first the specific deficits. Deficits in reproductive behaviors began to be identified about 1940 (Aronson, 1948; Noble, 1939; Noble & Borne, 1941; see Davis & Kassel, 1983, for review). Whether all of these are of significant interest here awaits the further determination of whether the observed deficits are a by-product of the loss of olfaction. We are interested only in those disruptions that are not primarily attributable to sensory loss.[1] In at least some species, the paradise fish, the deficit does not appear to be olfaction-based.

---

[1]The focus upon nonsensory processes is a personal bias. Much excellent work has been done on recovery of function following insults to the visual system, primarily the optic tracts and tectum (Davis & Schlumpf, 1984; Edwards & Grafstein, 1983; Giulian, 1984; Kohsaka, 1982; Leitner, Francis, & Gazzaniga, 1982; Northmore, 1981; Yolen & Hodos, 1976, as examples). These, however, have not explored factors that modulate the recovery of visual function, just the degree to which it does recover.

Deficits in associative learning began to be identified in the 1960s only after researchers began to focus upon avoidance learning (see Overmier & Hollis, 1983; Savage, 1980 for reviews). The limited body of research is in sharp contrast to the much more extensive and systematic data-base on these topics with mammals as reviewed elsewhere in this volume (see also, e.g., Lashley, 1929; Meyer & Meyer, 1977).

Some experimental contrasts useful in identifying functional deficits, instances of recovery, and the factors modulating these are sketched in Table 10.1. These "designs" are only illustrative because they are incomplete (e.g., E–1 vs. E–2) and necessarily imply additional control comparisons (e.g., E–1 vs. A–1). Nonetheless, the table does give substance to the host of issues and concerns. Consider some examples. Design A identifies sparing versus loss of functions critical to Test T. Design B assesses whether the preceding loss is permanent or whether rest time alone will result in recovery. Of course, a concern here might be regeneration of structures because Maron (1963) has reported an instance of telencephalon regeneration in young teleosts. However, other studies suggest such telencephalic regeneration is *at best* limited (Bernstein, 1967; Kirsche, 1965; Pflugfelder, 1965; Segaar, 1965) especially in adult fish of most species, including the commonly studied goldfish. Design C tests whether some specific "therapy" experience or change in the test conditions (e.g., increased motivation) will induce recovery relative to control procedures. Of course, one must have an instance of "recovery" before one can study the factors that modulate recovery. Design D tests whether postoperative retention of a task learned postoperatively is normal. Design E assesses whether preoperative enrichment provides protective immunization against loss of function. While Design F tests for loss or sparing of memory for task T, Designs A versus F may allow resolution of the nature of a functional loss as "storage" versus "retrieval." Design G (as extensions of E and F) tests for stimulated recovery, whereas Design H tests for sensitization to recovery therapy. Design I with its serial ablations is the experimental analog to "momentum of lesion," whereas Design J with its postoperative rest before test provides a control for length of time since first operation in Design I. Design K assesses the role of an interoperative experience (or therapy during the course of a "growing" lesion) upon sparing. The remaining designs (incomplete) assess the necessity of the existence of a preablation enrichment or association in order for an interoperation or a postablation treatment to be successful in inducing sparing. Although all of these and others could be useful, they have enjoyed only limited use in the research with teleosts, little of it systematic.

Review

Although not the focus of this chapter or volume, perhaps the first thing one should remark upon is the very significant sparing that follows total ablation of the teleost telencephalon. As we have briefly noted, a number of early experi-

TABLE 10.1
Basic Experimental Comparisons for Assessing Deficits and Recovery

Design/ Group	Training or Pretreatment	Operation	Training or Pretreatment or Recovery Treatment	Operation	Critical Test (T)	Recovery Therapy (rt) or Handle	Critical Test (T)
A-1				00	T		
A-2				ØØ	T		
B-1				00			T
B-2				ØØ			T
C-1				00		h	T
C-2				ØØ		rt	T
D-1				00	T		T
D-2				ØØ	T		T
E-1				ØØ	T		
E-2			rt	ØØ	T		
F-1				ØØ	T		
F-2			T	ØØ	T		
F-3			T	00	T		
G-1				ØØ			T
G-2			rt or T	ØØ			T
G-3			rt or T	00			T
H-1			rt or h	00		h	T
H-2			rt or T	ØØ		h	T
H-3			rt or T	ØØ		rt	T
I-1		00		ØØ	T		
I-2		Ø0		−Ø	T		
I-3		00		00	T		
J-1		00		ØØ			T
J-2		Ø0		−Ø			T
K-1		00	rt or T	ØØ	T		
K-2		Ø0	rt or T	−Ø	T		
K-3		00	rt or T	00	T		
L-1	rt or T	00		ØØ	T		
L-2	rt or T	Ø0		−Ø	T		
L-3	rt or T	Ø0	rt or T	−Ø	T		
L-4		Ø0		−Ø	T		
L-5	rt or T	00		00	T		
M-1	rt or T	00		ØØ		h or rt	T
M-2	rt or T	Ø0		−Ø		h or rt	T
M-3	rt or T	Ø0	rt or T	−Ø		h or rt	T
M-4		Ø0		−Ø		h or rt	T

Notes: 00 = sham operation
      ØØ = unilateral ablation
      −Ø = second stage of serial unilateral ablations
      ØØ = bilateral ablation

ments simply failed to detect any significant aberrations in behavior following the ablation. Researchers had to look carefully and quantitatively at complex "tasks" such as reproductive behaviors or instrumental avoidance response learning to find disturbances (Overmier & Gross, 1972, 1974). Simple swimming, feeding, and even discriminative instrumental learning for immediate food rewards were not impaired (Healey, 1957; Savage, 1969b). But striking disruptions of reproductive behaviors and impairments in avoidance behavior are now well established, although the underlying mechanisms are still matters of conjecture and experimentation (Flood, Overmier, & Savage, 1976; Hollis & Overmier, 1978).

Reproductive Behaviors.   Ablation of the telencephalon markedly disrupts and impairs the complex behaviors and their integration that underlie the reproductive success of a variety of teleost species. These impaired behaviors include territorial defense, courtship, nest building, spawning, and parenting (Davis & Kassel, 1983, for review). In some fish (e.g., goldfish, *Carassius auratus*), these impairments are now known to be at least in part attributable to the loss of olfaction (Kyle & Peter, 1982; Stacey & Kyle, 1983; but see Koyama, Satou, Oka, & Ueda, 1984). In other fish (e.g., paradise fish, *Macropodus opercularis*), the impairment is not a concomitant of the loss of olfaction (Schwagmeyer, Davis, & Kassel, 1977). Let us consider the latter instances further.

Using ethological analyses, Schwagmeyer et al., found that telencephalon ablation markedly decreased or eliminated males' frontal attack, display, nest building, and spawning as measured over the course of 5-day spawning tests. Moreover, the sequential integration of those reproductive behaviors which did occur (attack, display, chase, quiver, curve, clasp) was disrupted. Additional studies (Davis, Kassel, & Schwagmeyer, 1976; Kassel, Davis, & Schwagmeyer, 1976) used an "operant" technique to study the attack/display component. It is well known that anabantiod fish such as the Siamese fighting fish will perform a specific swimming act to get visual access to a conspecific to which they then direct attacks and displays. Davis and his associates reasoned that if ablation disrupts the normal mechanisms underlying the attack/display/nest/spawn sequences, then performance in this operant task should be impaired as well. Indeed, it was and the operant impairment was related to the previously demonstrated impairment in spawning. Sham-operated fish showed no reduction in the frequency of performing the operant response relative to the preoperative baseline, whereas the ablated fish (procedure F-2) made virtually no operant responses, although their ability to swim was unimpaired. Although these experiments didn't provide direct comparisons to preoperatively naïve fish, the "zero" levels of postoperative performances imply that the preoperative experiences provided little if any protection against the effects of the ablations.

Davis et al. tested whether additional spawning opportunities provided postoperatively (similar to procedure H-3) might result in recovery of the operant response for attack/display. Ten consecutive days with a female failed to result in recovery of the operant response. However, it must be noted that few if any reproductive behaviors actually occurred during the 10-day spawning opportunity, so the absence of "therapeutic" effects of spawning on sexually motivated instrumental behaviors is not certain.

In an extension of this research, Kassel et al. studied the postoperative relearning of the operant (procedure F-2) over an extended series of test sessions spaced several days apart. From preoperative baseline to postoperative tests, both ablated and sham-operated fish showed a decline in response rate, but whereas the ablated fish showed a 95% decline the sham fish showed only a 20% decline. Over the succeeding sessions, performances by both groups increased, but while the shams made full recovery, the ablated fish reached barely one-third of their preoperative baseline of responding and showed little persistence into extinction. Unfortunately, we cannot say whether the modest recovery that was seen in the ablated fish is attributable to the prior operant sessions or to the passage of time (30 days) over which the sessions were distributed. Finally, after these operant sessions, the males were given a spawning test like those in previous experiments. Again, no ablated fish spawned, but in the present experiment ablated fish interacted with the female, even making some frontal displays. This represents an improvement over that previously seen when tested immediately. Here again, we are unsure of the source of their very modest recovery, diaschisis and the passage of time, or the intervening postoperative operant experiences.

Further efforts to study factors that might result in sparing and/or recovery of reproductive functions were made by Kassel and Davis (1977). The factors they manipulated were (1) whether or not the fish had preablation spawning experience, (2) "momentum of lesion" through the serial ablation of each hemisphere with 5 weeks intervening between operations versus simultaneous bilateral ablation, and (3) postablation recovery time. The first two factors were combined in a 2 × 2 factorial (procedures F-1, F-2, K-1, K-2) in which the spawning experience preceded the final ablation by 3 weeks; the spawning test sessions followed the final ablation by 2 weeks. Because any increased reproductive behavior that might be observed in serially ablated males might reflect time-dependent recovery processes initiated by the *first* unilateral ablation, an additional naïve group underwent bilateral ablation 7 weeks prior to the spawning test session (procedure G-1). The data from this interesting experiment are shown in Table 10.2.

The importance of the three factors was a function of the particular reproductive behavior measured. A "serial lesion effect" (Finger, Walbran, & Stein, 1973) is clear when we use clasping and spawning as our index, but not with nest building as our index. This serial lesion effect does not interact with prior experience. Prior experience did not modulate postablation clasping and spawn-

TABLE 10.2
Effects of Intact, Unilateral, Serial, and Simultaneous Bilateral
Telencephalon Ablation on Reproductive Behavior

| Group | n | Behavior | | |
		Gathered nest	Clasp	Spawn
Simultaneous				
(2-week recovery)				
Inexperienced	6	0	17	17
Experienced	8	25	12	12
Serial				
(2-week recovery)				
Inexperienced	8	0	62	38
Experienced	8	12	50	25
Simultaneous				
(7-week recovery)				
Inexperienced	8	0	50	25
Unilateral	8	100	100	100
Intact	8	100	100	100

Data from Kassel and Davis, 1977.

ing. On the other hand, prior experience did appear to result in more postablation nest building as indexed by duration of nest building (not shown) or
percentage of gathered nests, although the effects are not significant with these
small ns.

Perhaps most intriguing is the consequence of the 7-week recovery manipulation relative to the Simultaneous and Serial 2-week recovery groups. Comparing
the 7-week and 2-week Simultaneous groups makes clear that the mere passage
of time contributed to recovery. This makes comparison of the 7-week Simultaneous group with the Serial groups most interesting because these groups are
equated on time since *first* ablation. Between these we see comparable performances suggesting that the serial lesion effect found here is attributable primarily
to time-based recovery. This led Kassel and Davis to conclude that removal of
the first hemisphere initiates alterations in nontelencephalic structures which
result in increased savings following removal of the second hemisphere.

The preceding results are intriguing but they do not reveal the mechanisms of
either the *suggested* savings in nest building after prior experience nor the savings
in the Serial and Simultaneous 7-week groups that appear to be time based.

In summary, neither preoperative nor postoperative experiences appear to
contribute much to recovery of function. There is evidence for a serial lesion
effect, but it may be the case that this is a by-product of the passage of time alone
rather than some more interesting process (cf. LeVere, 1975, 1980).

Avoidance Behavior.   Ablation of the telencephalon markedly impairs the ability of teleost fish to learn, retain, or relearn instrumental avoidance behaviors which are integral to the survival of the individual by ensuring the safety of the fish (Overmier & Hollis, 1983). This deficit has been reported for a wide variety of species over a variety of avoidance tasks of both passive and active forms. The observed impairment is especially surprising because avoidance behavior has often been viewed as in integration of two simpler forms of learning: (a) classical conditioning of fear, and (b) instrumental escape learning (Kimble, 1961; May, 1948). Both of these are *unimpaired* and are learned and retained normally in telencephalon ablated fish (Flood et al., 1976). Obviously those early simple theoretical views of avoidance behavior are wrong; nonetheless, the mystery of the deficit deepens given that the elementary building blocks of avoidance behavior are clearly intact.

All of the experiments we will discuss in this section used some form of "shuttlebox," which is typically an elongated apparatus divided by a partial partition into two separate chambers; upon presentation of a warning signal, the fish is required to swim from one compartment to the other within a specified short period of time (e.g., 10 seconds) or an aversive stimulus will be presented (tactile, Kovacevic, 1978; electrical, Horner, Longo, & Bitterman, 1961). Normal fish typically learn this task easily and quickly, and their asymptotic behavior is relatively stable and persistent.

The most common experiment, relevant to our discussion, has been one which compares normal (or sham-operated) fish with ablated fish on postoperative *de novo* learning or on relearning. Such a design, if factorial, should provide a reasonable assessment of sparing of learning capacity, retention of original learning, and/or sparing or recovery of *relearning* capacity. Unfortunately, most of those experiments available are not factorial and, moreover, some use postoperative training conditions that differ from those preoperatively (e.g., Kaplan & Aronson, 1967)!

One consistent series of experiments was carried out by Hainsworth, Overmier, and Snowdon (1967) using goldfish. Their first experiment compared (a) intact normal, (b) sham-operated (procedure A-1), and (c) telencephalon-ablated (A-2) fish on rates of original learning of the shuttlebox avoidance task. The normal and sham groups performed identically and reached the 70% avoidance criterion quickly (median 2.8 days) whereas the ablated fish took substantially longer (median 8.5 days) as shown in Fig. 10.2A. Not shown there is that the ablated group did eventually learn to criterion. Thus, some capacity for learning of the avoidance response is spared.

Was the learning achieved by the ablated fish, by whatever underlying mechanisms, functionally equivalent to that of the sham fish? Hainsworth et al. assessed this by testing persistence of the learned avoidance response without further reinforcer presentations (i.e., in extinction). Even though both groups exceeded the criterion level on the last day prior to extinction, they were not

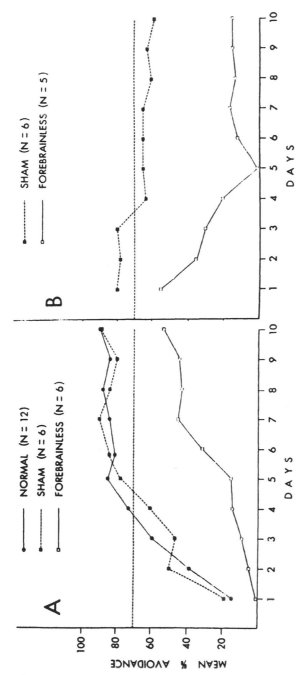

FIG. 10.2. Performance indexed by percentage avoidance responses during *de novo* acquisition (panel A) and, after all groups exceeded the 70% criterion, extinction (panel B) by normal, sham, and telencephalon-ablated ("forebrainless") fish. (After Hainesworth et al., 1967)

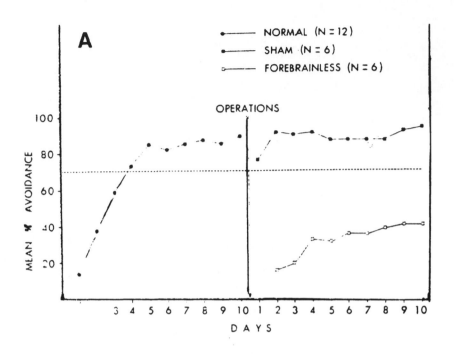

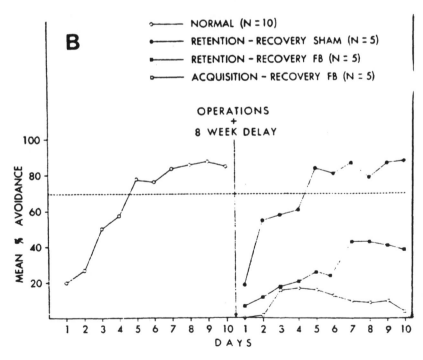

equally persistent, and the ablated fish's performances quickly fell to very low levels as shown in Fig. 10.2B. The quantitatively similar performances at asymptote were qualitatively different as revealed in the extinction test. The postoperative learning thus differs in a significant way from normal learning.

Hainsworth et al.'s second experiment compared sham-operated and ablated fish on postoperative retention and retraining (procedures F-3 vs. F-2). The results shown in Fig. 10.3A, reveal that the ablated fish show very poor retention of preoperatively learned avoidance and relearn very slowly.

Across experiment comparison of their ablated groups (all methods were identical) allows some assessment of whether the preoperative training experience facilitated relearning. The data are somewhat mixed in that the groups are equal on postoperative day 1, the relearning group is somewhat better through days 2–5 (means 20% vs. 10%), but the de novo learning group is somewhat better on days 7–10 (means 47% vs. 37%). If there is facilitation of postoperative avoidance learning as a result of preoperative avoidance training, it is not markedly obvious in this immediate postoperative retention/relearning test. The facilitation effect *appears* to become more clear when a simple 8-week recovery period is allowed before testing (H-1, H-2, A-2) as shown in Fig. 10.3B, because the relearning by the ablated fish is somewhat better than the de novo learning by ablated fish. However, this "effect" is attributable to the poorer de novo learning, not to improvement in relearning after a rest because the relearning curves for the ablated groups in Fig. 10.3A (no rest period) and Fig. 10.3B (8-week rest period) are virtually identical.

The issues of whether or not postoperative relearning relative to de novo postoperative learning begins at a higher level or proceeds faster or both are important for assessing whether there is savings through the ablative process, whether pretreatment facilitates later relearning, or both. The Hainsworth et al. results are generally, but not entirely, negative on these. However, others often cited have reported savings.

For example, Dewsbury and Bernstein (1969) compared postoperative relearning by sham and ablated fish with de novo learning by ablated fish in a special "shuttlebox"—one essentially without a barrier. They reported that the sham fish showed perfect retention postoperatively; the ablated fish did not; however, their performance returned to the original asymptotic level by the second day of retraining. The de novo learning group required 5 days of training to achieve the same level that the pretrained ablated fish reached in 2, and

FIG. 10.3. Performance indexed by percentage avoidances for de novo acquisition and then retention and relearning after 2 days (panel A) or 8 weeks (panel B) of postoperative rest. In panel B, group "Acquisition Recovery FB" shows de novo learning by fish ablated 8 weeks before by sham-operated and telencephalon-ablated ("forebrainless" or FB) fish. (After Hainesworth et al., 1967)

based upon this, these investigators concluded that preablation training results in postoperative savings.

However, I have substantial reservations about Dewsbury and Bernstein's data for two reasons. Firstly, the postoperative training for the groups differed in that those groups undergoing retraining received the sequence signal-habituation, train, ablate, and train again, while the *de novo* learning group received the sequence ablate–habituation–train. This means that only the latter group received habituation *immediately* preceding the final training, and such habituation trials—sometimes referred to as latent inhibition trials (Lubow & Moore, 1959)—are known to slow down learning. Secondly, in their shuttlebox, carefully directed movements were not required to achieve avoidances and, indeed, any significant increase in random activity could lead to an avoidance. Importantly, activity is known to be classically conditionable in fish (Overmier & Curnow, 1969), this conditioning can result in pseudoavoidances (Woodard & Bitterman, 1971), and classical conditioning of activity is not impaired by telencephalon ablation (Overmier & Savage, 1974).[2] Thus, the observed better performance of the retrained fish relative to that of the group learning *de novo* may very well be attributed to sampling the acquisition curves at different points in the course of classical conditioning. Hence, there are substantial reasons to doubt that Dewsbury and Bernstein's data can be taken as evidence that pretraining of *avoidance* behavior results in postablation savings and/or facilitated relearning of avoidance.

Savage (1969a) also compared relearning by sham and ablated fish with *de novo* learning in ablated fish in an experiment without the problems that have been noted. Again, sham fish showed perfect retention while the ablated fish did not; the ablated fish did relearn to some degree but their asymptotic level was well below that of the sham fish (55% vs. 90+ %). The *de novo* learning by ablated fish started at a somewhat lower level postoperatively but reached the same low asymptote on the same day as did those ablated fish being retrained. Thus, Savage's experiment offers some slight evidence for postablation retention savings from pretraining but this does not confer permanent advantage. There appears to be a permanent deficit in ability to master the avoidance task that is essentially the same whether the ablated fish are just learning the task or relearning the task.

Because pretraining to criterion seems to yield some limited, postoperative retention, one must now inquire as to whether additional postcriterion training preoperatively (so-called "overtraining") would result in even greater savings. Overmier and Papini (1986) tested this idea by comparing groups trained to the 70% avoidance criterion ($\bar{x} = 6.6$ sessions) and then either sham operated or

---

[2]Indeed, *de novo* learning by normal and ablated fish did not differ at all in Dewsbury and Bernstein's so-called avoidance task, suggesting that they were recording primarily classically conditioned responses.

ablated versus a group trained to the criterion plus 15 additional days of over-training (on average, 200% overtraining) and then ablated. Fig. 10.4A shows the results; although ablation clearly impairs retention and the postablation asymptote of relearning, the data suggest that preoperative overtraining does improve retention somewhat, although the effect is not statistically reliable ($p =$ .10, one-tailed).

Overmier and Papini (1986) also tested whether performance in retention tests was improved by increasing the level of motivation as Finger and Stein (1982) have suggested might be the case. Using a 2×2 factorial design they compared two pairs of sham and ablated groups of goldfish trained preoperatively and retrained postoperatively at two different motivational levels. These results are presented in Fig. 10.4B. The effect of level of motivation is clear and retention and relearning *performance* levels are significantly improved at the higher level of motivation. Unfortunately, the experiment did not include pre-to-post crossover *shifts* in motivational levels nor postasymptotic shifts in motivational levels (say, on day 10), and, thus, one cannot be certain whether the obtained results reflect differences in levels of learning and retention, per se, or merely differences in levels of activation of equal degrees of learning, retention, and relearning. It is the old "learning-versus-performance" question again. Nonetheless, the results are sufficiently suggestive that further research here is clearly warranted.

Further efforts to study factors that might result in sparing and/or recovery of avoidance behavior were made by Overmier and Papini (1985). The factors they manipulated here were (1) "momentum of lesions," again through serial ablation of hemispheres, and (2) whether or not the fish had *interoperative relearning* experience. In carrying out this experiment, the authors controlled for total amount of training before the final ablation; what differed is whether some of that training (10 sessions) took place between operations or before the first operation (overtraining). The design (a concatenation of variations on procedures F-3, K-1, L-1-2-3) is shown in Table 10.3. Their results were clear, simple, and disappointing. The first operation (sham or unilateral ablation) had no effect on retention or performance, and all groups performed identically at a high level (80%–90% avoidances). Following the second operation, the sham groups (S + S and S − S) continued to perform at the same high level. The ablated groups (S + B, U + U, U − U), however, all showed dramatic loss of the avoidance behavior; they did relearn to a degree, but to a level that was asymptotically less than that of the sham groups. Most importantly, the ablated groups did *not* differ from one another—although the serial group was better on a later reversal learning task (not shown in table). Thus, neither serial ablation nor interoperative retraining enhanced retention or relearning. It is, of course, possible that other interoperative training experiences might prove more successful in this regard, but it intuitively seems that training on the exact test procedures is the experience most likely to provide a basis for transfer of training.

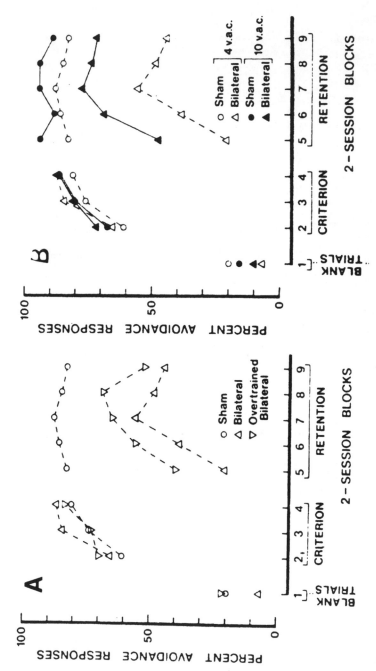

FIG. 10.4. Performances indexed by percentage avoidance of sham-operated and telencephalon-ablated ("bilateral") groups. Panel A shows effects of preablation overtraining on later retention and relearning. Panel B show the effects of level of motivation on retention and relearning. (After Overmier & Papini, 1986)

TABLE 10.3
Session Sequences to Test for Effects of Serial Ablations
With and Without Interoperative Training

Group	Criterion Sessions[*]	Overtrain Sessions	First Operation	Interoperative Training	Second Operation	Retrain
U + U	6	0	U_1	10	U_2	8
S + B	6	0	S	10	B	8
S + S	6	0	S	10	S	8
U − U	6	10	U_1	0	U_2	8
S − S	6	10	S	0	S	8

Note: U = unilateral ablation
       S = sham
       B = bilateral ablation
       + = had interoperative training
       − = without interoperative training
       [*] = mastery criterion of six successive sessions in which the percentage of avoidance equaled or exceeded 70%.

SUMMARY

Researchers have explored postablation deficits, sparing, and recovery of function in teleost fish with respect to two types of behaviors: reproductive and avoidance behaviors. Only in these two are dramatic deficits systematically seen following ablation of the telencephalon. In neither is the induced loss complete. In neither does prior relevant experience result in clinically significant increased sparing of functions or facilitate recovery of functions. Nor is recovery ever complete either. For both classes of behavior, there is a suggestion of a serial lesion effect, more so for reproductive behavior than avoidance behavior, but what evidence there is may be an artifact of total recovery time since the first lesion. When this is controlled for there is no evidence for a serial lesion effect.

Given that postablation behavior recovers at least partly, one wonders whether this postablation behavior is qualitatively similar to that seen in normal subjects. The data available from extinction tests of each suggest that the answer is "no" because the behaviors are distinctly less stable. Of course, this immediately then raises the question of the mechanisms mediating the observed recovery of behaviors. LeVere (1975, 1980) and Finger and Almli (1984) distinguished among a number of mechanisms. The present data do not permit any meaningful choices among these, except that the extinction data suggest that recovery of *function* may be an incorrect label for the recovery of behaviors seen here because the relative instability of the behaviors imply that the ablated fish now do function differently. As to whether active neuronal reorganization is the basis cannot be adjudicated properly. However, the fact that most forms of this process are time-based and the finding that "recovery" of the reproductive behaviors is time-based while recovery of avoidance behavior is not could imply that active neuronal reorganization is involved in the former but not the later. Recovered avoidance behavior may reflect rather behavioral compensatory shifts to a new but less efficient strategy.

Clearly, with respect to teleosts, more is unknown than known. The teleost model may yet be an interesting one for future research. The finding that level of motivation is a significant factor is of interest. Yet required are experiments to ascertain the locus of this effect of varying motivation; is it upon original learning, retention, relearning, or is it merely a performance factor? Future research also would be more likely to make significant contributions if a wider range of tasks were employed including, for example, spatial learning tasks (viz. Olton, 1985; Schenk & Morris, 1985) which are proving themselves so useful in assessing brain function in mammals. Perhaps we have been looking at too highly constrained behaviors and learning tasks to detect protective, or therapeutic effects or the serial lesion effect. To date the data base is simply too limited.

ACKNOWLEDGMENTS

Preparation of this manuscript was supported in part by grants from NICHD (HD-07151) and the University of Minnesota to the Center for Research in Learning, Perception, and Cognition.

REFERENCES

Aronson, L. R. (1948). Problems in the behavior and physiology of a species of African mouth-breeding fish. *Transactions of the New York Academy of Sciences, 11*, 33–42.

Aronson, L. R. (1981). Evolution of telencephalic function in lower vertebrates. In P. R. Laming (Ed.), *Brain mechanisms of behavior in lower vertebrates* (pp. 33–58). Cambridge, England: Cambridge University Press.

Bernstein, J. J. (1961a). Loss of hue discrimination in forebrain ablated fish. *Experimental Neurology, 3*, 1–17.

Bernstein, J. J. (1961b). Brightness discrimination following forebrain ablation in fish. *Experimental Neurology, 3*, 297–306.

Bernstein, J. J. (1962). Role of the telencephalon in color vision of fish. *Experimental Neurology, 6*, 173–185.

Bernstein, J. J. (1967). The regenerative capacity of the telencephalon of the goldfish and rat. *Experimental Neurology, 17*, 44–56.

Bernstein, J. J. (1970). Anatomy and physiology of the central nervous system. In W. S. Hoar & D. J. Randall (Eds.), *Fish physiology* (Vol. 4, pp. 1–90). New York: Academic Press.

Bitterman, M. R. (1975). The comparative analysis of learning. *Science, 188*, 699–709.

Colyer, S. W., & Jenkins, C. (1976). Pheromonal control of aggressive displays in Siamese fighting fish (*Betta splendens*). *Perceptual & Motor Skills, 42*, 47–54.

Davis, R. E., & Kassel, J. (1983). Behavioral functions of the teleostean telencephalon. In R. E. Davis & R. G. Northcutt (Eds.), *Fish neurobiology: Vol. 2. Higher brain areas and functions* (pp. 237–259). Ann Arbor: University of Michigan Press.

Davis, R. E., Kassel, J., & Schwagmeyer, P. (1976). Telencephalic lesions and behavior in the teleost, *Macropodus opercularis*: Reproduction, startle reaction, and operant behavior in the male. *Behavioral Biology, 18,* 165–177.

Davis, R. E., & Schlumpf, B. E. (1983). Circumvention of extra retinal photoresponses in assessing recovery of vision following optic nerve crush in goldfish. *Behavioral Brain Research, 7,* 65–79.

Desmoulins, A. (1825). *Anatomie des systemes nerveux des animaux vertebres appliqué à la physiologie et à la zoologie.* Paris: Mequignon–Marvis.

Dewsbury, D. A., & Bernstein, J. J. (1969). Role of the telencephalon in performance of conditioned avoidance responses by goldfish. *Experimental Neurology, 23,* 445–456.

Edwards, D. L., & Grafstein, B. (1983). Intraocular tetrodotoxin in goldfish optic nerve regeneration. *Brain Research, 269,* 1–14.

Finger, S., & Almli, C. R. (1984). Brain damage and neuroplasticity: Mechanisms of recovery or development? *Brain Research Reviews, 10,* 177–186.

Finger, S., & Stein, D. G. (1982). *Brain damage and recovery: Research and clinical perspectives.* New York: Academic Press.

Finger, S., Walbran, B., & Stein, D. (1973). Brain damage and behavioral recovery: Serial lesion phenomena. *Brain Research, 63,* 1–18.

Flood, N. B., Overmier, J. B., & Savage, G. E. (1976). The teleost telencephalon and learning: An interpretive review of data and hypotheses. *Physiology and Behavior, 16,* 783–798.

Giulian, D. (1984). Target regulation of protein biosynthesis in retinal ganglion cells during regeneration of the goldfish visual system. *Brain Research, 296,* 198–201.

Hainsworth, F. R., Overmier, J. B., & Snowdon, C. T. (1967). Specific and permanent deficits in instrumental avoidance responding following forebrain ablation in the goldfish. *Journal of Comparative & Physiological Psychology, 63,* 111–116.

Healey, E. G. (1957). The nervous system. In M. E. Brown (Ed.), *The physiology of fishes* (Vol. 2, pp. 1–119). New York: Academic Press.

Hodos, W., & Campbell, C. B. G. (1969). *Scala naturae:* Why there is no theory in comparative psychology. *Psychological Review, 76,* 337–350.

Hollis, K. L., & Overmier, J. B. (1978). The function of the teleost telencephalon in behavior: A reinforcement mediator. In D. I. Mostofsky (Ed.), *The behavior of fish and other aquatic animals* (pp. 137–195). New York: Academic Press.

Horner, J. L., Longo, N., & Bitterman, M. R. (1961). A shuttlebox for the fish and a control circuit of general applicability. *American Journal of Psychology, 74,* 114–120.

Jackson, H. (1873). Lectures on the diagnosis of tumors of the brain. II. *Medical Times Gazette, 2,* 195–197.

Janzen, W. (1933). Untersuchungen über Grosshirnfunktionen des Goldfisches (*Carassius auratus*). *Zoologische Jahrbucher abteilung fur Allgemeine Zoologie und Physiologie der Tiere, 52,* 591–628.

Kaplan, H., & Aronson, L. R. (1967). Effect of forebrain ablation on the performance of conditioned avoidance response in the teleost fish, *Tilapia h. macrocephala. Animal Behaviour, 15,* 438–448.

Kassel, J., & Davis, R. (1977). Recovery of function following simultaneous and serial telencephalon ablation in the teleost, *macropodus opercularis. Behavioral Biology, 21,* 489–499.

Kassel, J., Davis, R. E., & Schwagmeyer, P. (1976). Telencephalic lesions and behavior in the teleost, *Macropodus opercularis:* further analysis of reproductive and operant behavior in the male. *Behavioral Biology, 18,* 179–188.

Kimble, G. A. (1961). *Hilgard and Marquis' conditioning and learning.* New York: Appleton.

Kirsche, W. (1965). Regenerative Vorgange in Gehirn und Ruckenmark. *Ergebnisse der Anatomie und Entwicklungsgesch, 38,* 143–153.

Kleerekoper, H. (1969). *Olfaction in fishes.* Bloomington, IN: Indiana University Press.

Kohsaka, S. (1982). Dissociation of enhanced ornithine decarboxylase activity and optic nerve regeneration in goldfish. *Developmental Brain Research, 4,* 149–156.

Kovacevic, N. S. (1978). Fish avoidance with tactile reinforcement. *Bolletino di Zoologia, 45,* 41–44.

Koyama, Y., Satou, M., Oka, Y., & Ueda, K. (1984). Involvement of the telencephalis hemispheres and the preoptic area in sexual behavior of the male goldfish, carassius auratus: A brain-lesion study. *Behavioral & Neural Biology, 40,* 70–86.

Kyle, A. L., & Peter, R. E. (1982). Effects of forebrain lesions on spawning behaviour in the male goldfish. *Physiology & Behavior, 28,* 1103–1109.

Laming, P. R. (1981a). *Brain mechanisms of behaviour in lower vertebrates.* Cambridge, England: Cambridge University Press.

Laming, P. R. (1981b). An introduction to the functional anatomy of the brains of fish and amphibians. In P. R. Laming (Ed.), *Brain mechanisms of behavior in lower vertebrates* (pp. 7–32). Cambridge, England: Cambridge University Press.

Lashley, K. S. (1929). *Brain mechanisms and intelligence.* Chicago: University of Chicago Press.

Leitner, D. S., Francis, A., & Gazzaniga, M. S. (1982). Optic nerve regeneration in goldfish under light deprivation. *Brain Research Bulletin, 8,* 105–107.

LeVere, T. E. (1975). Neural stability, sparing, and behavioral recovery following brain damage. *Psychological Review, 82,* 344–358.

LeVere, T. E. (1980). Recovery of function after brain damage: Theory of the behavioral deficit. *Physiological Psychology, 8,* 297–308.

Lubow, R. E., & Moore, A. U. (1959). Latent inhibition: The effect of non-reinforced preexposure to the conditioned stimulus. *Journal of Comparative & Physiological Psychology, 52,* 415–419.

Maron, K. (1963). Endbrain regeneration in *Lebistes reticulatus. Folia Biologica, 11,* 3–10.

May, M. A. (1948). Experimentally acquired drives. *Journal of Experimental Psychology, 38,* 66–77.

Meader, R. G. (1939). Notes on the functions of the forebrain in teleosts. *Zoologica, 24,* 11–14.

Meyer, D. R., & Meyer, P. M. (1977). Dynamics and bases of recoveries of functions after injuries to the cerebral cortex. *Psychological Psychology, 5,* 133–165.

Nieuwenhuys, R. (1967). The interpretation of the cell masses in the teleostean forebrain. In R. Hassler & H. Stephan (Eds.), *Evolution of the forebrain* (pp. 32–40). New York: Plenum.

Noble, G. K. (1939). Neural basis of social behavior in vertebrates. *The Collecting Net, 14,* 121–124.

Noble, G. K., & Borne, R. (1941). The effect of forebrain lesions on the sexual and fighting behavior of *Betta splendens* and other fishes. *The Anatomical Record, 79*(Suppl. No. 138), 49.

Northcutt, R. G., & Bradford, M. R. (1980). New observations on the organization and evolution of the telencephalon of actinopterygian fishes. In S. O. E. Ebbesson (Ed.), *Comparative neurology of the telencephalon* (pp. 41–98). New York: Plenum.

Northmore, D. P. (1981). Visual localization after rearrangement of retinotectal maps in fish. *Nature, 293,* 142–144.

Olton, D. S. (1985). Memory: Neuropsychological and ethophysiological approaches to its classification. In L. G. Nilsson & T. Archer (Eds.), *Perspectives on learning and memory* (pp. 95–113). Hillsdale, NJ: Lawrence Erlbaum Associates.

Overmier, J. B., & Curnow, P. G. (1969). Classical conditioning, pseudoconditioning, and sensitization in "normal" and forebrainless goldfish. *Journal of Comparative & Physiological Psychology, 68,* 193–198.

Overmier, J. B., & Gross, D. M. (1972). Quantitative study of nest building activity of the East African mouthbreeding fish, *Tilapia mossambica. Zeitschrift für Tierpsychologie, 31,* 326–329.

Overmier, J. B., & Gross, D. M. (1974). Effects of telencephalic ablation upon nestbuilding and avoidance behavior in East African mouthbreeding fish, *Tilapia mossambica. Behavioral Biology, 12,* 211–222.

Overmier, J. B., & Hollis, K. L. (1983). Teleostean telencephalon in learning. In R. E. Davis & G. Northcutt (Eds.), *Fish neurobiology, Vol. 2: Higher brain areas and functions* (pp. 265–278). Ann Arbor: University of Michigan.

Overmier, J. B., & Papini, M. (1985). Serial ablations of the telencephalon and avoidance learning by goldfish (*Carassius auratus*). *Behavioral Neuroscience, 99,* 509–520.

Overmier, J. B., & Papini, M. (1986). Factors modulating the effects of teleost telencephalon ablation on retention, relearning, and extinction of instrumental avoidance behavior. *Behavioral Neuroscience, 100,* 190–199.

Overmier, J. B., & Savage, G. E. (1974). Effects of telencephalic ablation on trace classical conditioning of heart rate in goldfish. *Experimental Neurology, 42,* 339–346.

Pflugfelder, O. (1965). Reparative und regenerative prozesse nach partieller Zerstorung von Fischgehirnen. *Zoologische Jahrbucher Abteilung fur Allgemeine Zoologie und Physiologie der Tiere, 71,* 301–312.

Prosser, C. L., & Brown, F. A. (1961). *Comparative animal physiology.* Philadelphia: Saunders.

Savage, G. E. (1980). The fish telencephalon and its relation to learning. In S. O. E. Ebbesson (Ed.), *Comparative neurology of the telencephalon* (pp. 129–174). New York: Plenum.

Savage, G. E. (1969a). Telencephalic lesions and avoidance behaviour in the goldfish (*Carassius auratus*). *Animal Behaviour, 17,* 362–373.

Savage, G. E. (1969b). Some preliminary observations on the role of the telencephalon in food-reinforced behaviour in the goldfish, *Carassius auratus. Animal Behaviour, 17,* 760–772.

Scalia, R., & Ebbesson, S. O. E. (1971). The central projections of the olfactory bulb in a teleost (*Gymnothorax funebris*). *Brain, Behavior, & Evolution, 4,* 376–399.

Schenk, F., & Morris, R. G. M. (1985). Dissociation between components of spatial memory in rats after recovery from the effects of retrohippocampal lesions. *Experimental Brain Research, 58,* 11–28.

Schnitzlein, H. N. (1968). Introductory remarks on the telencephalon of fish. In D. Ingle (Ed.), *The central nervous system and fish behavior* (pp. 97–100). Chicago: University of Chicago Press.

Schwagmeyer, P., Davis, R. E., & Kassel, J. (1977). Telencephalic lesions and behavior in the teleost *Macropodus opercularis:* Effects of telencephalon and olfactory bulb ablation on sparing and foamnest building. *Behavioral Biology, 20,* 463–470.

Segaar, J. (1965). Behavioral aspects of degeneration and regeneration in fish brain: A comparison with higher vertebrates. *Progress in Brain Research, 14,* 143–231.

Stacey, N. E., & Kyle, A. L. (1983). Effects of olfactory tract lesions on sexual and feeding behavior in the goldfish. *Physiology & Behavior, 30,* 621–628.

Woodard, W. T., & Bitterman, M. R. (1971). Classical conditioning of goldfish in the shuttlebox. *Behavior Research Methods & Instrumentation, 3,* 193–194.

Yolen, N. M., & Hodos, W. (1976). Behavioral correlates of "tectal compression" in goldfish: I. Intensity and pattern discrimination. *Brain, Behavior, & Evolution, 13,* 451–467.

11

The Use of Overtraining in Striate/Extrastriate Lesion Deficit Analysis

Jeannette P. Ward
Department of Psychology
Memphis State University

Behavioral analysis of visual capacity following ablation of brain subdivisions has served to illuminate the functional organization of the visual system in relation to visually guided behavior for the past 100 years (Munk, 1881/1960). The method continues to be a principal route by which the structure and function of brain can be meaningfully related to visually guided behavior (e.g., Frommer, 1978; Glassman, 1978; Meyer, 1958). For most of this century, the design of behavioral studies and the interpretation of results have been based on the assumption that the neurons of adult mammalian organisms have no power of regeneration. This has resulted in a more or less static view of brain deficits with recovery of function attributed to compensation by spared tissue (Steele Russell, 1982).

Much of the visual lesion deficit analysis research has been conducted and interpreted from this more static perspective of brain. In these studies, preoperative training has often been incorporated into the design of research to permit within subject comparison because the number of subjects was small or because placement of identical lesions was not certain. Without benefit of preoperative comparison, a deficit in visually guided behavior is usually termed sensory or perceptual when the deficit is profound and criterion performance not achieved; when acquisition proceeds slowly for brain lesioned subjects as compared with intact subjects but the discrimination test is finally mastered, a deficit in learning ability is inferred. With preoperative training as a basis for comparison, the possibilities of behavioral analysis are expanded to include: (1) Immediate recognition of the preoperatively trained stimuli after ablation, that is, evidence for retention of function, and (2) No recognition after surgery but relearning of the same discrimination, that is, evidence for compensation or recovery of function. Thus, while postoperative training and testing gives information about sensory/perceptual and learning capacities retained, the use of preoperative training permits the assessment of the effects of brain damage on pre-existing visual discrimination habits.

Karl Lashley (1920) was the first to employ preoperative overtraining in order to investigate the possible effect of habit on brain organization. He had discovered that ablation of occipital cortex resulted in loss of a simple brightness discrimination. To determine if increased practice might result in a reorganization of the habit that would be resistant to cortical insult, Lashley (1921) employed preoperative overtraining. In this study, preoperatively trained and overtrained rats alike lost the brightness discrimination following ablation of visual cortex but re-established the discrimination with about the same amount of training as required prior to surgery. Despite the failure of this early manipulation of training to produce a behaviorally detectable reorganization of brain function, this and a later report (Lashley, 1935) composed the foundation for continuing study of the neural mediation of brightness discrimination as a function of lesion extent and training variables.

Lashley was also one of the founders of another literature, the study of what he called "detail vision," that is, epicritic visual function employed in the discrimination of patterns or forms (Lashley, 1939; Lashley & Frank, 1934). Integration of these two literatures is difficult because of somewhat different priorities and methodologies. For example, in the study of detail vision a principal concern has been the cytoarchitectonic subdivisions of brain involved in the perception and learning of rather complex visual stimuli. By comparison, the brightness discrimination literature has had as a principal concern identification of experiential factors associated with memory and performance of the discrimination. The emphases of the two areas may have been conditioned by early research that found capacity for simple brightness discriminations retained after large occipital lesions (Lashley, 1921, 1935) whereas capacity for the discrimination of form and pattern was lost (Kluver, 1942; Lashley & Frank, 1934). Still, the manipulation of training variables has had a role in both research areas. In the pages that follow, evidence is developed to show that the use of overtraining in the study of pattern and of brightness discriminations has contributed insights to the organization of visual function important to the understanding of loss, preservation, and recovery of visual function following damage to neocortex.

Though different in kind, the phenomena described by pattern and brightness studies may have in common neural mediation by the visual pathway to neocortex that parallels the classic geniculostriate system, that is, the tectocortical system. The possible contribution of this system to retention and recovery of visual function after damage to striate cortex can best be assessed after consideration of some facts about this second visual projection to neocortex.

TECTOCORTICAL STRUCTURE
AND FUNCTION

The fact of an anatomical pathway for visual impulses originating in the upper layers of the superior colliculi and relaying through the pulvinar nucleus of the thalamus to extrastriate posterior neocortex has been generally known for over 15 years (Abplanalp, 1970; Benevento & Fallon, 1975; Graham, 1977; Harting, Hall, & Diamond, 1972; Hughes, 1977; Lin & Kaas, 1979). The existence of a second pathway by which visual impulses ascend to posterior neocortex complicates interpretation of all previous studies of destriate animals since residual visual function may now be attributed either to the superior colliculi per se or to the tectocortical pathway of which the colliculi are a part.

Evidence from study of the destriate tree shrew (Tupaia glis) does, however, permit conclusions about the extent to which visually guided behavior is mediated by the superior colliculi alone or is dependent on the projection of this structure to neocortex. In the tree shrew the entire pulvinar nucleus receives a projection from the superior colliculus and in turn projects to lateral and posterior cortex adjacent to striate cortex. The striate and extrastriate projection systems are largely nonoverlapping in this species so that lesions in striate cortex result in retrograde degeneration in the dorsal lateral geniculate nucleus whereas lesions in extrastriate cortex result in corresponding degeneration in the pulvinar nucleus (Harting et al., 1972).

The tree shrew was selected for study because of its phylogenetic position as a presumed protoprimate and for its unique visual system that pairs extremely large superior colliculi with a cytoarchitectonically well-developed geniculostriate system as shown in Fig. 11.1. Early reports emphasized the surprising amount of visual function remaining to destriate tree shrews (Snyder & Diamond, 1968; Snyder, Hall, & Diamond, 1966). Subsequently, however, the ultimate dependence of residual visual capacity of destriate tree shrews on the tectocortical system as opposed to the superior colliculi alone was demonstrated by Ward and Masterton (1970). In this study three tree shrews suffered complete retrograde degeneration of neurons in both the dorsal lateral geniculate and pulvinar nuclei of the thalamus consequent to ablation of posterior neocortex. In a two-choice visual discrimination apparatus, these animals were able to discriminate between test stimuli that differed with respect to luminous flux but performed at chance when this cue was no longer available. The loss of visual capacity was comparable with that of Kluver's (1942) monkeys following occipital lobectomies or the profound loss of visual pattern discrimination capacity recently reported for the domestic cat with extensive cortical damage involving both striate and extrastriate systems (Antonini, Berlucchi, & Sprague, 1985).

In the study of Ward and Masterton (1970), tree shrews that had complete destruction of the geniculostriate system alone were still capable of brightness

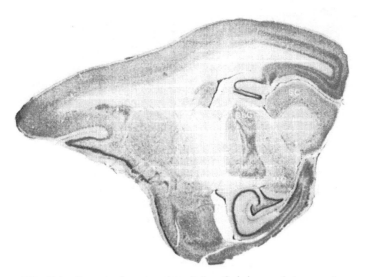

FIG. 11.1.   Parasagittal section through lateral thalamus of the tree shrew (*Tupaia glis*) showing principal structures of the visual system: DLG, dorsal lateral geniculate of the thalamus; Pul, pulvinar nucleus of the thalamus; SC, superior colliculus. Striate cortex is visible immediately above the superior colliculus and the ventral subdivision (unlabeled) of the lateral geniculate nucleus is the structure seen immediately anterior to (to the left of) DLG.

discrimination when stimuli were equated for luminous flux. Because extrastriate cortex was shown to be critical to visually guided discrimination in the absence of striate cortex, the question arose as to what type of visual capacity remained to the destriate tree shrew with the tectocortical system essentially preserved.

Certainly the pattern vision mediated by extrastriate cortex alone may be expected to be somewhat different than that of intact subjects. Ward, Frank, and Moss (1975) found that destriate tree shrews had a deficit in epicritic vision that was more specific to small area than to fineness of extended pattern and also reported that a decrease in stimulus display area was compensated by an increase in stripe width and a decrease in stripe width compensated by an increase in stimulus area. The phenomenon was reliable across many values of stripe width and area. These results suggest that the extrastriate system of the tree shrew has as one mode of operation the ability to summate information about area and contour. Trevarthen (1968) has proposed that visual function may be organized in two functional systems subserving two different types of visual behavior: (1) a focal visual system related to binocular and epicritic functions and (2) an ambient system important to the organism in action, that is, concerned with movement about the broad surfaces and extended patterns of the environment.

It may be that the geniculostriate system of tree shrew approximates Trevarthen's focal visual system whereas the extrastriate system processes information about large, patterned surfaces of the surround as a frame for the central content of acute vision.

Functional Significance of Visual Cortex

Behavioral study of the visual function of neocortical subdivisions in the lesser bushbaby (*Galago senegalensis*) was initiated in order to explore the functions of striate and extrastriate subdivisions in a species that might serve as a bridge, both phyletically and neuroanatomically, between the tree shrew and the anthropoid primates. The bushbaby is a prosimian similar, perhaps identical, to the earliest true primates (Napier & Napier, 1967). The brain of the bushbaby is intermediate in anatomical complexity between that of tree shrew and anthropoid primates (Fig. 11.2).

Effects of Striate Cortex Lesions.   Ablation of occipital cortex in the lesser bushbaby results in profound and enduring disruption of visually guided behavior (Atencio, Diamond, & Ward, 1975; Caldwell & Ward, 1982). Bushbabies with complete lesions of striate cortex retained capacity to discriminate extended area patterns of horizontal and vertical stripes but were unable to acquire the discrimination of two-dimensional forms (Atencio et al., 1975). It is useful to make the distinction between extended area stripes as patterns and restricted area bounded figures against a contrasting ground as forms, as suggested by Zusne (1970), because cortical lesions often differentially affect the discrimination of these two types of stimuli.

In a study by Caldwell and Ward (1982), bushbabies were evaluated after occipital lobectomy. One group had striate lesions similar to those of the Atencio et al. (1975) study, whereas lesions of a second destriate group included peristriate cortex. The principal differences in visual capacities for these groups were related to loss or retention of this lateral and ventral peristriate cortex. Destriate subjects that retained peristriate cortex retained pattern vision, whereas those without this area preserved did not. A similar critical role for extrastriate cortex of destriate *Macaca* has been proposed by Pasik, Pasik, Schilder, and Wininger (1973) and Campbell, Butter, and Leiby (1984). No destriate subject could master a form discrimination.

At this point the evidence for tree shrews and bushbabies may be compared. The larger lesion bushbabies of Caldwell and Ward (1982) performed like tree shrews after complete loss of both geniculostriate and tectocortical systems (Ward & Masterton, 1970) in that both species retained only the capacity for luminous flux discrimination. By contrast, the smaller lesion bushbabies of Caldwell and Ward (1982) and Atencio et al. (1975), and tree shrews with

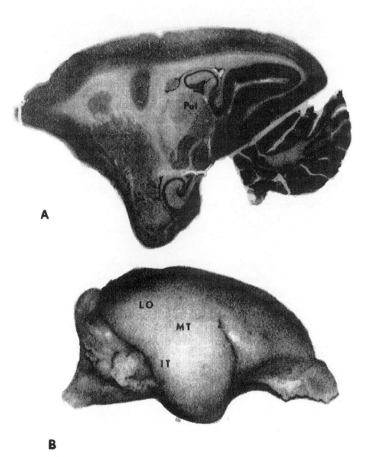

A

B

FIG. 11.2.   (A) Parasagittal section through the lateral thalamus of the lesser bushbaby (*Galago senegalensis*) showing some principal structures of the visual system. (Pul, pulvinar nucleus of the thalamus; MG, medial geniculate nucleus of the thalamus). For this species, the pulvinar is seen to be large with at least two subdivisions. The dorsal lateral geniculate nucleus is the elongated, striped structure immediately below the pulvinar and anterior to (to the left of) the medial geniculate nucleus. Striate cortex of the calcarine fissure and occipital lobe is visible in the upper right of the figure. (B) 45° view of the surface of one hemisphere of the lesser bushbaby brain showing general location of neocortical areas referred to in text: LO, lateral occipital; MT, middle temporal; IT, inferotemporal.

218

some tectocortical system remaining gave evidence of pattern vision. Thus, in bushbaby and tree shrew extrastriate cortex is necessary to learned pattern discrimination in the absence of the geniculostriate system.

Manipulation of preoperative training as a variable for analysis has not been an important feature of the studies which we have discussed or of earlier studies. It is difficult to discern from the literature consistent differences in form or pattern discrimination that might be attributed to preoperative training because studies of destriate subjects have rarely been designed for the analysis of preoperative training effects (however, see Dru, Walker, & Walker, 1975; Horel, Bettinger, Royce, & Meyer, 1966; Meyer, 1958; Spear & Barbas, 1975). The value of this type of analysis is illustrated subsequently.

Some Functions of Extrastriate Cortex

In the tree shrew, the pulvinar nucleus of the thalamus is a homogeneous unit and its projection field in extrastriate cortex is essentially undivided (Harting et al., 1972). Primates have a large and complex pulvinar with multiple subdivisions all of which are not equally engaged with the tectocortical pathway. Similarly, in primates subdivisions of posterior cortex proliferate and extrastriate cortex becomes a collective of cortices related to visual function by virtue of anatomical connection with the geniculostriate and/or tectocortical systems (Diamond, Fitzpatrick, & Sprague, 1985; Raczkowski & Diamond, 1980, 1981; Weller & Kaas, 1982). The inferotemporal, peristriate, and middle temporal cortices are three regions of extrastriate cortex that are terminals for the tectocortical pathway in bushbaby.

Inferotemporal Cortex. Study of the visual functions of the temporal lobe in the Rhesus monkey began with the report of "psychic blindness" following temporal lobectomy (Kluver & Bucy, 1939). The deficit has been demonstrated to be specific to vision, as opposed to other sense modalities, to occur in the absence of basic sensory deficit, to be specific to the learning of difficult visual stimuli, and to be modified by preoperative overtraining. The deficit is contingent on damage to the inferior temporal (IT) neocortex (for literature review, see Dean, 1982; Gross, 1973a, 1973b; Mishkin, 1972).

In the interest of exploring the correspondence between extrastriate visual function in bushbaby, compared with Rhesus monkey, a study was made of the visual capacity of bushbabies after ablation of IT cortex (Atencio et al., 1975). Two of the several stimulus sets employed in this study are shown in Fig. 11.3 and 11.4. The subjects were trained first with large, then medium, then small versions of the basic form stimuli shown in Fig. 11.3. The stimuli shown in Fig. 11.4 were used to assess the capacity for visual search. In this test the original form discrimination was maintained but for every trial each member of the pair was randomly assigned a position in one of the four corners of the display card.

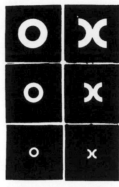

SUBJECT	ABLATION	TRIALS TO CRITERION
237	INTACT	530
	IT	360
241	INTACT	480
	IT	480
239	INTACT	280
	IT	330
185	IT	1500
186	IT	3120
168	LO	4300
166	LO	3130

FIG. 11.3.   Basic stimulus set used for form discrimination training with performance record as trials to criterion for set as a function of type of lesion. All subjects were first trained on the large, then medium, then small, versions of the form discrimination. Note that deficit was most severe for subjects with lateral occipital cortex removed bilaterally (LO), although lesions of inferotemporal cortex (IT) also retarded acquisition of the discrimination, especially in the absence of preoperative training.

Although overtraining of the preoperatively trained bushbabies was not specifically intended, the nature of these tests required repeated testing on the original form discrimination. One IT subject had 1,030 and the other 690 preoperative form training trials. The subjects did not recognize the form stimuli after surgery but did relearn the discrimination with about the same amount of training required initially. This represents a savings, if compared with postoperative scores of subjects not trained postoperatively (Fig. 11.3). All IT subjects achieved criterion on the visual search test. Three required extended training and preoperative overtraining also may have been helpful to this discrimination as the number of trials required was greater for subjects not trained prior to surgery (Fig. 11.4).

Lateral Occipital Lesions.   The lateral occipital (LO) lesion was employed initially for the bushbaby as a control lesion (Atencio et al., 1975) patterned after the lateral striate (LS) lesion often used in studies of Rhesus monkey. Unlike the monkey LS lesion, LO lesions of the bushbaby include both lateral striate and adjacent peristriate cortex.

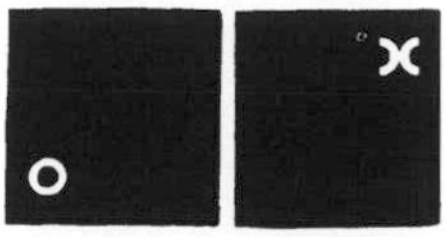

SUBJECT	ABLATION	TRIALS TO CRITERION
237	INTACT	20
	IT	50
241	INTACT	40
	IT	360
185	IT	760
186	IT	470
168	LO	500*
166	LO	1000*
MT-1	MT	80
MT-2	MT	140
MT-3	MT	20

FIG. 11.4. Example of stimuli used for visual search test and performance of the lesser bushbaby (G. *senegalensis*) as a function of type of neocortical lesion. Note that both subjects with lateral occipital (LO) lesions were not able to perform the discrimination; their performance was at chance for the number of trials shown. Subject 168 was discontinued after 500 trials of chance performance, due to refusal to attempt this task further.

*FAILED TO ACHIEVE CRITERION

In the Atencio et al. (1975) study, LO bushbabies were given the same discrimination tests postoperatively as the IT subjects discussed herein. These subjects required nine times the average trials of intact bushbabies to acquire the form discrimination (see Fig. 11.3). Although all other subjects in this study showed strong positive transfer from the large to the medium and small version of the form, the LO bushbabies did not. It required many more trials for them to master the medium than the large forms and again more trials for the small than the medium sized stimuli. LO bushbabies were completely unable to master the visual search test. They performed at a chance level when the forms they had discriminated successfully for hundreds of trials in the center of the stimulus cards appeared a short distance away in one of the four corner positions. In summary, the animals had great difficulty in learning a form discrimination, were unable to recognize forms when size was reduced, and were unable to maintain discrimination of forms whose position in space was altered. It is unlikely that the large deficit in visual discrimination was due solely to the small scotoma involving only 10 degrees of the lower central visual field (Jon Kaas, personal communication). The LO bushbabies were indistinguishable in performance from intact subjects in measured acuity and in food reaching accuracy.

In order to determine whether the LO deficit in bushbabies was indeed a form-learning deficit rather than a sensory deficit, Marcotte and Ward (1980) adopted the preoperative overtraining paradigm used to demonstrate this distinction for IT monkeys (Chow & Survis, 1958; Orbach & Fantz, 1958). Prior to any surgical procedure, an acuity estimate was obtained for each animal. Animals were then trained to criterion and overtrained for 300 trials on a form discrimination; additional subjects (O-OS) yoked to subjects in the form discrimination condition were trained for an equal number of trials on patterned stripes with area and position on the stimulus cards equivalent to that of the form stimuli. Form-trained subjects (O-OF) and their yoked controls (O-OS) received bilateral LO lesions. Other subjects pretrained on the form discrimination (I-OF) underwent no surgical procedures but remained in their home cages without additional training during the 6-week postoperative recovery period. All subjects were reintroduced to the two-choice apparatus by once again being tested for minimal separable acuities. Next a form discrimination problem, novel for all subjects, was given. This was followed by a second form discrimination problem that was a recognition or relearning test for the intact (I-OF) and LO bushbabies trained on form prior to surgery (O-OF) but was a second novel form problem for the yoked LO bushbabies preoperatively trained on equivalent area stripe patterns (O-OS).

The results of preoperative discrimination training are shown in Table 11.1. Postoperative training and testing scores are given in Table 11.2. Visual acuity estimates were unchanged from pre- to postoperative testing for all subjects. The main result of this study was that preoperative overtraining on a specific form discrimination problem protected the LO bushbabies from deficit in discrimination of that stimulus pair whereas a pronounced deficit in learning the discrimination of novel form pairs remained. Recognition of familiar stimuli was preserved whereas learning about new forms was impaired dramatically.

TABLE 11.1
Relative Efficiency of Performance
(as Percentage Correct) of Intact Bushbabies
in Training and Overtraining on Either a Form
Discrimination or an Equivalent Limited Area
Stripe Discrimination

Subjects & Stimuli	Training	Overtraining
Form		
100	71%	100%
101	68%	100%
300	71%	96%
301	65%	85%
302	66%	93%
Limited Area Stripes		
200	96%	100%
201	88%	98%

TABLE 11.2

Postoperative Form Discrimination Performance of Intact and Lateral Occipital
Lesion Bushbabies With and Without Training on Original Forms as Trials
and Errors to Criterion and as Percentage Correct

	Novel Form			Original Form		
	Trials	Errors	% Correct	Trials	Errors	% Correct
Subject & Stimuli						
Pretrained on Form						
I-OF						
100	100	7	93%	60	0	100%
101	100	9	91%	60	0	100%
O-OF						
300	560	217	61%	140	11	92%
301	460	104	77%	60	0	100%
302	240	44	82%	60	0	100%
Not Pretrained on Form						
O-OS						
200	1120	414	63%	540	178	67%
201	820	236	71%	740	269	64%

Middle Temporal Lesions. The middle temporal (MT) area of primates is
an anatomically and electrophysiologically distinct subdivision of extrastriate
visual cortex (Allman & Kaas, 1971; Allman, Kaas, & Lane, 1973; Montero,
1980; Spatz, 1977; Symonds & Kaas, 1978). This area has a first order representation of the contralateral visual hemifield with expansion of central field representation comparable with that of striate cortex. Although the MT area of the
lesser bushbaby has many cortical and subcortical afferent and efferent connections, as yet incompletely described, a principal relationship is a reciprocal one
with striate cortex. The neurons of MT have larger receptive fields than those of
striate cortex and are particularly responsive to directionally coded movement.
Some behavioral evidence has indicated that this area may be important to
visual capacities involving spatial or movement analysis (Keys, 1981; Wilson,
Keys, & Johnston, 1979). Keys (1981), however, suggested that the visual
deficits of his subjects may have been due to undercutting of fibers of passage to
LO cortex.

Silver, Caldwell, and Ward (1975) tested bushbabies with bilateral lesions of
MT cortex on the same tests given to IT and LO subjects as we have discussed.
The MT subjects were only trained and tested after surgery with performance
compared with that of intact bushbabies. The MT subjects were not different
than intact bushbabies in food retrieval, acuity, form learning, or the visual
search test. As this test involves changing spatial relations between figure and
ground from trial to trial, it was expected that bushbabies with MT lesions would

be deficient. The undisturbed performance of MT subjects stands in contrast to the total inability of LO lesion subjects to perform the visual search test and the performance deficit of IT subjects that was attenuated by preoperative overtraining.

Overview of Detail Vision Studies

The studies of striate and extrastriate cortex in tree shrew and bushbaby suggest a model of neural mediation of visual function wherein two parallel pathways from the eye proceed to adjacent and interconnected regions of the posterior neocortex and function together in the intact subject in support of normal visual function. Evidence indicates that striate cortex is especially important to epicritic and focal vision whereas peristriate cortex is a secondary system organized for the processing of contours over extended visual fields. The use of preoperative overtraining and ablation of LO cortex has shown that the cortical areas representing the center of gaze at the interface of these two systems has a special role in the encoding of form discriminations but is not necessary to form recognition. The LO deficit may be due to disruption of a visuomotor capacity important to a special use of central vision in the attentive inspection and encoding of novel form stimuli. It is proposed that this sensorimotor capacity is critical to the perceptual encoding of novel stimulus contours but less important once a discrimination has been acquired. The facilitating effect of stimulus familiarity in peripheral field discrimination is not a unique result; Bender and Furlow (1945) reported that familiar stimuli were recognized in peripheral visual fields when novel stimuli were not.

LO cortex may incorporate neural connections for special eye movements employed in inspection and encoding of behaviorally relevant figure contours. In the bushbaby many areas of the posterior neocortex project subcortically to the superior colliculus, a structure that has an important role in the control of eye movements. There is, however, an especially notable projection from the boundary regions of striate and peristriate cortex that subserve central vision, that is, the locus of the LO lesion (See, e.g., Fig. 6.19, Galago 1321L in Diamond, 1982, p. 131).

Preoperative overtraining facilitates the performance of IT lesion bushbabies in both visual search and form discrimination. The effect of preoperative overtraining on form discrimination is, however, different for IT than LO lesion subjects. Although LO lesion subjects recognize the preoperatively overtrained form pair immediately, IT lesion subjects must relearn the discrimination and do so with about the same amount of training as required initially. This suggests that the IT deficit may reflect a disruption of associative functions, for example, the coding of reward contingencies, as has been previously suggested for IT lesion monkeys by Gross (1973a). Test of this hypothesis could be accomplished by evaluating IT bushbabies in tasks that selectively affect IT lesion monkeys, such as concurrent discrimination learning, interpolated problems, sensitivity to shock punishment and partial reinforcement. Sanford and Ward (1986) have shown that concurrent visual discrimination learning is well within the capacity of intact bushbabies.

OVERTRAINING IN BRIGHTNESS DISCRIMINATION

Lashley's (1921) early finding that a learned brightness discrimination is not retained after bilateral removal of striate cortex but can be re-established with about the same amount of training has stood the test of time and replication (Barbas & Spear, 1976; Ghiselli, 1938; Hamilton & Treichler, 1968; Lashley, 1935; Thompson, 1960). In addition, the question of whether the re-establishment of the discrimination is due to new learning, that is, compensation by spared tissue, or to reaccess of traces of the original learning has generated a large literature. Meyer (1984) has maintained that memory engrams are established immediately and permanently and performance deficit after brain damage is essentially a memory access problem. His evidence that dl-amphetamine facilitates performance in retention testing but not in original learning supports this view (Braun, Meyer, & Meyer, 1966; Jonason, Lauber, Robbins, Meyer, & Meyer, 1970; Meyer, 1972). LeVere has found motivational variables important to retention of the brightness discrimination (LeVere, Chappell, & LeVere, 1984; LeVere & Davis, 1977; LeVere, LeVere, Chappell, & Hankey, 1984) and also has furnished evidence that the brightness discrimination performance is deficient after visual cortex damage due to competitive compensatory efforts of spared neural systems (LeVere, 1984; LeVere & LeVere, 1982). Finally, using a very simple conditioned shock avoidance response contingent on ambient light onset, Gavin and Isaac (1986) have reported that rats with both single-stage bilateral and serial lesions of striate cortex have no brightness discrimination deficit at all if allowed sufficient postoperative recovery time. This spontaneous recovery is explained as a release of inhibition of function.

Of particular interest to a consideration of overtraining are serial lesion studies. In these studies the unilateral ablation of striate cortex is followed by retention testing and retraining; a second unilateral lesion completes the serial ablation of striate cortex and a final test of retention is made. The final retention performance of subjects with serial lesions is compared with that of subjects with single-stage bilateral striate cortex ablation. Studies of this type often report the retention deficit much attenuated by serial lesions, compared with single-stage bilateral lesions (for a review, see Finger, Walbran, & Stein, 1973). The protective effects of the serial lesion procedure with its attendant interpolated retraining or other visual experience (Meyer, Isaac, & Maher, 1958; Petrinovich & Bliss, 1966) seems to represent the kind of neural reorganization that Lashley (1921) sought. Ades (1946) termed this compensatory reorganization.

If compensation or compensatory reorganization of spared neural systems occurs, the question would seem to be: What neural systems? Very little research effort has been directed to this question beyond suggesting that practice created subcortical connections at "lower levels" of the visual system (Thompson, 1960). In the only study that has explored this question in relation to the tectocortical system, Hughes (1977) found that subjects with large lesions of striate and peristriate cortex were not able to relearn a simple pattern discrimination and that destriate rats with lesions of the lateral posterior nucleus (pulvinar) of the thalamus had a profound deficit in the relearning of pattern, compared with rats with ablation of striate cortex alone. Most visual cortex studies have not reported on degeneration in the lateral posterior nucleus (pulvinar) of the thalamus, but even striate lesions termed large do not appear to encompass sufficient lateral and posterior neocortex to eliminate the cortical projection area of this thalamic nucleus completely (Hughes, 1977; Montero, Rojas, & Torrealba, 1973). An effect of striate cortex lesion size was reported by Petrinovich and Carew (1969), who found postoperative savings for smaller lesion rats with nonspecific experience whereas subjects with larger striate lesions required task-specific interoperative training. Thus, it seems likely that in many cases the visual function retained after serial lesions and interspersed retraining was mediated by the spared visual cortex of the tectocortical system.

Some of the test paradigms in the brightness discrimination literature use stimuli that do not require a brightness discrimination, that is, the discrimination of one illuminated surface from another in an organized visual field, but only require the detection of the presence of some light as opposed to no light or of simple light onset, that is, luminous flux discriminations. Discriminations of the latter sort can be supported by the nucleus of the accessory optic tract in the absence of all visual cortex and the superior colliculi if the response requirements are sufficiently undemanding (Pasik & Pasik, 1973; Urbaitis & Meikle, 1968). By contrast, brightness/area discriminations for which luminous flux has been equated require some intact visual neocortex (Caldwell & Ward, 1982; Kluver, 1942; Pasik et al., 1973; Ward & Masterton, 1970). Use of true brightness discrimination tests would permit evaluation of the compensatory reorganization hypothesis. For example, placement of unilateral striate lesions with and without section of the corpus callosum followed by retraining and subsequent removal of striate and lateral posterior neocortex of the undamaged hemisphere would permit evaluation of the compensatory reorganization hypothesis. The lateral posterior cortices are connected through the corpus callosum and, if residual function is mediated by this neocortical subdivision, the brightness discrimination would be spared for subjects that were trained with the callosal fibers intact but impaired for subjects without this source of communication between hemispheres during training.

Although there are many lines of evidence supporting the fact that engrams of preoperative brightness training are retained after striate cortex lesions, the experimental design of LeVere (1984) is most elegant. Intact rats trained on compound brightness and haptic cues transferred equally well to either cue presented alone. After bilateral ablation of striate cortex, rats mastered the compound cue problem quickly but transfer tests indicated that the solution was based on the haptic cue. When subjects were trained on a brightness discrimination prior to surgery, mastery of the compound cue problem was retarded for destriate rats, although transfer tests indicated that haptic cues were most relevant to its solution. The preoperative training retained by spared neural tissue served as an impediment to mastery of the compound cue problem. If the lateral posterior neocortex, which is the terminus of the tectocortical system, is the relevant spared neural tissue, then a larger lesion of neocortex that removes both striate and extrastriate visual cortex should eliminate that impediment and improve performance on the compound cue problem.

Evidence for the participation of extrastriate visual cortex in brightness discrimination is found in the research of Barbas and Spear (1976) who used a different type of serial lesion. In addition to the unilateral serial lesion usually employed, they also made bilateral partial lesions that were placed either first in the lateral half of the striate cortices and then completed serially by removing the medial halves or executed in the reverse order. The rats were trained prior to the first surgery and then tested for retention after each serial lesion. They found that rats with ablation of lateral striate cortex had a significantly greater loss of the brightness discrimination than those with lesions of the medial half. Not only would lesions of lateral striate cortex be most likely to invade the projection areas of the tectocortical system directly, but projection from the entire striate cortex to extrastriate visual cortex is principally by a lateral route. It is proposed that the greater deficit following the lateral striate lesion was due to the disconnection of the extrastriate visual cortex from striate cortex influence.

In lesion deficit analysis there are many training and testing factors to be considered. Not the least of these are the task demands placed on the animal in terms of the response required. Schneider (1969) clearly demonstrated this point for assessment of visual function by showing that simple visual orientation was possible with the superior colliculi alone whereas visually guided behavior in a two-choice discrimination apparatus depended on intact visual cortex. More recently, Mishkin, Malamut, and Bachevalier (1984) have made a distinction between noncognitive habits and cognitive memories and offered evidence that these are mediated by different subsystems of brain. It is apparent that task demands, motor as well as sensory, are important to this distinction.

To the present overtraining has been useful in providing insights about functional specialization of subdivisions of the visual system. It is too soon to dismiss the possibility that overtraining may contribute to retention or facilitation of recovery of behavioral function by promoting dynamic reorganization of brain as hopefully pursued by Lashley (1921). However, if the overtraining procedure is to contribute to the understanding of brain function, it must do so in consideration of the brain subdivisions involved and of the demands of the particular test situation used.

SUMMARY

Preoperative overtraining has been employed profitably in the study of both brightness and pattern discrimination. However, as has been reviewed, the questions for which this technique has been enlisted have differed considerably. Studies of brightness discrimination have largely used the training technique in pursuit of possible neural compensatory reorganization phenomena, whereas studies of form and pattern discrimination have successfully employed preoperative overtraining to assist in characterization of the deficit as to type and in identification of the source of performance deficit.

In the study of bushbaby striate and extrastriate cortical function use of preoperative overtraining made possible the determination that the visual deficit following lesions in the lateral occipital cortices was, in fact, a form discrimination learning deficit, a deficit restricted to the process of inspecting and/or encoding the contours of novel figures with recognition of familiar figure pairs undisturbed. Because the cortical regions that the LO lesion involves represent an interface between the geniculostriate and tectocortical systems in the cortical representation of central vision, because this area of interface gives rise to a substantial projection to the superior colliculus, and because bushbabies sustaining this LO lesion also have a profound deficit in a simple visual search test, it is suggested that the form discrimination learning deficit following bilateral lesions of LO cortex is essentially a sensorimotor deficit. The dissociation between the ability to recognize familiar forms and the ability to inspect and encode the contours of novel forms is evidence for somewhat separate pathways and perhaps special neural mechanisms for these functions. It is proposed that LO cortex incorporates a special sensorimotor function for the integration of eye movements and perceptual encoding in central visual fields. Creutzfeldt (1985) has observed "that in the various visual areas not only different features of a stimulus are represented, but also different responses to stimuli. The different visual fields could then also be understood as a co-operative of various sensorimotor links between the eye and visually guided behavior" (p. 76).

Lashley's (1921) original decision to employ preoperative overtraining was based on his interest in "the automatization of habits through long practice," that is, the concept that behaviors when practiced become habits and that these habits are different than the unpracticed behaviors from which the habit is composed and thus perhaps differently organized in brain processes. Although Lashley chose to study a "visual habit," the automatization of which he wrote is most clearly seen in motor skill acquisition as discussed by Miller, Galanter, and Pribram (1960, p. 6). Thus, practice, training, or overtraining could be expected to affect the organization and function of motor or sensorimotor systems preferentially. For the LO lesion bushbaby preoperatively overtrained form discriminations remain familiar whereas novel discriminations are established only with great difficulty just because the sensorimotor function required for the "practiced" discrimination is different than that required to inspect and encode the novel contours. Ultimately, preoperative overtraining may find its best use as a strategy to assist behavioral lesion deficit analysis in discovery of the "various sensorimotor links" of Creutzfeldt (1985).

REFERENCES

Abplanalp, P. (1970). Some subcortical connections of the visual system in tree shrews and squirrels. *Brain Behavior and Evolution, 3,* 155–168.

Ades, H. W. (1946). Effect of extirpation of parastriate cortex on learned visual discrimination in monkeys. *Journal of Neuropathology and Experimental Neurology,* 60–65.

Allman, J. M., & Kaas, J. H. (1971). Representation of the visual field in striate and adjoining cortex of the owl monkey (*Aotus trivirgatus*). *Brain Research, 35,* 89–106.

Allman, J. M., Kaas, J. H., & Lane, R. H. (1973). The middle temporal visual area (MT) in the bushbaby, *Galago senegalensis. Brain Research, 57,* 197–202.

Antonini, A., Berlucchi, G., & Sprague, J. M. (1985). Cortical systems for visual pattern discrimination in the cat as analyzed with the lesion method. In C. Chagas, R. Gattass, & C. Gross (Eds.), *Pattern recognition mechanisms* (pp. 153–164) New York: Springer–Verlag.

Atencio, F. W., Diamond, I. T., & Ward, J. P. (1975). Behavioral study of the visual cortex of *Galago senegalensis. Journal of Comparative and Physiological Psychology, 89,* 1109–1135.

Barbas, H., & Spear, P. D. (1976). Effects of serial unilateral and serial bilateral visual cortex lesions on brightness discrimination relearning in rats. *Journal of Comparative and Physiological Psychology, 90,* 279–292.

Bender, M. B., & Furlow, L. T. (1945). Visual disturbances produced by bilateral lesions of the occipital lobes with central scotomas. *Archives of Neurology and Psychiatry, 53,* 165–170.

Benevento, L. A., & Fallon, J. H. (1975). The ascending projections of the superior colliculus in the rhesus monkey (*Macaca mulatta*). *Journal of Comparative Neurology, 160,* 339–362.

Braun, J. J., Meyer, P. M., & Meyer, D. R. (1966). Sparing of a brightness habit in rats following visual decortication. *Journal of Comparative and Physiological Psychology, 61,* 79–82.

Caldwell, R. B., & Ward, J. P. (1982). Central visual field representation in striate-peristriate cortex as a functional unit of pattern discrimination in the bushbaby (*Galago senegalensis*). *Brain Behavior and Evolution, 21,* 161–174.

Campbell, A., Butter, C., & Leiby, C. (1984). Effects of inferior temporal lesions on visual discrimination performance in monkeys with complete and incomplete striate cortex ablations. *Behavioral Neuroscience, 98,* 935–945.

Chow, K. L., & Survis, J. (1958). Retention of overlearned visual habit after temporal cortical ablation in monkey. *AMA Archives of Neurology and Psychiatry, 79,* 640–646.

Creutzfeldt, O. (1985). Comparative aspects of representation in the visual system. In C. Chagas, R. Gattass, & C. Gross (Eds.), *Pattern recognition mechanisms* (pp. 53–81). New York: Springer–Verlag.

Dean, P. (1982). Analysis of visual behavior in monkeys with inferotemporal lesions. In D. J.

Ingle, M. A. Goodale, & R. J. W. Mansfield (Eds.), *Analysis of visual behavior* (pp. 587–628). Cambridge, MA: MIT Press.

Diamond, I. T. (1982). The functional significance of architectonic subdivisions of the cortex: Lashley's criticism of the traditional view. In J. Orbach (Ed.), *Neuropsychology after Lashley* (pp. 101–136). Hillsdale, NJ: Lawrence Erlbaum Associates.

Diamond, I. T., Fitzpatrick, D., & Sprague, J. M. (1985). The extrastriate visual cortex: A historical approach to the relation between the "visuo-sensory" and "visuo-psychic" areas. In A. Peters & E. G. Jones (Eds.), *Cerebral cortex, Vol. 4, Association and auditory cortices* (pp. 63–87). New York: Plenum.

Dru, P., Walker, J. B., & Walker, J. P. (1975). Recovery of pattern vision following serial lesions of striate cortex. *Brain Research, 88,* 353–356.

Finger, S., Walbran, B., & Stein, D. G. (1973). Brain damage and behavioral recovery: Serial lesion phenomena. *Brain Research, 63,* 1–18.

Frommer, G. P. (1978). Subtotal lesions: Implications for coding and recovery of function. In S. Finger (Ed.), *Recovery from brain damage: Research and theory* (pp. 217–280). New York: Plenum.

Gavin, M. R., & Isaac, W. (1986). Recovery of function of a conditioned avoidance response in rats with serial and single-stage bilateral occipital ablation. *Physiological Psychology, 14,* 31–35.

Ghiselli, E. E. (1938). Mass action and equipotentiality of the cerebral cortex in brightness discrimination. *Journal of Comparative and Physiological Psychology, 25,* 273–287.

Glassman, R. B. (1978). The logic of the lesion experiment and its role in the neural sciences. In S. Finger (Ed.), *Recovery from brain damage: Research and theory* (pp. 4–31). New York: Plenum.

Graham, J. (1977). An autoradiographic study of the efferent connections of the superior colliculus of the cat. *Journal of Comparative Neurology, 173,* 629–654.

Gross, C. G. (1973a). Inferotemporal cortex and vision. In E. Stellar & J. M. Sprague (Eds.), *Progress in physiological psychology* (pp. 77–123). New York: Academic Press.

Gross, C. G. (1973b). Visual functions of inferotemporal cortex. In R. Jung (Ed.), *Handbook of sensory physiology, Vol. 2, 3B.* Berlin: Springer–Verlag.

Hamilton, D. M., & Treichler, R. F. (1968). Multiple-stimulus dimensions in brightness discrimination learning by rats with striate lesions. *Journal of Comparative and Physiological Psychology, 66,* 363–368.

Harting, J. K., Hall, W. C., & Diamond, I. T. (1972). Evolution of the pulvinar. *Brain Behavior and Evolution, 6,* 424–452.

Horel, J. A., Bettinger, L. A., Royce, G. J., & Meyer, D. R. (1966). Role of neocortex in the learning and relearning of two visual habits by the rat. *Journal of Comparative and Physiological Psychology, 61,* 66–78.

Hughes, H. G. (1977). Anatomical and neurobehavioral investigations concerning the thalamocortical organization of the rat's visual system. *Journal of Comparative Neurology, 175,* 311–335.

Jonason, K. R., Lauber, S. M., Robbins, M. J., Meyer, P. M., & Meyer, D. R. (1970). Effects of amphetamine upon relearning pattern and black–white discriminations following neocortical lesions in rats. *Journal of Comparative and Physiological Psychology, 73,* 47–55.

Keys, W. (1981). Behavioral analyses of visual cortex of the Galago. *Journal of Comparative and Physiological Psychology, 95,* 288–303.

Kluver, H. (1942). Functional significance of the geniculostriate system. *Biological Symposium, 7,* 253–299.

Kluver, H., & Bucy, P. C. (1939). Preliminary analysis of functions of the temporal lobe in monkeys. *Archives of Neurology and Psychiatry, 42,* 979–1000.

Lashley, K. S. (1920). Studies of cerebral function in learning. *Psychobiology, 2,* 55–135.

Lashley, K. S. (1921). Studies of cerebral function in learning. II. The effects of long continued practice upon cerebral localization. *Journal of Comparative Psychology, 1,* 453–468.

Lashley, K. S. (1935). The mechanism of vision. XII. Nervous structures concerned in habits based on reactions to light. *Comparative Psychology Monographs, 11,* 43–79.

Lashley, K. S. (1939). The mechanism of vision. XVI. The functioning of small remnants of the visual cortex. *Journal of Comparative Neurology, 70,* 45–67.

Lashley, K. S., & Frank, M. (1934). The mechanism of vision. X. Postoperative disturbances of habits based on detail vision in the rat after lesions in the cerebral visual areas. *Journal of Comparative Psychology, 17,* 355–391.

LeVere, N. D., & LeVere, T. E. (1982). Recovery of function after brain damage: Support for the compensation theory of the behavioral deficit. *Physiological Psychology, 10,* 165–174.

LeVere, T. E. (1984). Recoveries of function after brain damage: Variables influencing retrieval of latent memories. *Physiological Psychology, 12,* 73–80.

LeVere, T. E., Chappell, E. T., & LeVere, N. D. (1984). Recovery of function after brain damage: On deposits to the memory bank. *Physiological Psychology, 12,* 209–212.

LeVere, T. E., & Davis, N. D. (1977). Recovery of function after brain damage: The motivational specificity of spared neural traces. *Experimental Neurology, 57,* 883–899.

LeVere, T. E., LeVere, N. D., Chappell, E. T., & Hankey, P. (1984). Recovery of function after brain damage: On withdrawals from the memory bank. *Physiological Psychology, 12,* 275–279.

Lin, C. S., & Kaas, J. H. (1979). The inferior pulvinar complex in owl monkeys: Architectonic subdivisions and patterns of input from the superior colliculus and subdivisions of visual cortex. *Journal of Comparative Neurology, 187,* 655–678.

Marcotte, R. R., & Ward, J. P. (1980). Preoperative overtraining protects against form learning deficits after lateral occipital lesions in *Galago senegalensis. Journal of Comparative and Physiological Psychology, 94,* 305–312.

Meyer, D. R. (1958). Some psychological determinants of sparing and loss following damage to the brain. In H. F. Harlow & C. N. Woolsey (Eds.), *Biological and biochemical bases of behavior* (pp. 173–192). Madison, WI: University of Wisconsin Press.

Meyer, D. R. (1972). Access to engrams. *American Psychologist, 27,* 124–133.

Meyer, D. R. (1984). The cerebral cortex: Its role in memory storage and remembering. *Physiological Psychology, 12,* 81–88.

Meyer, D. R., Isaac, W., & Maher, B. (1958). The role of stimulation in spontaneous reorganization of visual habits. *Journal of Comparative and Physiological Psychology, 51,* 546–548.

Miller, G. A., Galanter, E., & Pribram, K. H. (1960). *Plans and the structure of behavior.* New York: Holt, Rinehart & Winston.

Mishkin, M. (1972). Cortical visual areas and their interaction. In A. G. Karczmar & J. C. Eccles (Eds.), *The brain and human behavior.* New York: Springer–Verlag.

Mishkin, M., Malamut, B., & Bachevalier, J. (1984). Memories and habits: Two neural systems. In G. Lynch, J. L. McGaugh, & N. M. Weinberger (Eds.), *Neurobiology of learning and memory.* New York: Guilford Press.

Montero, V. M. (1980). Patterns of connections from striate to cortical visual areas in superior temporal sulcus of macaque and middle temporal gyrus of owl monkey. *Journal of Comparative Neurology, 189,* 45–59.

Montero, V. M., Rojas, A., & Torrealba, F. (1973). Retinotopic organization of striate and peristriate visual cortex in the albino rat. *Brain Research, 53,* 197–201.

Munk, H. (1960). On the functions of the cortex (G. von Bonin, trans.). In G. von Bonin (Ed.), *The cerebral cortex* (pp. 97–117). Springfield, IL: C. C. Thomas. (Original work published 1881)

Napier, J. R., & Napier, P. H. (1967). *A handbook of living primates.* New York: Academic Press.

Orbach, J., & Fantz, R. L. (1958). Differential effects of temporal neocortical resections on overtrained and nonovertrained visual habits in monkeys. *Journal of Comparative and Physiological Psychology, 51,* 126–129.

Pasik, T., & Pasik, P. (1973). Extrageniculostriate vision in the monkey: IV. Critical structures for light vs. nolight discrimination. *Brain Research, 56,* 165–182.

Pasik, T., Pasik, P., Schilder, P., & Wininger, J. (1973). Extrageniculostriate vision in the monkey: Effect of circumstriate cortex or superior colliculi ablations. Paper presented at the meeting of the International Congress of Neurology, Barcelona. *Exerpta Medica International Congress Series No. 296.*

Petrinovich, L., & Bliss, D. (1966). Retention of a learned brightness discrimination following ablations of the occipital cortex in the rat. *Journal of Comparative and Physiological Psychology, 61,* 136–138.

Petrinovich, L., & Carew, T. J. (1969). Interaction of neocortical lesion size and interoperative experience in retention of a learned brightness discrimination. *Journal of Comparative and Physiological Psychology, 68,* 451–454.

Raczkowski, D., & Diamond, I. T. (1980). Cortical connections of the pulvinar nucleus in *Galago. Journal of Comparative Neurology, 193,* 1–40.

Raczkowski, D., & Diamond, I. T. (1981). Projections from the superior colliculus and cortex to the pulvinar nucleus in *Galago. Journal of Comparative Neurology, 200,* 231–254.

Sanford, C. G., & Ward, J. P. (1986). Mirror image discrimination and hand preference in the bushbaby (*Galago senegalensis*). *Psychological Record, 36,* 439–449.

Schneider, G. E. (1969). Two visual systems. *Science, 163,* 895–902.

Silver, B. V., Caldwell, R. B., & Ward, J. P. (1975). *Behavioral study of the middle temporal (MT) visual area in the bushbaby (Galago senegalensis).* Unpublished manuscript.

Snyder, M., & Diamond, I. T. (1968). The organization and function of the visual cortex in the tree shrew. *Brain Behavior and Evolution, 1,* 244–288.

Snyder, M., Hall, W. C., & Diamond, I. T. (1966). Vision in tree shrews (*Tupaia glis*) after removal of striate cortex. *Psychonomic Science, 6,* 243–244.

Spatz, W. B. (1977). Topographically organized reciprocal connections between areas 17 and MT (visual area of superior temporal sulcus) in marmoset, *Callithrix jacchus. Experimental Brain Research, 27,* 91–108.

Spear, P. D., & Barbas, H. (1975). Recovery of pattern discrimination ability in rats receiving serial one-stage visual cortex lesions. *Brain Research, 94,* 337–346.

Steele Russell, I. (1982). Some observations on the problem of recovery of function following brain damage. *Human Neurobiology, 1,* 68–72.

Symonds, L. L., & Kaas, J. H. (1978). Connections of striate cortex in the prosimian, *Galago senegalensis. Journal of Comparative Neurology, 181,* 477–512.

Thompson, R. (1960). Retention of a brightness discrimination following neocortical damage in the rat. *Journal of Comparative and Physiological Psychology, 53,* 212–215.

Trevarthen, C. B. (1968). Two mechanisms of vision in primates. *Psychologische Forschung, 31,* 299–337.

Urbaitis, J. C., & Meikle, T. H., Jr. (1968). Relearning a dark–light discrimination by cats after cortical and collicular lesions. *Experimental Neurology, 20,* 295–311.

Ward, J. P., Frank, M., & Moss, M. (1975). Visual acuity deficits in destriate tree shrews as a function of stimulus area and stripe separation. *Society of Neuroscience Abstracts, 1,* 104.

Ward, J. P., & Masterton, R. B. (1970). Encephalization and visual cortex in the tree shrew (*Tupaia glis*). *Brain Behavior and Evolution, 3,* 421–469.

Weller, R. E., & Kaas, J. H. (1982). The organization of the visual system in *Galago*: Comparisons with monkey. In D. E. Haines (Ed.), *The lesser bushbaby as a laboratory animal* (pp. 107–135). Boca Raton, FL: CRC Press.

Wilson, M., Keys, W., & Johnston, T. D. (1979). Middle temporal cortical visual area and visuospatial function in *Galago senegalensis. Journal of Comparative and Physiological Psychology, 93,* 247–259.

Zusne, L. (1970). *Visual perception of form.* New York: Academic Press.

12

Experimental Amnestic Sensory Agnosia: Preoperative Modulation

J. Jay Braun
Department of Psychology
Arizona State University

Memory-related disorders are perhaps the most common consequences of neo-cortical damage. In their pure forms, these disorders range from disruptions of memory for the learned significance of specific environmental stimuli (sensory agnosia), to disruptions, on the output side, of learned behavioral sequences (apraxia). Agnosia and apraxia are defined on the basis of acquired, life history, knowledge; these disorders represent apparent losses of such knowledge, losses that often are overcome with specific retraining.

This chapter focuses on sensory agnosia as a symptom of localized ablation of sensory neocortex. Controlled research is emphasized, as flagged in the present title by the word, "experimental." The modifier, "amnestic," acknowledges the important view that the kinds of sensory agnosias discussed here represent deficits in "remembering" rather than losses of specific memories (see D. R. Meyer, 1972, 1984).

Apparently complete loss of certain sensory-specific, preoperatively instated habits, followed by recovery with retraining, is an ubiquitous consequence of bilateral ablation of sensory neocortex. The conditions under which the apparent loss may be revealed as less than complete, with emphasis on the effects of preoperative manipulations, will be examined.

SOME HISTORICAL OBSERVATIONS

Hermann Munk (1890) can be credited with the first clear description of one form of amnestic sensory agnosia. He called it *seelenblindheit* (psychic blindness, mind blindness), and he observed the phenomenon in dogs following posterior neocortex ablations: The dogs seemed to have lost the ability to respond appropriately to visual cues that had become associated with certain responses prior to surgery, yet they appeared nonetheless capable of "seeing" insofar as they avoided bumping into things and displayed a capacity to relearn visually guided responses. For example, Munk noted that tricks the dogs had learned to perform to hand signals would not be performed following posterior cortical ablation, yet the dogs would perform the same tricks to previously associated vocal commands. Coupled with observations by clinical neurologists of visual perception disturbances in humans with posterior cortical damage, Munk's observations were among those that led to the initial identification of the occipital pole as a visual projection area of the brain (see Benton, 1978, for a thoughtful presentation of the early history of the visual agnosia concept).

In his classic monograph on the aphasias, Freud (1891) coined the word, "agnosia," to identify the effects of brain injury that resulted in impaired recognition not based on a fundamental loss or disruption of a basic sensory ability. Memory-specific sensory losses following brain damage were indicated by the kinds of observations that led Freud to consider agnosia as a taxonomically distinct category of brain-damage consequences, and by the observations which led to Munk's concept of "mind blindness." Extensive research correlating experimental brain damage with behavior in nonhuman mammals during the first half of the present century revealed recoverable sensory agnosia to be a highly predictable outcome of modality-specific sensory neocortex ablations across neocortical areas, and across species (Morgan, 1951).

Lashley (e.g., 1920, 1921, 1935) provided what has become the most thoroughly researched experimental model of sensory agnosia: the loss of a brightness discrimination habit in rats following ablation of posterior (principally visual) neocortex. Lashley (1935) found that such ablation was followed by complete amnesia (no retention) for a preoperatively instated brightness discrimination, but that the posterior neocortex was *not* necessary for the original learning of the same habit. He found the mean performances of untrained normal rats, untrained rats lacking visual neocortex, and *preoperatively trained* rats lacking visual neocortex to be virtually identical on the two-choice brightness discrimination task. This highly replicable fundamental observation became an important model for modern research and theory concerned with memory, amnesia and the neocortex (e.g. see D. R. Meyer, 1984, 1988; D. R. Meyer & P. M. Meyer, 1977; P. M. Meyer & D. R. Meyer, 1982), and it provides the notochord for this chapter.

Ubiquity

By 1951, agnosia with subsequent recovery had been observed for sensory specific habits in rats following ablations of auditory neocortex (Pennington, 1937) and somatosensory neocortex (D. E. Smith, 1939; Zubek, 1951) as well as for visual neocortex. Rounding out the picture for rats, recent studies have shown that bilateral ablation of gustatory neocortex, the "taste-nerve area" originally identified by Benjamin and Pfaffmann (1955), results in complete agnosia for preoperatively instated discriminative taste habits (Braun, Kiefer, & Ouellet, 1981).

Within the last few decades it became apparent that the basic pattern of results now documented so thoroughly for brightness discrimination habits in the rat following ablation of visual neocortex (e.g., Horel, Bettinger, Royce, & D. R. Meyer, 1966) holds for many other kinds of learned visual habits as well. Light avoidance habits in the shuttlebox (D. R. Meyer, Isaac, & Maher, 1958), simple visual placing behaviors (Braun, 1966), and rewarded visual depth discriminations (Braun, Lundy, & McCarthy, 1970) all appear to be lost (no apparent retention) but recoverable with retraining following one-stage, bilateral removal of posterior neocortex.

Sensory agnosia also had been demonstrated extensively in mammals other than rats. For example, agnosia for brightness discrimination habits was observed in cats (K. U. Smith, 1937), dogs (Marquis, 1934) and monkeys (Kluver, 1936), and in all instances the brightness habits were found to be readily recoverable with retraining.

Finally, loss followed by subsequent recovery with retraining is evident also for species other than rats following *nonvisual* sensory cortical ablations. In cats, for example, Diamond and Neff summarized the results of studies of intensity, frequency, tonal pattern, and sound localization discrimination as revealing in general that "In a one-stage, bilateral ablation [of auditory neocortex], amnesia for the learned habit usually occurs, but the discrimination can be relearned" (Diamond & Neff, 1957, p. 300).

Theoretical Considerations

A great deal of literature supports the broad generality of amnestic sensory agnosia as a symptomatic consequence of sensory neocortical damage. Rarely, however, is the generality of this finding presented as the most fundamental observation to be defined and explained. To be sure, sometimes the observed losses appear to be irrevocable, such as observed for certain visual pattern discrimination habits following visual cortex ablation (e.g., Lashley & Frank, 1934; Lavond & Dewberry, 1980), and sometimes there is no appreciable loss as found for tactile "form" (Zubek, 1952) or cutaneous temperature discriminations (Finger, Scheff, Warshaw, & Cohen, 1970) following ablation of somatosensory neocortex in rats. But most of the results clearly lie between these two extremes, forming a basis for the empirical generalization emphasized here. The outstanding generality of this finding has received very little modern publicity, as previously lamented (Kiefer, Leach, & Braun, 1984).

Acknowledging that one must be wary of using brain lesion consequences as bases for inferences of the functions of localized brain areas, it is believed nonetheless that understanding associative sensory agnosia is an important key to understanding sensory neocortical function in general (Braun et al., 1981; Kiefer et al., 1984). Functional support for a broad category of what Warren and Kolb (1978) identified as "class common" neural mechanisms is provided by the generality of recoverable sensory agnosia as a symptom of sensory neocortex ablation.

Retrieval of Latent Preoperative Memories

Here I wish to describe some observations that simultaneously illustrate the perils of interpreting brain-damage effects in functional localization terms, and that lead to an interpretation of associative sensory agnosia as a retrieval disorder rather than a memory loss. These observations concern what LeVere (1984) has called "latent memories," preoperatively instated memories that normally appear dormant, but which under some circumstances influence postoperative retraining performances. Theoretical and other implications of these findings have been treated elsewhere, and the interested reader is invited to peruse these sources for more information (e.g., Braun, 1978; LeVere, 1984; D. R. Meyer, 1972; D. R. Meyer, 1984; D. R. Meyer, 1987; D. R. Meyer & P. M. Meyer, 1977; P. M. Meyer & D. R. Meyer, 1982). The present intent is to describe briefly two of the research circumstances that led to the discovery, and confirmation, of "latent memories" for the black–white discrimination habit following ablation of visual neocortex.

Consider the observation that preoperative black–white discrimination training appears to have absolutely no influence on the number of trials required for postoperative retraining following complete ablation of visual neocortex: Trials required for normal learning = trials required for learning in rats lacking visual neocortex = trials required for retraining in preoperatively trained rats lacking visual neocortex. Furthermore, there was no significant correlation between preoperative and postoperative trials-to-criterion measures (Horel et al., 1966). In addition, extensive preoperative overtraining—to be discussed in detail—does not typically lead to improved postoperative performances: Rats so trained generally behave postoperatively as though they are naïve (Lashley, 1921). Such a pattern of results would seem strongly to suggest normal localization of the black–white discrimination engram within the visual neocortex, an observation challenging the generality of Lashley's support for "mass action" and "equipotentiality" as describing neocortical involvement in learning and retention of maze habits (Lashley, 1929).

It is to Lashley's credit that despite the overwhelming evidence for a functional localization conclusion for habits guided by specific sensory cues, he remained firm in his belief that amnesia from brain damage is not due to the destruction of specific engrams (Lashley, 1950). His stubbornness in this regard was vindicated by the finding that rats lacking visual neocortex displayed postoperative sparing of the black–white habit when retrained under the influence of mild doses of amphetamine (Braun, P. M. Meyer, & D. R. Meyer, 1966). The drug treatment appeared to have tapped preoperatively induced changes because the acquisition performances of naïve rats lacking visual neocortex were not improved by amphetamine treatments —*drug-facilitated performances depended on the rats having been trained prior to surgery*. This observation supported the view that associative sensory agnosia following sensory neocortex ablation represents a retrieval problem rather than a memory loss (D. R. Meyer, 1972; D. R. Meyer & P. M. Meyer, 1977).

Amphetamine treatments previously had been shown to facilitate behaviors thought permanently lost following various kinds of damage to the central nervous system, including righting behaviors following low decerebration in cats (Maling & Acheson, 1946), and visual placing behaviors following extensive neocortical damage (Macht, 1950; P. M. Meyer, Horel, & D. R. Meyer, 1963). But the Braun et al. (1966) study was the first demonstration of amphetamine-induced retrieval of a specific habit acquired under controlled conditions in the laboratory, a habit that heretofore had appeared to be lost completely following complete ablation of visual neocortex.

Subsequent research by LeVere and Morlock (1973,1974) added substantial support to the view that preoperatively instated memories for the black–white habit were spared following visual cortex lesions. Using a reversal paradigm, LeVere and Morlock found that rats lacking visual neocortex showed a clear deficit when they were retrained on the *reversal* of the problem that they had learned prior to surgery. In other words, preoperative training to run through the white door interfered with postoperative retraining to run through the black door of the discrimination apparatus. Rats retrained on the same problem they had learned prior to surgery showed the usual amnesia (no savings), but not the excessive difficulty displayed by those trained on the reversal. Thus, LeVere and Morlock (1973,1974) demonstrated a latent influence of a preoperatively instated engram in reversal learning while affirming Lashley's general observation of apparent complete loss of the habit when its retention is directly tested. In addition, this research identified the latent engram as specific to the visual cue. The results of amphetamine facilitation (Braun et al., 1966) had left open the possibility that the drug had facilitated nonspecific aspects of the training paradigm.

It is apparent from these studies that despite a seeming lack of relationship between normal and postoperative engrams for the black–white habit, traces of the normally instated engram persist, and can influence, postoperative behavior. Why they remain so latent, however, is a difficult question (but see T. E.

LeVere & N. D. LeVere, 1982). As most experiments cited in the ensuing discussion will show, even very extensive preoperative overtraining on the black–white habit fails to register on postoperative retraining.

PREOPERATIVE OVERTRAINING
EFFECTS

That highly established habits such as verbal identification or visual recognition of objects and/or people should seem sometimes to disappear following a stroke or head injury certainly suggests that "overtraining" does not protect long-established habits from appearing to be totally lost following certain kinds of cortical damage. But to what degree, if any, might such habits recover more quickly as a function of practice prior to brain damage?

Answering this question requires parametric comparisons of recovery following different amounts of preoperative practice with a task, and only a handful of studies have explored the issue. From the limited data available it appears that the answer is, as usual, "it depends." It depends on the neocortical area damaged, on the extent of the brain lesion giving rise to the sensory agnosia symptom in the first place, and on the nature of the task.

Levels of Preoperative Criteria

Operationally, one researcher's idea of "criterion" performance levels can be another's idea of overtraining. Certainly the wide variety of learning criteria employed as reference points for concluding that learning has taken place ("trials-to-criterion" measures) potentially constitute many different levels of preoperative training. As shown by Spear and Braun (1969), conclusions regarding the relative *learning* efficiencies of normal rats and rats lacking visual neocortex can vary substantially, depending on the criterion level selected for measuring performance. Rats lacking visual neocortex were "superior" at low criterion levels on a brightness discrimination habit, equivalent to normal at moderate levels and "inferior" at high criterion levels. Similar ambiguity originally led Horel et al. (1966) to present their data as learning curves displaying successive criteria as a function of mean trials to each criterion.

Lashley (e.g., 1922,1935) typically trained his rats to the very stringent criterion levels of 20 or 30 consecutive correct responses on a discrimination problem having, as near as can be deduced from his apparatus descriptions, a high brightness differential between the two stimuli. Horel et al. (1966), on the other hand, employed a relatively modest criterion requirement of 9 correct out of 10 consecutive responses and used a black–white discrimination problem based on reflected light and shiny black or white plexiglas doors. Despite these differences, the two sets of studies came to essentially the same conclusions.

There appeared to be a relatively complete dissociation between pre- and post-operatively instated engrams for the brightness and the black–white discrimination habits. This conclusion was reinforced by the lack of correlation between pre- and postoperative trials to criterion measures in rats following ablation of posterior neocortex (Horel et al., 1966).

The lack of influence of preoperative training on postoperative retraining is a result that has been replicated many times for brightness and black–white discrimination habits following extensive posterior neocortical ablation (e.g. Barbas & Spear, 1976; Bauer & Cooper, 1964; Spear & Braun, 1969). But these observations do not address the question of extreme habit automatization that might be produced by extensive overtraining. It could be argued that simply training the animals to a criterion level of performance and stopping results in weakly consolidated memories that might be especially susceptible to brain lesion-induced disruption. The first set of studies to be reviewed here suggests that this is not the case, because highly extensive overtraining did not obviously modulate the degree of postoperative loss.

Results for Massive Visual Neocortex Ablations

Testing the hypothesis that habit "automatization" might be reflected in diminished cortical involvement, Lashley (1921) provided a group of six normal rats with more than 1,200 trials of overtraining on the brightness discrimination task after having trained them to a criterion of 30 consecutive errorless trials. Prior to ablation of posterior (visual) neocortex these rats had displayed up to 500 consecutive errorless trials! Lashley found that the postoperative trials to criterion scores (mean = 85.6) were equal to the preoperative training scores (mean = 85.0) suggesting that the overtraining was without effect. He concluded that "the cortical or subcortical representation is determined at the time of learning and is not modified by subsequent practice" (Lashley, 1921, p. 467). The highly overtrained rats behaved as though they had never before experienced the brightness discrimination problem but, Lashley mentioned, the same rats often would orient immediately to the demands of the training apparatus; this implied kinesthetic-motor familiarity with both the apparatus and the general task. Thus the agnosia, specific to the brightness discrimination per se, was not overcome to an appreciable degree by very extensive (roughly 1400%) overtraining.

Other studies employing less stringent learning criteria, and using a different kind of training apparatus, essentially confirmed Lashley's conclusions regarding the lack of effect of overtraining on postoperative retention. For example, as part of the basic training procedure, Braun et al. (1966) provided their rats with 100% overtraining (on the average, twice as many trials were provided as required to reach the 9-out-of-10 learning criterion). This was done in order to ensure well-consolidated preoperative learning. Once again the performances of rats lacking visual neocortex were the same, regardless of whether or not they had been preoperatively trained, and these performances were also essentially identical to the training scores of normal rats. Similar control groups run by Glendenning (1972) resulted in the same results for the black–white discrimination habit.

It should be noted here that Lashley's 1935 study is most frequently cited as making the case for agnosia of the brightness discrimination habit after posterior neocortex ablation, and Lashley routinely employed preoperative overtraining in the groups reported in this study. All of the rats were initially trained to a criterion of 20 consecutive errorless trials, and this was followed by a "preoperative retention" measure during which the rats were brought once again to criterion before surgery. So it can be said that the original conclusions regarding lack of apparent retention of the habit were based on performances of highly trained, then overtrained, rats.

Having reviewed the studies cited, thus far, one would hesitate to suggest that overtraining might produce sparing of a habit for which animals are typically amnestic following localized ablation of sensory neocortex. But other results exist with which one can take exception to such a conclusion.

A study by Gray and D. R. Meyer (1981) provides one such set of results. This study was conducted in the same laboratory, using very similar procedures, as two of the studies (Braun et al., 1966; Glendenning, 1972) which support the conclusion in the first place. The training paradigm employed was identical to that of Glendenning (1972) except that Gray and Meyer gave their rats 300% overtraining for a total of 100 preoperative trials, compared with approximately 50 preoperative trials in the Glendenning study. The group overtrained in "experiment 2" of the Gray and Meyer study displayed modest savings, calculated here to be about 27%, for the black–white discrimination habit; their retraining scores were significantly less than the scores obtained for control subjects that had been preoperatively trained on a different habit. Comparing their results with previous failures to observe an overtraining effect, Gray and D. R. Meyer (1981) concluded that "*extensive* preoperative overtraining conveys some protection of postoperative performance" (p. 54, abstract, italics added). No explanation was offered concerning the lack of an overtraining effect in the original Lashley (1921) study in which, as described previously, the preoperative overtraining had been far more extensive than that employed by Gray and Meyer. In addition, comparing the Gray and D. R. Meyer (1981) results to those of Glendenning (1972), it is difficult to understand how a difference of only about 40 trials of overtraining on a task that requires about 25 for acquisition could have such an impact on reacquisition.

Unfortunately, the Gray and D. R. Meyer (1981) experiment did not include a control group that had been treated identically except for the overtraining, and histology was not presented for the rats in this experiment. Noting that the first of these criticisms could also be leveled at Lashley's 1921 study, my tentative conclusion nonetheless is that the Gray and Meyer finding represents either a statistical anomaly, or some of the rats in the critical group had substantially incomplete, or otherwise unusual, lesions. The ambiguity presented by these results ultimately creates few problems. It is clear that preoperative overtraining has no blatant effect on postoperative retention. The issue raised by the contradictory result of Gray and D. R. Meyer (1981) would not warrant replication for clarification, because the general conclusion would be little swayed by any conceivable outcome. Clear proof of overtraining effects in the specific experimental situation described is very difficult to find.

In any case, as described in a prior section, in view of the discovery of circumstances leading to clear evidence of survival of preoperative engrams after complete sensory neocortical extirpations (e.g., see LeVere, 1984; P. M. Meyer & D. R. Meyer, 1982), the question of whether such engrams might have slightly more impact following overtraining is a moot issue. Interesting, and enigmatic, however, remains the question of why preoperative engrams that reveal themselves in reversal training fail to have an impact on straightforward retraining following surgery.

Partial Ablations of Visual Neocortex

Rarely in the real world of accidental brain injury do the accompanying lesions neatly include the bilateral representation of a particular sensory area, as in the studies outlined previously, without considerable and asymmetrical damage to other areas. In this regard, systematic studies of partial ablations having profound consequences on a measurable behavioral capacity, as in a study by Marcotte and Ward (1980), should be especially encouraged.

Lateral occipital lesions in bushbabies disrupt principally the macular projection area from the retina, and are associated with severe retardation of "form" discrimination abilities (Atencio, Diamond, & Ward, 1975). Such lesions leave peripheral retinal projections essentially intact. Marcotte and Ward (1980) reported that preoperative *overtraining* prevented form learning deficits following surgery. In reviewing this study, it is important to note first that preoperative *training*, not "overtraining," is the independent variable. The title is misleading in this regard. Marcotte and Ward found that operated bushbabies readily performed a form discrimination that had been learned (plus extensive overtraining) prior to surgery, but displayed greatly retarded acquisition of a new form discrimination. There were no groups that had been trained, but not overtrained, against which to assess the effects of overtraining per se.

Therefore, the study shows that preoperative experience with a specific form discrimination task (a capital H vs. an inverted capital A) is followed by postoperative retention of the discrimination, but that acquisition of a new form (annulus vs. reversed split annulus) discrimination is nonetheless severely disrupted relative to normal acquisition. It would appear that after learning a relatively subtle form discrimination with the macular projection area intact, the problem can be readily re-created and addressed by the rest of the visual field following lateral occipital lesions. The lateral occipital area would seem to be important for identification of subtle discriminative details between forms during the learning phase, but not necessary for retention once the critical discriminative details have been learned.

With regard to the issues upon which we focus in this book, the observations outlined herein reinforce an old observation, but with a new twist. The old observation is that incomplete sensory neocortical lesions are often accompanied by sparing of habits that are lost following complete lesions (Frommer, 1978). In an extreme case, Lashley (1939) estimated that retention of a horizontal-versus-vertical stripe discrimination problem in rats could be observed when only one-fiftieth of their geniculostriate system was left intact, as determined from cell counts in the dorsal lateral geniculate nucleus. That is, roughly 700 cells could sustain a pattern discrimination which, according to Lashley's data, could not be performed when visual neocortex was completely ablated.

Likewise of interest in this regard is the observation that cats sustaining between 98% and 99% optic tract destruction reacquired skilled form discriminations (Galambos, Norton, & Frommer, 1967) which could not be performed by cats having 99% or greater destruction of the optic tracts (Norton, Galambos, & Frommer, 1967). Once again it is evident that very small remnants of a system can sustain impressive discriminative performance capacities. However, the studies attesting to this were not designed to address the issue of the impact of preoperative overtraining on the efficacy of the recovery of discriminative capacities.

Emphasizing the disruptive effects of a partial lesion on fine-grained discrimination *learning*, Marcotte and Ward (1980), found a clear effect of the lesion: the same lesion had no effect on similar fine-grained discrimination task that had been preoperatively learned. Thus—the new twist—discrimination *learning*, rather than *retention*, was shown to be a victim of the partial ablation of visual neocortex. Visual agnosia was not evident in this experiment, as it has not been evident in other experiments employing incomplete lesions. However, the role of overtraining per se in the postoperative sparing of the preoperatively acquired discrimination, observed by Marcotte and Ward (1980), remains unclear.

Somatosensory Neocortex

Weese, Neimand, and Finger, (1973) tested retention for tactile discrimination habits in rats following ablation of somatosensory neocortex. Three levels of preoperative training were given to three groups of blinded rats: none, training to criterion, and training to criterion plus 100% overtraining. The mean outcome for the overtraining group suggested a mild improvement of retention for this group, relative to sham-operated control groups, and this was the conclusion stressed in the Weese et al. (1973) paper. However, it is noted that *the overtraining group did not differ significantly from the group that had been simply trained to criterion preoperatively.* Therefore, the results of this study were ambiguous with regard to the effects of overtraining.

Overall, the Weese et al. study can be taken to suggest the possibility of a mild influence; it also may be that complete amnesia for somatosensory habits following somatosensory neocortex ablations is not as reliably obtained as it is for visual or gustatory habits in rats (e.g., Finger, Lennard, Hammer, & Ehrman, 1971), most likely because of task variables.

If preoperative overtraining or experience does indeed influence postoperative recovery following the somatosensory neocortex lesion, practice on the specific task is necessary. Finger (1978b) found that extensive experience by blind rats, from weaning to 60 days of age, in an enriched tactual environment, did not influence tactual discrimination recovery following such an ablation. Therefore, generalized enriched somatosensory experience was without impact on postoperative somatosensory agility.

Gustatory Neocortex

Benjamin (1959) reported a preoperative practice effect for two-bottle taste threshold assessments in rats lacking gustatory neocortex. He presented groups of normal rats with 0, 1, 2, or 8 preoperative taste threshold determinations for quinine hydrochloride solutions, ablated the gustatory neocortex, and then conducted another taste threshold determination. Curiously, the two groups that displayed "normal" thresholds postoperatively were groups 0 and 8—the two extremes! There was no *systematic* influence of preoperative experience on postoperative performance. Both of the middle groups, 1 and 2, showed elevated thresholds relative to normal, whereas having had no preoperative experience at all resulted in "normal" behavior.

Benjamin's results probably were due to performance variables. Taste threshold determinations in rats lacking gustatory neocortex tend to be somewhat unstable, and they are highly dependent on conditions of testing and deprivation. In extensive tests using large numbers of rats, employing several kinds of assessment paradigms and assessing thresholds for the four basic classes of taste stimuli, we were unable to find evidence for threshold differences between normal and operated rats (Braun, Lasiter et al., 1982). But our rats had been subjected to considerably more training trials than had been used by Benjamin. It is quite possible that the differences reported by Benjamin in the 1959 study were based on nontaste task variables—for example, differences in learning to switch drinking spouts when confronting the quinine taste stimulus, or the possible use of odor cues by the inexperienced group (or by the highly experienced group) of operated rats.

Whatever the explanation for Benjamin's results, they bear only remotely on the central issue of this chapter—recovery from sensory agnosia in cases where a clear relationship between a distinctive sensory cue and a behavior has been learned. Benjamin (1959) was examining hedonic responses to different concentrations of quinine solutions, effectively studying "reactive thresholds" rather than the "associative salience" of taste stimuli (Braun, Lasiter et al., 1982).

With regard to specific taste–behavior associations, one study has noted that extensive preoperative overtraining on a taste habit, in conjunction with an odor stimulus, did not protect the taste habit from being lost following gustatory neocortex ablation (Kiefer et al., 1984). So with regard to a habit clearly guided by a taste stimulus, the data so far collected agree with the bulk of the results for visual habits following visual neocortex ablation: no overtraining effect.

Intrinsic Neocortex

Readily demonstrable effects of overtraining on recovery have been found following ablations of *intrinsic* neocortex. While these studies fall outside of the class of studies focused upon in this document, they are mentioned here in order to show that the somewhat pessimistic conclusions which have been emphasized for sensory neocortex ablation do not generalize to nonsensory neocortex.

Orbach and Fantz (1958) authored one of the first studies showing an undisputed overtraining enhancement of recovery in monkeys following temporal neocortex ablations. Six monkeys were trained on three different kinds of visual discrimination problems (color, brightness, and pattern). All of the monkeys received overtraining on one of the problems, and regular training on the other two problems, such that two different monkeys received extensive (approximately 400%) overtraining on each of the discrimination tasks. Five of the six monkeys showed complete sparing of the overtrained tasks (0 to 2 trials to criterion) but no retention of either of the two tasks for which there had been no overtraining. This efficiently designed experiment provided a convincing single-dissociation demonstration of an impact of overtraining on recovery following neocortical damage. This was not an isolated result (e.g., Chow & Survis, 1958). Therefore, visual agnosia that may accompany ablation of temporal association cortex, sparing primary sensory neocortex, can be completely overcome using extensive preoperative overtraining such as that employed by Orbach and Fantz.

Likewise, though somewhat further removed from classic sensory agnosia studies, preoperative overtraining has been demonstrated to enhance recovery of delayed alternation following prefrontal lesions in the rat (Wilcott, 1986) and was associated with sparing of habituated heart rate to immersion of the tail in cold water following prefrontal lesions in rats (Glaser & Griffin, 1962).

TASK VARIABLES

Consider the following thought experiment: Blind rats have a small photocell affixed to the tops of their heads, and the leads from the photocell, with properly modulated output, are implanted in the rats' brains. The rats successfully learn a brightness discrimination habit of the sort employed by Lashley (e.g., 1935) presumably on the basis of some difference in brain stimulation produced by swinging the head back and forth between dark and light discriminanda. Then the locations of the implanted leads are changed (i.e., from medial geniculate to, say, ventrobasal complex). Would the rats display retention of the habit? Probably not. A new differential pattern of brain activity would accompany swinging the head from side to side in the discrimination apparatus, and the blind rats would have to learn this new discrimination just as they would have to if tactual cues replaced auditory cues in a similar experiment.

Would the habit, once learned, be properly identified as a "brightness discrimination habit"? Operationally, yes. In terms of the rats' perception of the situation, however, the question seems somewhat vacuous. The important point to be made for the traditional brightness, taste, auditory, and so forth, discrimination experiments addressed by this chapter, is as follows: What the experimenter defines as the discriminanda may not correspond to the subject's perception of the situation. This is a salient underlying theme of the studies briefly summarized here under "task variables."

About 25 years ago, David Yutzey (now at the University of Connecticut) and I, while graduate students at Ohio State University, considered the possibility that rats lacking visual neocortex may relearn a black–white discrimination problem on the basis of differential feedback from the response of the iris to changing brightnesses. This possibility had been suggested to us by a neuroanatomy professor (one of our teachers) who did not believe that mammals could "see" without visual neocortex. We somewhat informally tested the iris-feedback hypothesis by applying atropine to the eyes of several operated rats that already had been retrained, and subjecting them to further retraining. Atropine treatment—the accompanying mydriasis—did not disrupt discrimination performances, and we concluded that the postoperative engram was not based on differential feedback from the iris to light. While nothing was found to challenge the belief that the "engram" was based on central representation of the differential radiant energy in the training apparatus, I remained uneasy in this belief because the door to a credible alternative explanation—feedback from pupillary fluctuation—had been opened by the challenge of our fine teacher.

In a similar vein, but more subtle, Kluver (1942) had found that monkeys lacking visual cortex seemed to use different cues than normal to relearn a so-called "brightness" discrimination. Monkeys readily learned to discriminate between panels differing in the total amount of light (flux), but not the amount of light per square unit of the stimulus (brightness). In other words, when flux was

245

held constant by varying the sizes of stimulus panels of different brightnesses, monkeys lacking striate cortex were unable to discriminate the panels.

In an especially innovative experiment, Bauer and Cooper (1964) reasoned that if rats, like monkeys, lost the ability to discriminate brightness, but retained the ability to discriminate on the basis of flux cues, than forcing the rats to learn preoperatively on the basis of flux would prevent loss when visual neocortex is ablated. They tested this hypothesis by fitting normal rats with translucent eye occluders, effectively eliminating pattern vision and leaving only the possibility of luminous flux (density) differences as a basis for discriminative responses. Rats so trained displayed substantial savings postoperatively on the "brightness" discrimination habit. Therefore, the loss of the habit by rats trained without occluders appeared to be related to loss of pattern discrimination ability. Indeed, supporting this finding, Hamilton and Treichler (1968) found that while confounded pattern cues (stripes) actually facilitated original learning of a brightness discrimination task in normal rats, such cues had no effect on relearning the task following ablation of visual neocortex.

Tryggvason and Tees (1974) confirmed and extended the Bauer and Cooper (1964) results without the complicating factor of the occluders. They found that rats trained to discriminate on the basis of luminous flux retained the flux problem following posterior neocortex ablation, but that rats so prepared appeared permanently incapacitated on "luminance" (brightness) discriminations. Thus, the loss displayed following visual neocortex ablation can be regarded as due to disruption of an associative sensory ability, and recovery can be regarded as based on normally less salient, but usually confounded, flux cues. From an operational standpoint, the traditional brightness discrimination tasks employed by Lashley (1935) and by Horel et al. (1966) can be regarded as the same task pre- and postoperatively. But the rat may see things differently. From its standpoint, flux stimuli would appear to have consequences for brain activity different from the consequences of brightness stimuli; this is perhaps similar conceptually to the differences between the consequences of the different placements of electrodes as described in the "thought experiment" that I outlined in the introduction to this section of the chapter.

Likewise, as shown by Finger et al. (1970), fine-grained temperature discrimination habits are essentially untouched by massive somatosensory neocortex ablations, a result suggesting a separate integrative basis for these, as opposed to light tactile (roughness) discriminations such as those originally employed by Zubek (1951) and by D. E. Smith (1939), which are lost.

More blatantly, it is no surprise that a learned, compound taste-odor aversion survives either ablation of gustatory neocortex or removal of the olfactory bulbs (but not both) being sustained by the cue for which the primary sensory mechanism remains relatively intact (Kiefer et al., 1984). However, more similar to the brightness-flux distinction is the situation in taste discrimination learning experiments when the taste cue is clearly dominant (intense) relative to a subtle associated odor cue: in this case, ablation of gustatory neocortex is alone sufficient to produce profound agnosia for the compound cue as though the subtle odor cue had not registered during normal training (Braun, Farber, & Hunt, 1982).

Conceptually similar to the taste-odor example in the preceding paragraph, but more difficult to accept intuitively, may be the distinction between flux and brightness stimuli from the standpoint of the organization of the mammalian brain. Thompson (1965) has argued that the visual neocortex of the rat does not respond to variations in diffuse light; that this is the province of subcortical visual systems. When brightness and flux cues are confounded, as they are with virtually any brightness discrimination task, normal rats appear to rely on the brightness differences, and ignore the flux differences, as a basis for discriminative performances. Lacking visual neocortex, however, they attend to the flux component. Likewise, lacking gustatory neocortex they may turn to more subtle odor cues as a basis for discriminating sapid solutions (Braun, Farber et al., 1982).

The observations emphasized here lead to the important suggestion that the sensory agnosia being discussed is in the first place due to loss of a highly specific informational processing capacity, and that recovery is based on residual capacities which remain relatively unaffected by the ablation. Not all dimensions of a mode of sensory input appear to be equally dependent on sensory neocortical processes. This conclusion is supported by LeVere and LeVere (1982) and by the results, described previously, of the studies by Kluver (1942) and by Tryggvason and Tees (1974). According to these analyses, preoperative learning based on input to a particular sensory system would appear to have a higher probability of surviving sensory neocortical damage following extensively generalized training with many facets of the stimuli, under a broad range of contextual conditions. LeVere (1984) came to a similar conclusion regarding the influence of preoperative training under different kinds of motivational conditions.

EXPERIENCES BETWEEN
SEQUENTIAL LESIONS

Research exploring the effects of postinjury experiences upon recovery following subsequent *increases* in injury extent provides a model for the important problem of adjustment to repeated stroke injuries. In general, with regard to sensory agnosia, sparing of a habit accompanies interoperative practice on the habit between sequential lesions of relevant sensory neocortex. But this is a conditional conclusion, and the purpose here is to identify the defining conditions as they relate to the central issue of this book—preoperative experience and recovery—leaving historical and general discussion of the phenomenon to other reviews (e.g., Finger, 1978a).

Rats retrained on a brightness or black–white discrimination task between successive unilateral ablations of the visual neocortex clearly retain the habit following the second lesion (Thompson, 1960). This effect is highly replicable (e.g., Kircher, Braun, D. R. Meyer, & P. M. Meyer, 1970) and can be obtained also following successive, subtotal *bilateral* lesions of visual neocortex (Barbas & Spear, 1976). Likewise, interoperative training is associated with more rapid recovery of visual placing behavior in rats following successive ablations of posterior neocortex (Braun, 1966), and it facilitates recovery of tactile discrimination performances following sequential unilateral ablations of somatosensory neocortex in rats (Finger et al., 1971).

Without specific interoperative training, rats do not show spared recovery of a black–white discrimination following large sequential unilateral lesions. As originally shown by Meyer, Isaac, and Maher (1958), for a light avoidance habit, Petrinovich and Carew (1969) found that home-cage experience in the light was sufficient to promote sparing of the black–white habit. But this was observed only when very *small* lesions were successively produced, 9 days apart. With larger lesions, general visual stimulation by itself was insufficient; however, training on the specific habit was clearly effective.

The serial lesion phenomenon is discussed here because it contributes to a perspective on the degree to which rehabilitation following initial brain damage might protect a victim from subsequent losses following further damage. The "rehabilitation" in such a case represents a preoperative manipulation relative to the "further damage." Of particular interest in this regard is whether the serial lesion effect with interoperative (re)training depends on the habit having been learned prior to brain damage of any kind, and very little research addresses this issue.

Bodart, Hata, D. R. Meyer, and P. M. Meyer (1980) found that interoperative training, by itself, was not followed by sparing of the black–white habit following the second lesion. A replication of this result led them to conclude that the previously described facilitative results of interoperative (re)training depended on the fact that the rats had been trained prior to the first lesion.

The Bodart et al. (1980) result contradicts Thompson's (1960) finding that serially ablated rats lacking preoperative training nonetheless exhibited some retention as a function of *interoperative* training. It is not possible to discern, from among many possibilities, specific differences in procedure that may account for these differences in results. But the experimental question is certainly an interesting one, for it addresses the issue of the viability of new sensory-guided learning based on a neural system that is, in effect, undergoing progressive degradation. The degree to which facilitative effects of interoperative experiences depend on preoperative instatement of relevant engrams deserves much further study.

REPRISE

Amnestic sensory agnosia following ablation of sensory neocortex is the subject of this chapter. The phenomenon is characterized, an historical perspective is presented, and the deficit is presented as based on a retrieval problem rather than as loss of a memory trace. The discussion then focuses on the impact of preoperative events on postoperative sparing of habits guided by specific sensory cues: Preoperative "overtraining," various task variables, and experiences between spaced successive lesions are the preoperative factors examined as they may influence the degree of postoperative loss.

With regard to protecting modality specific habits from loss following complete ablation of relevant sensory neocortical areas, the weight of the evidence favors the conclusion that there is no profound effect of preoperative overtraining on recovery from amnestic sensory agnosia. Once a habit has been clearly learned, additional overtraining is not likely to confer a special resistance to degradation and apparent loss of the habit following complete ablation of relevant sensory neocortex.

However, overtraining may convey some protection following partial damage to a sensory neocortical area, a possibility that should be more thoroughly studied. Such research is especially important in light of the fact that accidental brain damage probably never bilaterally and symmetrically includes an entire sensory neocortical area as do most of the studies cited herein.

Likewise, similarly important, studies of the influence of special training and other experiences between successive lesions (i.e., experience during progressive brain damage) of sensory neocortex should be encouraged. In particular, the degree to which the facilitative effects of interoperative experiences may rely upon a habit having been learned prior to surgery should be investigated.

Presurgical enrichment (or, pretrauma education) may not necessarily turn out to mean more resources with which to recover from the brain damage, but may mean, simply, that subjects from the enriched preoperative environmental conditions have much more to lose. To the degree that habits guided by specific sensory cues have associative salience tied to intact, relevant sensory neocortex, loss of the sensory neocortex results in apparent loss of the habit. The better the sensory-specific education, the greater the apparent loss following ablation of relevant sensory neocortex.

However, highly generalized preoperative training may yet prove to enhance postoperative recovery in some cases, and this most likely will be due to the increased probability of tapping an associative sensory dimension during normal training that is relatively independent of cortical sensory systems. Favoring this possibility are the data presented in the "Task Variables" section. Differences in the relative associative salience of intramodal sensory cues, and the differences between such cues in their dependence for associative effectiveness on the presence of sensory neocortex, are noted. One can train rats preoperatively on

249

"brightness," "tactual," "taste," and probably, "tone" discriminations, and probably find near-complete postoperative retention of such habits, following relevant sensory neocortex ablation, *if the rats originally learn the discrimination on the basis of cues that are postoperatively salient.* This simple statement is perhaps the most parsimonious generalization that can be extracted from the entire literature reviewed and summarized in the present document.

REFERENCES

Atencio, F. W., Diamond, I. T., & Ward, J. P. (1975). Behavioral study of the visual cortex of *Galago senegalensis. Journal of Comparative and Physiological Psychology, 89,* 1109–1135.

Barbas, H., & Spear, P. D. (1976). Effects of serial unilateral and serial bilateral visual cortex lesions on brightness discrimination relearning in rats. *Journal of Comparative and Physiological Psychology, 90,* 279–292.

Bauer, J. H., & Cooper, R. M. (1964). Effects of posterior cortical lesions on performance of a brightness discrimination task. *Journal of Comparative and Physiological Psychology, 58,* 84–93.

Benjamin, R. M. (1959). The absence of deficits in taste discrimination following cortical lesions as a function of the amount of preoperative practice. *Journal of Comparative and Physiological Psychology, 52,* 255–258.

Benjamin, R. M., & Pfaffmann, C. (1955). Cortical localization of taste in the albino rat. *Journal of Neurophysiology, 18,* 56–64.

Benton, A. (1978). The interplay of experimental and clinical approaches in brain lesion research. In S. Finger (Ed.), *Recovery from brain damage: Research and theory* (pp. 49–70). New York: Plenum.

Bodart, D. J., Hata, M. G., Meyer, D. R., & Meyer, P. M. (1980). The Thompson effect is a function of the presence or absence of preoperative memories. *Physiological Psychology, 8,* 15–19.

Braun, J. J. (1966). The neocortex and visual placing in rats. *Brain Research, 1,* 381–394.

Braun, J. J. (1978). Time and recovery from brain damage. In S. Finger (Ed.), *Recovery from brain damage: Research and theory* (pp. 165–198). New York: Plenum.

Braun, J. J., Farber, N., & Hunt, D. (1982) Olfactory mediated recovery from taste agnosia following gustatory neocortex ablation. *Bulletin of the Psychonomic Society, 20,* 156 (Abstract).

Braun, J. J., Kiefer, S., & Ouellet, J. (1981). Psychic ageusia in rats lacking gustatory neocortex. *Experimental Neurology, 72,* 711–716.

Braun, J. J., Lasiter, P. S., & Kiefer, S. W. (1982). The gustatory neocortex of the rat. *Physiological Psychology, 10,* 13–45.

Braun, J. J., Lundy, E. G., & McCarthy, F. (1970). Depth discrimination in rats following removal of visual neocortex. *Brain Research, 20,* 283–291.

Braun, J. J., Meyer, P. M., & Meyer, D. R. (1966). Sparing of a brightness habit in rats following visual decortication. *Journal of Comparative and Physiological Psychology, 61,* 79–82.

Chow, K. L., & Survis, J. (1958). Retention of overlearned visual habit after temporal cortical ablation in monkey. *Archives of Neurology and Psychiatry, 79,* 640–646.

Diamond, I. T., & Neff, W. D. (1957). Ablation of temporal cortex and discrimination of auditory patterns. *Journal of Neurophysiology, 20,* 300–315.

Finger, S. (1978a). Lesion momentum and behavior. In S. Finger (Ed.), *Recovery from brain damage: Research and theory,* (p. 135–164). New York: Plenum.

Finger, S. (1978b). Postweaning environmental stimulation and somesthetic performance in rats sustaining cortical lesions at maturity. *Developmental Psychobiology, 11,* 5–11.

Finger, S., Lennard, P. R., Hammer, R., & Ehrman, R. (1971). Retention of tactile discriminations following somatosensory cortical lesions in the rat. *Experimental Brain Research, 12,* 354–360.

Finger, S., Scheff, S., Warshaw, I., & Cohen, K. (1970). Retention and acquisition of fine temperature discriminations following somatosensory cortical lesions in the rat. *Experimental Brain Research*, 10, 340–346.

Freud, S. (1891). *Sur Affassung der Aphasien*. Leipzig, Vienna: Denticke.

Frommer, G. P. (1978). Subtotal lesions: Implications for coding and recovery of function. In S. Finger (Ed.), *Recovery from brain damage: Research and theory* (pp. 217–280). New York: Plenum.

Galambos, R., Norton, T. T., & Frommer, G. P. (1967). Optic tract lesions sparing pattern vision in cats. *Experimental Neurology*, 18, 8–25.

Glaser, E. M., & Griffin, J. P. (1962). Influences of the cerebral cortex on habituation. *Journal of Physiology* (London), 160, 429–455.

Glendenning, R. L. (1972). Effects of training between two unilateral lesions of visual cortex upon ultimate retention of black-white discrimination habits by rats. *Journal of Comparative and Physiological Psychology*, 80, 216–229.

Gray, T. S., & Meyer, D. R. (1981). Effects of mixed training and overtraining on recoveries from amnesias in rats with visual cortical ablations. *Physiological Psychology*, 9, 54–62.

Hamilton, D. M., & Treichler, R. F. (1968). Multiple-stimulus dimensions in brightness-discrimination learning by rats with striate lesions. *Journal of Comparative and Physiological Psychology*, 66, 363–368.

Horel, J. A., Bettinger, L. A., Royce, G. J., & Meyer, D. R. (1966). Role of neocortex in the learning and relearning of two visual habits by the rat. *Journal of Comparative and Physiological Psychology*, 61, 66–78.

Kiefer, S., Leach, L., & Braun, J. J. (1984). Taste agnosia following gustatory neocortex ablation: Dissociation from odor and generality across taste qualities. *Behavioral Neuroscience*, 98, 590–608.

Kircher, K. A., Braun, J. J., Meyer, D. R., & Meyer, P. M. (1970). Equivalence of simultaneous and successive neocortical ablations in production of impairments of retention of black–white habits in rats. *Journal of Comparative and Physiological Psychology*, 71, 470–475.

Kluver, H. (1936). An analysis of the effects of the removal of the occipital lobes in monkeys. *Journal of Psychology*, 2, 49–61.

Kluver, H. (1942). Functional significance of the geniculo-striate system. In H. Kluver (Ed.), *Visual Mechanisms* (pp. 253–299). Lancaster, PA: Jacques Cattell.

Lashley, K. S. (1920). Studies of cerebral function in learning. *Psychobiology*, 2, 55–135.

Lashley, K. S. (1921). Studies of cerebral function in learning. II. The effects of long-continued practice upon cerebral localization. *Journal of Comparative Psychology*, 1, 453–468.

Lashley, K. S. (1922). Studies of cerebral function in learning. IV. Vicarious function after destruction of the visual areas. *American Journal of Physiology*, 59, 44–71.

Lashley, K. S. (1929). *Brain mechanisms and intelligence*. Chicago: University of Chicago Press.

Lashley, K. S. (1935). The mechanism of vision: XII. Nervous structures concerned in habits based on reactions to light. *Comparative Psychology Monographs*, 11, 43–79.

Lashley, K. S. (1939). The mechanism of vision: XVI. The function of small remnants of the visual cortex. *Journal of Comparative Neurology*, 70, 45–67.

Lashley, K. S. (1950). In search of the engram. *Society of Experimental Biology Symposium No. 4: Physiological Mechanisms in Animal Behavior*, pp. 478–505. Cambridge, England: Cambridge University Press.

Lashley, K. S., & Frank, M. (1934). The mechanism of vision: X. Post-operative disturbance of habits based on detail vision in the rat after lesions in the cerebral visual areas. *Journal of Comparative Psychology*, 17, 355–391.

Lavond, D. G., & Dewberry, R. G. (1980). Visual form perception is a function of the visual cortex: II. The rotated horizontal-vertical and oblique-stripes pattern problems. *Physiological Psychology*, 8, 1–8.

LeVere, T. E. (1984). Recoveries of function after brain damage: Variables influencing retrieval of latent memories. *Physiological Psychology*, 12, 73–80.

LeVere, T. E., & LeVere, N. D. (1982). Recovery of function after brain damage: Support for the compensation theory of the behavioral deficit. *Physiological Psychology, 10*, 165–174.

LeVere, T. E., & Morlock, G. W. (1973). The nature of visual recovery following posterior decortication in the hooded rat. *Journal of Comparative and Physiological Psychology, 83*, 62–67.

LeVere, T. E., & Morlock, G. W. (1974). The influence of preoperative learning on the recovery of a successive brightness discrimination following posterior neodecortication in the hooded rat. *Bulletin of the Psychonomic Society, 4*, 507–509.

Macht, M. B. (1950). Effects of d-amphetamine on hemidecorticate, decorticate, and decerebrate cats. *American Journal of Physiology, 163*, 731–732.

Maling, H. M., & Acheson, G. H. (1946). Righting and other postural activity in low decerebrate and in spinal cats after d-amphetamine. *Journal of Neurophysiology, 9*, 379–386.

Marcotte, R. R., & Ward, J. P. (1980). Preoperative overtraining protects against form learning deficits after lateral occipital lesions in *Galago senegalensis*. *Journal of Comparative and Physiological Psychology, 94*, 305–312.

Marquis, D. G. (1934). Effects of removal of the visual neocortex in mammals with observations on the retention of light discrimination in dogs. *Proceedings of the Association for Research in Nervous and Mental Diseases, 13*, 558–592.

Meyer, D. R. (1972). Access to engrams. *American Psychologist, 27*, 124–133.

Meyer, D. R. (1984). The cerebral cortex: Its roles in memory storage and remembering. *Physiological Psychology, 12*, 81–88.

Meyer, D. R. (1988). Bases of inductions of recoveries and protections from amnesias. In, S. Finger, T. LeVere, R. Almli, & D. Stein (Eds.), *Brain injury and recovery: theoretical and controversial issues*. New York: Plenum.

Meyer, D. R., Isaac, W., & Maher, B. (1958). The role of stimulation in spontaneous reorganization of visual habits. *Journal of Comparative and Physiological Psychology, 51*, 546–548.

Meyer, D. R., & Meyer, P. M. (1977). Dynamics and bases of recoveries of functions after injuries to the cerebral cortex. *Physiological Psychology, 5*, 133–165.

Meyer, P. M., Horel, J. A., & Meyer, D. R. (1963). Effects of d-amphetamine upon placing responses in neodecorticate cats. *Journal of Comparative and Physiological Psychology, 56*, 402–404.

Meyer, P. M., & Meyer, D. R. (1982). Memory, remembering and amnesia. In R. L. Isaacson & N. E. Spear (Eds.), *Expression of knowledge*. New York: Plenum.

Morgan, C. T. (1951). The psychophysiology of learning. In S. S. Stevens, (Ed.), *Handbook of experimental psychology*, (pp. 758–788). New York: Wiley.

Munk, H. (1890). *Über die Functionen der Grosshirnrinde*. Berlin: August Hirschwald.

Norton, T. T., Galambos, R., & Frommer, G. P. (1967). Optic tract lesions destroying pattern vision in cats. *Experimental Neurology, 18*, 26–37.

Orbach, J., & Fantz, R. L. (1958). Differential effects of temporal neo-cortical resections on overtrained and non-overtrained visual habits in monkeys. *Journal of Comparative and Physiological Psychology, 51*, 126–129.

Pennington, L. A. (1937). The function of the brain in auditory localization. *Journal of Comparative Neurology, 66*, 415–442.

Petrinovich, L., & Carew, T. J. (1969). Interaction of neocortical lesion size and interoperative experience in retention of a learned brightness discrimination. *Journal of Comparative and Physiological Psychology, 68*, 451–454.

Smith, D. E. (1939). Cerebral localization in somesthetic discrimination in the rat. *Journal of Comparative Psychology, 28*, 161–188.

Smith, K. U. (1937). Visual discrimination in the cat: V. The postoperative effects of removal of the striate cortex upon intensity discrimination. *Journal of Genetic Psychology, 51*, 329–370.

Spear, P., & Braun, J. (1969). Non-equivalence of normal and posteriorly neodecorticated rats on two brightness discrimination problems. *Journal of Comparative and Physiological Psychology, 67*, 235–239.

Thompson, R. (1960). Retention of a brightness discrimination following neocortical damage in the rat. *Journal of Comparative and Physiological Psychology, 53*, 212–215.

Thompson, R. (1965). Centrencephalic theory and interhemispheric transfer of visual habits. *Psychological Review, 72*, 385–398.

Tryggvason, S., & Tees, R. C. (1974). Retention of three brightness discriminations by rats following posterior cortical lesions. *Journal of Comparative and Physiological Psychology, 86*, 637–647.

Warren, J. M., & Kolb, B. (1978). Generalizations in neuropsychology. In S. Finger (Ed.), *Recovery from brain damage: Research and theory,* (pp. 36–48). New York: Plenum.

Weese, G., Neimand, E., & Finger, S. (1973). Cortical lesions and somesthesis in rats: Effects of training and overtraining prior to surgery. *Experimental Brain Research, 16*, 542–550.

Wilcott, R. C. (1986). Preoperative overtraining and effects of prefrontal lesions on delayed alternation in the rat. *Physiological Psychology, 14*, 87–89.

Zubek, J. (1951). Studies in somesthesis. I. Role of the somesthetic cortex in roughness discrimination in the rat. *Journal of Comparative and Physiological Psychology, 44*, 339–353.

Zubek, J. (1952). Studies in somesthesis. IV. Role of somatic areas 1 and 2 in tactual "form" discrimination in the rat. *Journal of Comparative and Physiological Psychology, 45*, 438–442.

13

The Effects of Preoperative Overtraining on Interhemispheric Transfer

Franco Lepore
Groupe de Recherche en Neuropsychologie Experimentale
Université de Montréal

The nervous system is made up of two symmetrical halves, each of which controls, for proximal sensory systems and for the motor system, the contralateral part of the body and, for distal receptors, the contralateral field. Yet sensory experience is unique and bilateral motor output is generally well coordinated. It has been shown during the last 30 years that this bilateral coordination is largely mediated by a series of commissures, the most important of which is, in higher mammals including humans, the corpus callosum. It is generally accepted that much of the work attempting to understand interhemispheric communication derives from the pioneering studies of Nobel laureate Roger Sperry and his student and collaborator, Ronald E. Myers in the late 1950s and early 1960s. Their "split-brain" paradigm is now well established (Myers, 1956,1962). For the visual system, cats were trained on a number of pattern discriminations using one eye, the other being occluded with an opaque patch. Once learning was established, the patch was transferred to the opened eye and the naïve eye was tested for interocular transfer. Results indicated that the animal performed almost as well with this eye as when using the trained eye. Because each eye projected to the two hemispheres, the next step consisted of splitting the optic chiasm, so that each eye would connect to only one hemisphere. The operation had little effect on the animal's ability to learn the original pattern discrimination using either eye and interocular transfer was also nearly perfect. The interocular transfer demonstrated in these experiments was in fact interhemispheric transfer. This was elegantly confirmed by transecting, besides the optic chiasm, the corpus callosum. These "split-brain" animals also had no problem in learning to discriminate monocularly the various patterns. However, when the patch was switched to the trained eye, recall through the naïve eye was completely absent: The animals required as many trials to relearn the discrimination as they needed during original learning. As a matter of fact, using a rather ingenious training procedure, Trevarthen (1962) was able to show that contradictory discrimination tasks could be simultaneously taught to the two eyes, without any apparent interference of one over the other.

These results, which have been replicated innumerable times, using a variety of species and most of the sensory modalities, show that the interhemispheric commissures are necessary and sufficient to allow lateralized information to become accessible to the other side. The objective of this chapter is to determine whether one important variable, namely, overtraining during original learning, has an effect on the nature of this interhemispheric transfer. A number of researchers have introduced this variable in their preoperative training schedule with a stated or implied premise: Overtraining, because it generates redundant neuronal activity, strengthens the synaptic mechanisms underlying learning so that recall, either through the directly stimulated or the commissurally activated hemisphere, is more easily evoked. This, however, raises one important question: How is the memory trace which is established during original learning accessed during transfer testing? The apparently simple answer is that this can be achieved in one of two ways. The first suggests that during original learning, the resulting engram is stored only in the hemisphere which is directly stimulated. When a subject is asked to solve the problem using the other hemisphere, the latter simply "reads out," via the commissural system, the required information (the readout mode). The second proposes that during original learning both hemispheres are immediately instructed, one via the thalamocortical pathway and the other through the latter's extension in the commissural system, about all the elements of the solution. The secondary engram thereby established in, or "written onto," the indirectly stimulated hemisphere is then directly accessed during transfer testing (the write-in mode).

It is not immediately obvious how overtraining could differentially affect interhemispheric transfer under either mode of functioning in the normal subject. The intuitive expectation that more learning means stronger trace formation and better transfer performance would probably prevail. If lateralized training is given prior to commissural transection, however, the effects of overtraining may be dramatically different for the two functional modes. In the readout mode, overtraining ensures that the unilateral trace layed down in the directly stimulated hemisphere is more robust. Following the commissurotomy, however, the naïve hemisphere has no longer access to this trace, irrespective of its strength, and would be unable to solve the problem. In the write-in mode, where bilateral traces are formed during learning, strengthening the trace through overtraining in the primary hemisphere also reinforces the trace in the secondary hemisphere. Hemispheric disconnection would not affect this secondary trace and transfer performance should be directly related to the amount of preoperative training.

The next section will examine which of these two mechanisms are used by the brain to ensure that lateralized learning becomes accessible to the other side. The experimental results which will be presented will show that many of the intuitive expectations which derive from these two modes of functioning will be confirmed. They will also show, however, that these two modes are neither mutually exclusive nor that they can account for all the results obtained. They will also expose some rather counterintuitive observations, the most important of which being that the commissural influence on engram formation in the contralateral hemisphere can be inhibitory rather than excitatory or null and that overtraining can, under certain conditions, be detrimental to subsequent recall.

WRITE-IN OR READOUT

Myers (1959, 1962) was the first to try to examine this problem. The experimental paradigm was straightforward; chiasm-split cats were trained monocularly to discriminate between pairs of two-dimensional patterns. Two sets of discriminations were examined, using pairs of patterns of uneven difficulty. Their relative difficulty was attested to by the fact that the animals required many more trials to attain criterion with one pair (the "hard" discrimination) than with the other (the "simple" discrimination). Once the animal reached criterion with one eye (i.e., hemisphere), the corpus callosum was transected and transfer was evaluated using the other eye (or hemisphere). Results indicated that transfer was excellent for the easy discrimination but nearly absent for the more difficult one. This result would tend to indicate that easy discriminations are immediately transcribed in the two hemispheres, whereas more difficult ones produce only unilateral traces. Myers (1962) arrived at the same conclusion using a slightly different paradigm. Split-chiasm cats were also monocularly trained to solve a "simple" (horizontal vs. vertical bars) and a "difficult" (disk vs. ring) problem. Once criteria were attained on both problems, the primary visual cortex in the trained hemisphere was ablated. During transfer testing, where the animals could only use the normal, untrained hemisphere to make their discrimination, performance was quite good on the "easy" task, but poor on the more "difficult" task.

Even though the memory record in the "easy" task was laid down bilaterally, however, the callosally determined engram was shown to be more labile than that generated through the sensory pathway (Myers, 1956, 1962). In one of these experiments (1956), he taught split-chiasm animals to discriminate between a horizontal and a vertical bar with one eye. Upon attaining criterion, a different but closely related discrimination (two horizontal vs. two vertical bars) was established with the other eye, the reinforcement valencies of the bars being reversed. When each eye was later tested, the animals invariably chose the pattern used during learning in preference to the one which presumably transferred through the callosum.

A number of other researchers have also suggested that the engram may be laid down unilaterally. Gazzaniga (1963), for example, trained normal monkeys to point, using one or the other hand, to one of two patterns. Upon splitting the commissures and the chiasm, he showed that in all cases recall was only excellent on one side, despite the fact that the animals were completely normal during learning. Downer (1962) used a similar transfer paradigm and showed that only the trained side retained the original pattern discrimination. Butler (1966) trained split-chiasm monkeys on one discrimination, lesioned the trained hemisphere and tested for transfer using the other. No carryover effects of the original learning were seen. To do the same experiment in the rat, whose optic pathways are more than 90% crossed, it is not necessary to section the optic chiasm; the ensuing detrimental effects on visual acuity and the bitemporal hemianopia are thereby avoided. Monocular testing, in conjunction with spreading cortical depression (SCD) of the ipsilateral hemisphere, has shown that the engram is lateralized, since SCD of the trained hemisphere during transfer testing perturbed the learned discriminative response (Nadel & Buresova, 1968; Steele Russell & Morgan, 1979). However, the response could be established in the previously depressed hemisphere in as few as one rewarded trial (Bures & Buresova, 1960; Steele Russell & Ochs, 1963). The previous study (Steele Russell & Morgan, 1979) also supported, in some sense, Myers's original contention that simple traces were bilaterally stored as opposed to the unilateral representation of more difficult discriminations, since rats taught to bar press in a fixed ratio paradigm (FR 15) retained this habit after hemidecortication of the trained hemisphere but lost the ability to associate this to a brightness discrimination, which they had also previously learned.

In humans, comparable studies cannot be carried out for obvious reasons. The closest experimental verification of engram formation during lateralized learning comes from Risse and Gazzaniga (1978) using patients submitted to amobarbital anesthesia of one hemisphere. While the left hemisphere was anesthetized, various objects were placed in the left hand, out of sight. Upon recovery, the subjects were unable to name the objects although they were able to recognize them by touch using the same hand. The results resemble closely those obtained using the SCD paradigm with rats. In general, however, it is clear that a number of functions, such as language, spatial organization, and possibly emotion and facial recognition, are highly lateralized in humans.

Although most of the studies cited herein concur to suggest that lateralized learning remains in the hemisphere which received the original training and that any carryover to the other hemisphere is weak and limited to simple tasks, a number of studies also arrive at quite different conclusions. Butler (1968), for example, using the paradigm consisting of training one hemisphere, splitting the callosum and then testing for transfer, did find bilateral engrams. The critical factor, it was suggested, was the training procedure. Training the naïve eye on a new pattern discrimination after the callosotomy was particularly important. A number of reasons were advanced to explain why training before transfer testing improved the performance in the latter condition. It gave the opportunity to the animal to learn nonspecific response contingencies with the naïve eye and allowed it to relearn the discrimination with a different temporal hemianopic field. Bilateral trace formation has also been demonstrated in a number of other studies using monkeys (Noble, 1968; Sullivan & Hamilton, 1973) and cats (Lepore, Phaneuf, Samson, & Guillemot, 1982; but see following). Also in partial support of Butler's hypothesis is a revealing study by Steele Russell, Bookman, and Mohn (1979), although the authors do not interpret it as confirming the bilateral storage hypothesis. They trained rats' monocularly on a brightness discrimination in a three-choice avoidance apparatus. Once criterion was attained, a "decoupling" procedure was followed whereby stimuli irrelevant to the learned discrimination were affixed onto the choice doors. The animal was forced to use the naïve eye (the other being occluded) to go through these doors, only one being open on any particular trial in a pseudorandom order. When this eye was tested for transfer on the original discrimination, its performance was perfect. They attributed the success of this procedure to the fact that the animal was forced to use the naïve eye during decoupling and thus was instructed in the oculomotor habits necessary to access any stored visual information, including that generated by the original learning.

Possibly the most original and significant studies on this problem have been carried out by Robert Doty and his collaborators (Doty, 1984; Doty, Lewine, & Ringo, 1985; Doty & Negrao, 1973; Doty, Negrao, & Yamaga, 1973; Doty, Overman, & Negrao, 1979). One summary experiment illustrates some of their findings. In this experiment, a number of monkeys were trained to negotiate a five-choice maze. The chiasm, anterior commissure, and the rostral part of the corpus callosum were then cut. The splenium, on the other hand, was ensnared in fine surgical wire. The surgery had little effect on the performance of the animals. When the snare was pulled, however, performance was good when the animals used both eyes or one of the two eyes (e.g., the left in the case of one monkey). When this animal used the right eye, performance was poor and extensive retraining was required to bring the monkey up to its original abilities.

The conclusions that were drawn from this and the other experiments by Doty and collaborators were numerous, but only the main one will be retained for the present discussion: When the splenium was intact and all other commissures were cut, only unilateral traces were produced. This occurred even if the animal has no chiasm transection and the two eyes were open during training, as in the maze learning experiment described previously. The main arbiter for this lateralization of the memory trace, it was suggested, was the corpus callosum, which must actively *inhibit* the establishment of secondary traces, possibly to increase mnemonic capacity. It is the only way one can explain why normal animals appear to have learned the maze with only one hemisphere even though both eyes were open (see also the experiment by Gazzaniga, 1963, described previously and one by Kaas, Axelrod, & Diamond, 1967, on the auditory system, which also appear to support this view).

In conclusion, therefore, it appears that our rather simple problem as to how lateralized learning becomes accessible to the two hemispheres is not so simple after all. A number of somewhat mutually exclusive points of view seem to emerge from the studies presented in this section. On the one hand, as exemplified by Myers, lateralized learning appears to result in the formation of unilateral engrams, except in cases where rather simple material is to be stored. In the latter case, however, the trace generated through the commissures is labile and subjugated to traces established through direct sensory pathways. Butler and, to a certain point, our own results to be discussed subsequently, suggest that bilateral engrams can be established under appropriate training conditions. The work of Doty and collaborators, on the other hand, mainly support the unilateral engram hypothesis; they moreover suggest that the callosum has as one of its roles the inhibition of potential engram duplication. Steele Russell and collaborators' position is somewhat more difficult to circumscribe. The results obtained in the hemidecortication experiment described are interpreted by the authors as indicating that the two hemispheres act in a unified manner so that interference with either leads to a generally degraded performance.

How would overtraining affect interhemispheric transfer within the context of each of these hypotheses? It is clear that its effects on transfer performance could be quite different; if bilateral traces are formed during original learning, then overtraining should have a beneficial effect on eventual transfer behavior; if original learning only transforms the primary hemisphere, then overtraining should have little effect on readout performance once this hemisphere is disconnected by a commissurotomy; if callosal activity inhibits contralateral trace formation, then overtraining may actually be detrimental to subsequent transfer performance. Before looking at the data relevant to this problem, however, it may be of some interest to examine the few studies which have attempted to evaluate the effects of overtraining on learning behavior in general.

EFFECTS OF OVERLEARNING ON PERFORMANCE IN ANIMALS

There are a substantial number of studies by experimental psychologists and learning theorists which have looked at the effects of overtraining on learning and extinction (see Mackintosh, 1974). However, most researchers doing biologically based experiments have been generally satisfied with the attainment of a more or less strict learning criterion in their solution of some other problem. In general, the expectation is that overtraining further consolidates or strengthens the synaptic mechanisms underlying learning so that the appropriate response is subsequently more easy to evoke, or more difficult to perturb or extinguish.

Most studies do in fact support this prediction. However, contrary to this expectation, others have shown that performance decreases with increased training or that extinction is easier to achieve (see discussion in Mackintosh, 1974). A number of reasons have been advanced to explain this effect. These include increased frustration generated during extinction by the withdrawal of reinforcement to well-established response patterns (when extinction is used to evaluate the strength of the learned response). This results from the generally longer training and the ensuing greater development of anticipated reward; boredom in carrying out the same response for a long period of time; the narrowing of stimulus generalization so that small changes are more disruptive of the performance (Miller, 1965). At the neurophysiological level, Bures (1965) postulated that as learning is prolonged, there is a reduction in the population of neurons which are recruited to carry out a particular performance. He showed, for example, that about half the units in the reticular formation can be trained to respond to a conditioned stimulus within about 10 to 20 conditioning trials. For most of these units, however, if stimulation were continued, the response decreased or disappeared completely after about 30 to 50 trials. This was interpreted as indicating that the units were only transitorily activated in some auxiliary, possibly attentional circuits which were involved in the formation of a new trace.

At the functional level, an hypothesis somewhat related to these neurophysiological speculations was advanced by Marshall (1973). He suggested, based on the animal experimental literature, that the effects of learning and overlearning depends on the hierarchical structure of what has to be learned. The overlearning of a simple, single habit may be immune to the effects of focal injury because its neurological substrate is quite diffuse. More complex habits ("learning sets"), which have correspondingly larger ranges of application, are neurologically more focalized and sensitive to injury. He considered that the sparing of automatic language in aphasics, which generally concerns overlearned verbal habits, is a manifestation of this principle.

Another factor which has been shown to be important when considering the effects of overlearning concerns not simply the total amount of overtraining but the type of overtraining within the context of a specific experimental situation. Miller (1965) looked at an approach-avoidance conditioning paradigm in which hungry rats had to run to the end of a runway to obtain food reinforcement. A painful electric shock was then introduced at the goal, which resulted among other things in increased running time. Important for the present discussion, it was not the total amount of exposure to the shock which was the critical factor in determining the adaptation of the approach response but rather the manner in which it was administered.

The few studies which have looked specifically at the effects of overtraining on the performance of brain-lesioned animals have, however, generally confirmed the intuitive expectation. Orbach and Fantz (1958), for example, found that preoperative overtraining substantially attenuated the effects of a temporal neocortical lesion on recall of a number of visual habits. Similar results were found by Chow and Survis (1958). They compared overtrained with non-overtrained monkeys in a series of learned pattern discriminations after temporal neocortical ablations. These lesions had been shown to affect substantially recall of the preoperatively learned visual habits. Chow and Survis confirmed this for the nonovertrained animal but found that the additional training following criterion attainment protected the animals from the perturbing effects of the lesion: they manifested near-perfect recall of the previously learned discriminations.

In conclusion, therefore, psychologists in general, and a few biologically oriented researchers in particular, have used overtraining to strengthen or stabilize performance (i.e., the underlying engram). This procedure has been adopted, as we shall see in the next section, quite routinely by those working on interhemispheric transfer. However, the experimental literature which we have presented has produced both the expected and some rather counterintuitive results. The effects of overtraining may depend on the context in which it is given and, more surprisingly, in some situations continued training can be detrimental to performance.

EFFECTS ON
INTERHEMISPHERIC TRANSFER

Many researchers working on the problem of interhemispheric transfer have given a variable amount of overtraining to the side undergoing the original learning before testing for transfer. In one of the very first papers published by Myers (1955), which examined interocular transfer in split-chiasm cats, it was stated that "When the cats attained a performance level of 34 or more correct in 40 trials after the pattern had been equated for brightness, the discrimination was *stabilized* by overtraining . . .". (p. 471, italics mine). However, Myers did not appear to attribute any special quality to overtraining other than the one stated since neither in this nor in most of the succeeding papers was there any systematic manipulation of this variable to see if it affected the amount of transfer. In fact as few as 120 and as many as 560 overtraining trials were given to different subjects within the same experimental group.

This procedure, and its underlying justification, seems to have been adopted by most of the researchers working on the problem of interhemispheric transfer. Nearly all the studies reported in the literature, whether carried out on the visual system, which accounts for the vast majority of these types of experiments, or the somatosensory system, terminate the section on original learning by stating that a certain number of overtraining trails were given to stabilize performance before testing for transfer.

It is immediately obvious from even a cursory examination of these studies that despite the overtraining, split-brain subjects (cats, monkeys, chimpanzees, and humans) that have been subjected to the learning of whole slates of complex sensory discriminations postcommissurotomy fail to show any interhemispheric transfer. In the few cases where transfer of postoperatively learned discriminations has been demonstrated in split-brain subjects, its manifestation has been attributed either to the quality of the stimulus (e.g., its simplicity or aversive nature) or to the motivational state of the animal (Lepore, Ptito, Provençal, Bédard, & Guillemot, 1985; Meikle, 1960; Sechzer, 1963; Voneida & Sperry, 1961).

Two series of studies examining interhemispheric transfer did introduce overtraining as one of the principal independent variables. Nadel and Buresova (1968) trained rats monocularly in a visual discrimination task while the ipsilateral hemisphere was depressed. On the next day, the animals were given a number of retraining trials on the same patterns, also monocularly, one subgroup using one eye and the second subgroup using the other eye, but with both hemispheres functional. On the third day, they were again trained using either the previously instructed hemisphere or the naïve hemisphere, the other being depressed. Results indicated that the interdepression training on the second day did not affect trace formation in the naïve hemisphere since very little transfer was evident when testing for transfer using this hemisphere. This suggested to the authors that when the relevant memory trace present in one hemisphere could be accessed directly, as occurred during the second day when both were functional, communication with the other hemisphere was redundant and not activated. The authors tested this hypothesis in a subsequent rather complex experiment (Buresova & Nadel, 1970), the general idea being that the presence of a strong trace in one hemisphere reduces the amount of communication it engages in with the other hemisphere. In summary, results indicated that overtraining had only a small positive effect on performance when the originally trained hemisphere was retested. More significantly, however, they also showed that continued training had a slight but *negative* effect on the strength of the secondary trace. This effect was also confirmed in a subsequent experiment attempting to evaluate the effects of Piracetam (a substance which supposedly facilitates learning) on interhemispheric transfer (Buresova & Bures, 1976). Again, 5 days of overtraining produced a slight detrimental effect on secondary trace formation in the commissurally informed hemisphere.

This negligible, or even slightly detrimental, effect of overtraining on transfer performance might have resulted from the cessation or even the active inhibition of transcommissural write-in onto the secondary hemisphere following the establishment of a strong trace in the primary hemisphere. It might also be due to the fact that the weak secondary trace formed through commissural systems could not be strengthened by repeated training. The researchers tried to distinguish between these two possibilities by modifying somewhat the first experiment described here (Buresova, Bures, & Rustova, 1971). During the second day, when both hemispheres were functional, retraining to criterion was carried out using the previously exposed eye. If the primary trace were to interfere with trace formation in the naïve hemisphere, then the retraining should not form a secondary trace in this hemisphere. Otherwise, a secondary trace should be formed in the latter hemisphere in which the strength might be equivalent to that which would be formed if this hemisphere were trained directly. The results obtained during transfer testing showed that a limited amount of saving was present in the overtrained group. This suggested to the authors that there was no active inhibition by the hemisphere containing the original trace to the establishment of a secondary trace in the second hemisphere. It also showed, however, that despite increased training, the secondary trace could not attain the strength of the primary one.

An experiment carried out in our own laboratory was specifically designed to evaluate the effects of overtraining on trace formation in the commissurally activated hemisphere (Lepore et al., 1982). The rationale for carrying out this study stemmed mainly from results obtained in a number of electrophysiological experiments also carried out in our laboratory. Single-cell activity was recorded in areas 17, 18, 19, and lateral suprasylvian of split-chiasm cats (Lepore & Guillemot, 1982; Lepore, Ptito, & Guillemot, 1986). For this preparation, responses evoked through the ipsilateral eye represented activity generated through the direct sensory pathway whereas those evoked through the contralateral eye were assumed to be conveyed through the callosum. Close to 30% of all cells recorded in the vicinity of the vertical meridian representation of areas 17, 18, and 19 were binocularly driven. This proportion was even higher in studies carried out in other laboratories in these areas (Cynader, Gardner, Dobbins, Lepore, & Guillemot, 1986) and in our laboratory on the lateral suprasylvian area (Lepore, Ptito, Samson, & Guillemot, 1981). This indicates that nearly half the cells in this region of central vision, which must be critical for pattern discrimination, were in part influenced by fibers coming from the contralateral hemisphere.

Two receptive field properties were particularly pertinent to the object of the present essay. First, receptive field properties of the neurons in the callosal zone, whether determined through the ipsilateral or contralateral (i.e., via the callosum) eye, were similar on all parameters tested: size, orientation, directionality, velocity tuning, and intrinsic organization. The callosal pathway resembled, at this level at least, the interhemispheric equivalent and extension of the direct sensory pathway. There was therefore every reason to expect that it should be sufficient to create a structured engram in the recipient hemisphere. However, ocular dominance, which represents the relative strength of each eye's influence on a receiving cell, nearly always favored the direct thalamocortical pathway. If engram formation requires that activity in a particular group of cells be repeated a critical amount of time, then the ocular dominance results suggest that stimulation through the callosum must be continued for a longer period of time if this level is to be reached. In the case of Myers's cats, a few hundred overtraining trials might have been sufficient to produce the amount of redundancy necessary for trace formation in the secondary hemisphere for a pattern which only took about 300 trials to learn originally (the "easy" patterns). The more "difficult" patterns, instead, which required about 800 trials to learn, might have generated a bilateral trace if given sufficient time.

All these factors were thus taken into consideration in designing the experiment which will be described (Lepore et al., 1982). Thus, only "difficult" patterns were used since "easy" patterns had already been shown to develop a secondary trace in the hemisphere contralateral to the trained side with little overtraining. The patterns making up the discriminative pairs consisted of (1) a circle and a cross and (2) two equilateral triangles, one having its apex at the top and the other at the bottom, both enclosed in a square. These pairs were considered difficult both on configurational grounds and because in other experiments they had been shown to require a substantial number of trials to be successfully discriminated (e.g., Ptito & Lepore, 1983). The experiment was carried out in split-chiasm cats using the classical transfer paradigm: monocular training after splitting the chiasm, followed by a callosal transection, and then transfer testing using the naïve eye (and hemisphere). Each eye learned one pattern discrimination and was tested for transfer, using the other eye. Training was carried out in a two-choice discrimination apparatus using appetitive reinforcement.

Two groups of split-chiasm cats were used. The subjects of one group learned a discrimination with one eye until they attained the strict learning criterion (36 correct responses in two consecutive sessions of 40 trials). Each animal then learned the other discrimination, using the other eye until it reached the same criterion. Criterion performance was re-established with the first eye and pattern after which the corpus callosum was transected (see histological reconstruction in Fig. 13.1). Subjects of the second group learned one of the discrimination to criterion, after which it received 1,600 overtraining trials in one or two daily sessions of 40 trials each. This arbitrary figure was chosen so as to represent about twice the number of trials which each animal required to learn the original discrimination. At the end of the period of overtraining, the animals were trained, using the second eye on the other pattern discrimination and, upon attaining criterion, were given 1,600 trials of overtraining. Criterion responding was re-established with the first eye, after which the callosum was sectioned.

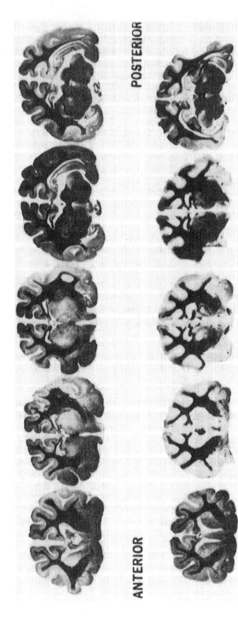

ANTERIOR

POSTERIOR

FIG. 13.1. Selected coronal sections of the brains of two cats used in the experiment. Sections were taken at different anteroposterior planes to illustrate that both the chiasma and corpus callosum were transected. They were stained using the Kluver–Barrera method.

The animals of the two groups were then tested for transfer using the eye which had not seen a particular pattern. The results were quite revealing (Fig. 13.2). Original learning for all subjects on the two patterns took on the average about 1,066 trials. This definitively placed the patterns in the "difficult" category. As far as transfer was concerned, neither group showed immediate transfer. Performance during the first transfer session was generally poorer than that during the last training or overtraining session. If performance on the first session were taken as the measure of transfer, as is often done in these types of studies, one would have concluded that no memory trace had been established through the commissural system, even in extensively overtrained animals.

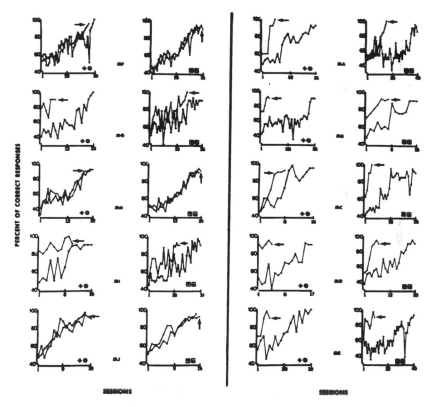

FIG. 13.2.   Individual learning curves for the five subjects constituting the non-overtrained group (two left-hand columns) and for the five subjects making up the overtrained group (two right-hand columns). On the abscissa are indicated the number of sessions and on the ordinate, the percentage of correct responses obtained during a particular session of 40 trials. The arrows point to the transfer curves (i.e., those obtained when the animal was tested with the second eye).

Further training, however, revealed quite a different picture. Many of the animals having received no overtraining required as many trial to re-establish criterion performance as during original learning with a particular pattern. Very little saving was shown by this group (19%; 188 trials fewer than the 1,016 required for original learning). But even under these conditions, some animals relearned much more rapidly at least one of the pattern discriminations (subjects MG and MI). The overall results obtained with this group nonetheless appear to confirm Myers's original contention that difficult pattern discriminations only result in unilateral traces.

All the animals which had been overtrained showed a substantial amount of saving. Whereas they took on the average 1,116 trials to achieve criterion during learning they only required 316 trials (a saving of 72%) to solve the problem using the second eye.

These results were also analyzed statistically using paired t-tests. Learning with the second eye, irrespective of the pattern, was faster than during original learning in the overtrained group. No such statistical difference was found in the nonovertrained animals. Moreover, although no cat showed near-perfect performance on the 40 trials of the first transfer testing session, three cats on a total of five discriminations had 9 correct responses in 10 consecutive trials within this session. This performance is significantly different from chance and has a probability of occurrence in an untrained animal of less than 0.01 (Runnells, Thompson, & Runnells, 1968). No cat obtained comparable results during initial learning, although two subjects from the nonovertrained group also reached this level of performance on three discriminations.

A number of conclusions can be drawn from these results. In agreement with the expectations derived from electrophysiological studies of the commissural system, sensory input to an hemisphere coming through this system from the opposite side can establish a memory trace which can then be accessed through normal sensory channels. However, learning through the callosal pathway appears to be slower than through the thalamocortical pathway. Overtraining, possibly because it produces redundant activity in the directly stimulated hemisphere, facilitates the process of transcallosal write-in onto the opposite hemisphere. As a matter of fact, it appears that this redundancy is essential to contralateral trace formation, since the nonovertrained group showed almost no saving, despite a fairly long period of original training.

The fact that performance in the first session of 40 trials during transfer testing was good but not perfect even for the overtrained animals indicates that the trace stored in the receiving hemisphere had to be reorganized within the context of their new visual reality: different seeing hemifield, new approach and motor strategies, modified scanning behavior, and so on. In this sense, the results, and their interpretation, generally agree with those of Butler (1968).

They do not, however, confirm the hypothesis formulated by Doty and collaborators. Not only were bilateral traces found in the present experiment but, more significantly, the postulated transcallosal inhibition which should have reduced trace formation in the contralateral hemisphere, particularly of the overtrained animals, did not manifest itself.

The conclusions which can be drawn from the data, as obtained in the present experiment, must nonetheless be made with caution. During monocular learning in split-chiasm cats, as was the case before the callosotomy, the second hemisphere was essentially functionally deafferented. Cortical cells, which would normally be active if no patch blocked input to the eye, may have been extremely receptive to any stimulation, which came through the callosum in this case. In the normal state, the callosal input must compete with the direct and maybe incompatible thalamocortical input to a particular cell. In such competitive situations only one type of input would prevail, namely, the more dominant direct input. It is possible that the *raison d'être* of the lower efficacy of the callosal route is to ensure that potentially incongruent information coming through the callosum does not interfere with trace formation of material coming from the direct pathway. In this sense one need not postulate an active inhibitory mechanism. This has the added advantage that it does not preclude the possibility of bilateral storage of complementary or congruent information coming through the callosum. Overtraining, because it increases redundancy, facilitates transcallosal write-in mechanisms in cases where callosal input does not have to compete with direct sensory input.

EFFECTS OF OTHER TRAINING STRATEGIES

A number a researchers working on the general problem of transfer have used training strategies which, though not exactly equivalent to overtraining, have sufficient characteristics in common with this procedure that they merit some mention in this chapter. The first stems from an observation of Myers (1955), who showed that split-chiasm cat were capable of interhemispheric transfer of visual pattern discriminations, but that this transfer was not as perfect as for normal cats. Berlucchi and collaborators (Berlucchi, Buchtel, Marzi, Mascetti, & Simoni, 1978), therefore, designed an experiment to see if experience with transfer tasks would improve interocular transfer in split-chiasm cats. In the same experiment, they also tried to evaluate whether repeated testing before splitting the forebrain commissures in these split-chiasm animals would result in the maintenance of some transfer ability in these now split-brain animals. They thus trained two groups of split-chiasm cats on a series of eight pattern discriminations. The corpus callosum and anterior commissure of the subjects in the first group were sectioned after they had learned and had been tested for transfer on four of these pattern discriminations and of those in the second group before any learning had taken place. It is interesting to note that after attaining criterion on each discrimination, five overtraining sessions were given (presumably to stabilize performance).

The results indicated that transfer performance of subjects in the first group (i.e., having only a chiasm section) was better on problems 3 and 4 than on problems 1 and 2. This indicated that experience with transfer facilitated its subsequent manifestation on similar problems. When the two groups of split-brain subjects were compared on transfer performance for the second series of four problems, the results indicated that there was no difference between the eyes, that is, original learning versus transfer, for the subjects of the second group (chiasm and commissural split before beginning of training) and a marginally significant superiority of the second eye (the one used for transfer testing) in the first group. This suggested to the authors that as a consequence of their experience with transfer, "the capacity for inter-ocular communication was largely but perhaps not completely eliminated by forebrain commissurotomy" (p. 536).

Mascetti and Mancilla (1986) also tried to improve interocular transfer in split-chiasm cats, using a special training program. They used a technique called Fading, which had previously been successfully used in a number of experimental and clinical settings. Essentially, this technique consisted of presenting the two stimuli which have to be discriminated in such a way that they differed maximally at the beginning of testing. As training continued, the differences were reduced in steps so that they came to differ minimally along the dimension which had to be discriminated. Split-chiasm cats trained to criterion in the classical two-way discrimination apparatus (they also received five sessions of overtraining) demonstrated, as had been shown by Myers (1955), that transfer was present but imperfect. Animals tested using the Fading method showed perfect interocular transfer. The authors postulate that the method improves callosal transmission and stabilizes and organizes the memory traces in the second hemisphere.

A third experiment, also remotely related to the theme of this chapter concerns the effects of serial disconnection of the commissures on interhemispheric transfer. Tieman and Hamilton (1973) sectioned, besides the optic chiasm, all the forebrain commissures except the splenium in two monkeys. These animals were given extensive training in pattern discrimination and generally showed very good transfer performance. Two other animals, which were similarly prepared, except that the spared callosum was slightly more anterior, also showed good learning performance but no transfer. The remaining callosum was then sectioned in the four animals. They were, as expected, able to learn new pattern discriminations. More importantly, however, all four also showed a substantial amount of transfer. A fifth monkey which had the prespenial callosum intact received, at the time at which this part was cut, a section of the posterior, habenular, and collicular commissures. This animal did not show transfer. Similarly, five other monkeys which received the chiasm and commissural transections in one stage, and who were given a substantial amount of training, also did not show transfer. The latter results indicate that the total amount of training was not the principal factor which determined the subsequent amount of transfer. Rather, the critical factor appeared to be the surgical procedure. The authors postulate that the experience received during the interval between the first and second lesion permitted the monkeys to develop alternate mechanisms for transfer which remained despite the subsequent splenial or presplenial sections. Based on the results of the fifth monkey, this mechanism might involve the midbrain commissures. However, experimental considerations suggested that this conclusion be taken with some caution.

TRANSFER IN SUBMAMMALIAN SPECIES

A few studies have looked at the effects of overtraining on interhemispheric transfer in submammalian species. By far the greatest amount of work on interhemispheric transfer and on the identification of the structures through which it is mediated has been carried out in the pigeon and the fish. Overtraining was invoked as a potential factor in explaining differences in results obtained in the pigeon. Levine (1952) trained pigeons monocularly in a modified Lashley jumping stand to discriminate a number of visual stimuli. When tested for transfer using the other eye, only stimuli presented close to the bird and below its head were recognized. Interocular transfer was absent for stimuli presented in front of the animal. Catania (1965), on the other hand, showed that pigeons trained on an operant VI schedule to peck at stimuli also presented in front of its head showed very good interocular transfer. Among the various reasons Catania gave to explain the differences in results with Levine was the fact that his operant conditioning paradigm required that the pigeons emit several thousand responses before being tested for transfer whereas those trained using the jumping stand technique only respond a few hundred times prior to being examined with the naïve eye. The overtraining inherent in the operant task was thus responsible for the high level of transfer demonstrated by the pigeons.

This hypothesis was specifically tested by Goodale and Graves (Goodale & Graves, 1982; Graves & Goodale, 1979). They designed an experiment which was, on the one hand, similar to Catania's, in the sense that the pigeon was required to peck a key placed in front of its head to discriminate a red from a green key. However, instead of using an operant VI schedule, which implied that the animal had to emit a large number of responses to receive a reward (i.e., thereby resulting in overtraining), they reinforced the subject on each peck. Moreover, to make the training situation more comparable with that of the jumping stand, they used a two-choice simultaneous discrimination instead of the successive discrimination employed by Catania. The results indicated that criterion on initial learning was attained in approximately the same number of trials as in the jumping stand. Moreover, performance with the untrained eye was also of high level. The authors conclude that overtraining was probably not a factor in explaining the differences between Catania and Levine's results. They favored an explanation which took into account the manner in which the pigeons used their eyes, given that sensitivity to the various stimuli used in the different experiments was not homogeneous across the retina (Goodale & Graves, 1982).

In the fish, Ingle and Campbell (1977) attempted to evaluate the relative importance of the various commissures for interocular transfer. They found that neither the anterior nor posterior commissures were particularly important since their transection did not block transfer of a simple pattern discrimination. A section of the postoptic commissure appeared to be the most detrimental for transfer, since performance with the untrained eye was nearly always close to chance on a series of discriminations. The results obtained for the tectal commissure were of particular interest. Its transection abolished transfer when the fish learned only a pattern discrimination. If, on the other hand, the fish practiced in performing a color discrimination with each eye before undergoing testing on a horizontal–vertical discrimination, its transfer performance on this pattern discrimination was of very high level. The authors postulated that sensory information transferred in tectal commissurotomized fish. However, in order for the animal to make the appropriate response, it must also have at its disposal in the untrained hemisphere the motor patterns which would guide its behavior when the stimulus was presented to this hemisphere. They suggested that the effect of pretraining the animals in the color discrimination was to instruct the untrained hemisphere such that it would "know what to do" (p. 333) with the sensory information which it received through the remaining commissural systems. This is also the position adopted by Yeo and Savage (1975) following their results which showed normal levels of interocular transfer in tectal commissurotomized goldfish, using differential classical conditioning of heart rate.

CONCLUDING REMARKS

The effects of overtraining on interhemispheric transfer are somewhat ambiguous. This ambiguity derives from a number of factors, not the least being the relative paucity of experiments which have directly addressed this point. No experiment has specifically looked at the effects of postoperative overtraining on interhemispheric transfer in split-brain humans or animals. However, converging results using this preparation would lead us to postulate that the use of overtraining would not much improve the rather poor transfer generally observed with these clinical or experimental subjects (although see Berlucchi et al., 1978). Preoperative overtraining, on the other hand, produces effects which are more difficult to categorize into a well-defined class. As was the case with the extensive animal literature which examined how overtraining affects learning in general, some rather unexpected results have been obtained by those working on transfer. Overtraining may not only have no effect but actually have a negative effect on subsequent transfer performance. In fact, such detrimental effects on transfer from continued training might be the only logical hypothesis which could be advanced by those who suggest that one of the functions of the callosum is actively to inhibit bilateral trace formation. In humans, such contralateral inhibition has often been invoked as one of the potential mechanisms through which lateralization of function is developed.

Our own experimental results have generally confirmed the intuitive expectation. However, we have suggested that this conclusion be taken with caution, since the results have been obtained under conditions which favored callosal write-in processes. We also advanced the hypothesis that there is no reason to postulate an active callosal inhibitory mechanism since the latter system is by its nature organized to limit the type of material which can be bilaterally stored. Only congruent or complementary information could effectively activate a cell which is receiving near-simultaneous direct and callosal inputs. Because the callosal input is generally weaker than the direct sensory input, the latter would probably dominate under competitive conditions. Overtraining, on the other hand, because it produces redundant activity, might facilitate contralateral transcription of appropriate but weaker callosal information, and this would be reflected by superior transfer performance.

ACKNOWLEDGMENTS

The studies reported in this chapter were carried out in part with grants from the Natural Sciences and Engineering Research Council of Canada, the Medical Research Council of Canada and the Ministry of Education of the Province of Quebec (program FCAR). The help of colleagues and graduate students must also be underlined.

REFERENCES

Berlucchi, G., Buchtel, E., Marzi, C. A., Mascetti, G. G., & Simoni, A. (1978). Effects of experience on interocular transfer of pattern discriminations in split-chiasm and split-brain cats. *Journal of Comparative and Physiological Psychology, 92,* 532–543.

Bures, J. (1965). Discussion. In D. P. Kimble (Ed.), *The anatomy of memory.* Palo Alto, CA: Science and Behavior Books.

Bures, J., & Buresova, O. (1960). The use of Leao's spreading depression in the study of interhemispheric transfer of memory traces. *Journal of Comparative and Physiological Psychology, 53,* 558–563.

Buresova, O., & Bures, J. (1976). Piracetam-induced facilitation of interhemispheric transfer of visual information in rats. *Psychopharmacologia, 46*, 93–102.

Buresova, O., Bures, J., & Rustova, M. (1971). Conditions for interhemispheric transfer of initially lateralized visual engrams in hooded rats. *Journal of Comparative and Physiological Psychology, 75*, 200–205.

Buresova, O., & Nadel, L. (1970). Interhemispheric transfer in the rat. *Physiology and Behavior, 5*, 849–853.

Butler, C. R. (1966). Cortical lesions and interhemispheric communication in monkeys (*Macaca mulatta*). *Nature (London), 209*, 59–61.

Butler, C. R. (1968). A memory-record for visual discrimination habits produced in both cerebral hemispheres of monkey when only one hemisphere has received direct visual information. *Brain Research, 10*, 152–167.

Catania, A. C. (1965). Interocular transfer of discriminations in the pigeon. *Journal of the Experimental Analysis of Behavior, 8*, 147–155.

Chow, K. L., & Survis, J. (1958). Retention of overlearned visual habit after temporal cortical ablation in monkey. *AMA Archives of Psychiatry, 79*, 640–646.

Cynader, M., Gardner, H., Dobbins, A., Lepore, F., & Guillemot, J.-P. (1986). Interhemispheric communication and binocular vision: Functional and developmental aspects. In F. Lepore, M. Ptito, & H. H. Jasper (Eds.), *Two hemispheres-one brain: Functions of the corpus callosum* (pp. 189–210). New York: Alan Liss.

Doty, R. W. (1984). Some thoughts and some experiments on memory. In L. R. Squire & N. Butters (Eds.), *Neuropsychology of memory* (pp. 330–339). New York: Guilford.

Doty, R. W., & Negrao, N. (1973). Forebrain commissures in vision. In R. Jung (Ed.), *Handbook of sensory physiology. VII/3. Central visual information* (pp. 543–582). Berlin: Springer-Verlag.

Doty, R. W., Negrao, N., & Yamaga, K. (1973). The unilateral engram. *Acta Neurobiologica Experimentalis, 33*, 711–728.

Doty, R. W., Lewine, J. D., & Ringo, J. L. (1985). Mnemonic interaction between and within cerebral hemispheres in macaques. In D. L. Alkon & C. D. Woody (Eds.), *Neural mechanisms of conditioning* (pp. 223–231). New York: Plenum.

Doty, R. W., Overman, W. H., & Negrao, N. (1979). Role of forebrain commissures in hemispheric specialisation and memory in macaques. In I. Steele Russell, M. W. van Hof, & G. Berlucchi (Eds.), *Structure and function of cerebral commissures* (pp. 333–342). Baltimore: University Park Press.

Downer, J. L. de C. (1962). Interhemispheric integration in the visual system. In V. B. Mountcastle (Ed.), *Interhemispheric relations and cerebral dominance* (pp. 87–100). Baltimore: John Hopkins Press.

Gazzaniga, M. S. (1963). Effects of commissurotomy on a preoperatively learned visual discrimination. *Experimental Neurology, 8*, 14–19.

Goodale, A., & Graves, J. A. (1982). Retinal locus as a factor in interocular transfer in the pigeon. In D. J. Ingle, M. A. Goodale, & R. M. Mansfield (Eds.), *The analysis of visual behavior* (pp. 211–240). Cambridge: MIT Press.

Graves, J. A., & Goodale, M. A. (1979). Do training conditions affect interocular transfer in the pigeon. In I. Steele Russell, M. W. van Hof, & G. Berlucchi (Eds.), *Structure and function of cerebral commissures,* (pp. 73–86), Baltimore: University Park Press.

Ingle, D., & Campbell, A. (1977). Interocular transfer of visual discriminations in goldfish after selective commissure lesions. *Journal of Comparative and Physiological Psychology, 91*, 327–335.

Kaas, J., Axelrod, S., & Diamond, I. T. (1967). An ablation study of the auditory cortex in the cat using binaural tonal patterns. *Journal of Neurophysiology, 30*, 710–724.

Lepore, F., & Guillemot, J.-P. (1982). Visual receptive field properties of cells innervated through the corpus callosum in the cat. *Experimental Brain Research, 46*, 413–424.

Lepore, F., Ptito, M., & Guillemot, J.-P. (1986). The role of the corpus callosum in midline fusion. In F. Lepore, M. Ptito, & H. H. Jasper (Eds.), *Two hemispheres-one brain: Functions of the corpus callosum* (pp. 211–229). New York: Alan Liss.

Lepore, F., Phaneuf, J., Samson, A., & Guillemot, J.-P. (1982). Interhemispheric transfer of visual pattern discrimination: evidence for the bilateral storage of the engram. *Behavioral Brain Research, 5,* 359–374.

Lepore, F., Ptito, M., Provençal, C., Bédard, S., & Guillemot, J.-P. (1985). Le transfert interhémisphérique d'apprentissages visuels chez le chat à cerveau divisé: effets de la situation expérimentale. [Interhemispheric transfer of visual pattern discriminations in the split-brain cat: effects of te experimental context.] *Canadian Journal of Psychology, 39,* 400–413.

Lepore, F., Ptito, M., Samson, A., & Guillemot, J.-P. (1981). The influence of the contralateral hemisphere on the receptive field properties of cells in the visual cortex of the cat. *Revue Canadienne de Biologie, 40,* 60–66.

Levine, J. (1952). Studies in interrelations of central nervous structures in binocular vision. III. Localization of memory trace as evidenced by lack of inter and intra-ocular habit transfer in the pigeon. *Journal of Genetic Psychology, 67,* 19–27.

Mackintosh, N. J. (1974). *The psychology of animal learning.* New York: Academic Press.

Marshall, J.C. (1973). Language, learning and laterality. In R. A. Hinde & J. Stevenson-Hinde (Eds.), *Constraints on learning* (pp. 445–456). New York: Academic Press.

Mascetti, G. G., & Mancilla, F. (1986). Perfect interocular transfer of visual pattern discriminations in split-chiasm cats trained by Fading. *Behavioral Brain Research, 8,* 321–330.

Meikle, T. H. (1960). Role of corpus callosum in transfer of visual discriminations in the cat. *Science, 132,* 1496.

Miller, N. E. (1965). Learning resistance to pain and fear: effects of overlearning, exposure and rewarded exposure in context. *Journal of Experimental Psychology, 60,* 137–145.

Myers, R. E. (1955). Interocular transfer of pattern discriminations in cats following section of crossed optic fibres. *Journal of Comparative and Physiological Psychology, 48,* 470–473.

Myers, R. E. (1956). Function of corpus callosum in interocular transfer. *Brain, 79,* 358–363.

Myers, R. E. (1962). Transmission of visual information within and between the hemispheres: A behavioral study. In V. B. Mountcastle (Ed.), *Interhemispheric relations and cerebral dominance* (pp. 52–73). Baltimore: John Hopkins Press.

Myers, R. E. (1959). Interhemispheric communication through corpus callosum: Limitations under conditions of conflict. *Journal of Comparative and Physiological Psychology, 52,* 6–9.

Nadel, L., & Buresova, O. (1968). Monocular input and interhemispheric transfer in the reversible split-brain. *Nature, 220,* 914–915.

Noble, J. (1968). Paradixical interocular transfer of mirror-image discriminations in the optic chiasm sectioned monkey. *Brain Research, 10,* 127–151.

Orbach, J., & Fantz, R. L. (1958). Differential effects of temporal neo-cortical resection on overtrained and non-overtrained visual habits in monkeys. *Journal of Comparative and Physiological Psychology, 51,* 126–129.

Ptito, M., & Lepore, F. (1983). Effects of unilateral and bilateral lesions of the lateral suprasylvian area on learning and interhemispheric transfer of pattern discrimination in the cat. *Behavioral Brain Research, 7,* 221–227.

Risse, G. L., & Gazzaniga, M. S. (1978). Well-kept secrets of the right hemisphere: A carotid amytal study of restricted memory transfer. *Neurology, 28,* 950–953.

Runnells, L. K., Thompson, R., & Runnells, P. (1968). Near perfect runs as a learning criterion. *Journal of Mathematical Psychology, 5,* 362–368.

Sechzer, J. A. (1963). Successful interocular transfer of pattern discrimination in "split-brain" cats with shock avoidance motivation. *Journal of Comparative and Physiological Psychology, 58,* 76–83.

Steele Russell, I., & Ochs, S. (1963). Localization of a memory trace in one cortical hemisphere and transfer to the other hemisphere. *Brain, 86,* 37–54.

Steele Russell, I., & Morgan, S. C. (1979). Some studies of interhemispheric integration in the rat. In I. Steele Russell, M. W. van Hof, & G. Berlucchi (Eds.), *Structure and function of cerebral commissures* (pp. 181–194). Baltimore: University Park Press.

Steele Russell, I., Bookman, J. F., & Mohn, G. (1979). Interocular transfer of visual habit in the rat. In I. Steele Russell, M. W. van Hof, & G. Berlucchi (Eds.), *Structure and function of cerebral commissures* (pp. 164–180). Baltimore: University Park Press.

Sullivan, M. V., & Hamilton, C. R. (1973). Memory establishment via the anterior commissure of monkeys. *Physiology and Behavior, 11,* 873–879.

Tieman, S. B., & Hamilton, C. R. (1973). Interocular transfer in split-brain monkeys following serial disconnection. *Brain Research, 63,* 368–373.

Trevarthen, C. B. (1962). Double visual learning in split brain monkeys. *Science, 136,* 258–259.

Voneida, T. J., & Sperry, R. W. (1961). Central nervous pathways involved in conditioning. *Anatomical Record, 139,* 287–288.

Yeo, C. H., & Savage, G. E. (1975). The tectal commissure and interocular transfer of a shape discrimination in the goldfish. *Experimental Neurology, 49,* 291–298.

14

Premorbid Effects Upon Recovery From Brain Injury in Humans: Cognitive and Interpersonal Indices

Jordan Grafman
Francois Lalonde
Irene Litvan
Paul Fedio
National Institutes of Health

INTRODUCTION

The issue of premorbid cognitive functioning can be quite interesting for neuropsychological research. Presumably, premorbid functioning indicates cognitive and behavioral knowledge representation and use. This knowledge representation can take the form of context-free (e.g., semantic) information or context-dependent (e.g., episodic) information which can be accessed by consciously mediated (e.g., declarative) or nonconsciously mediated (e.g., procedural) production systems. Although a patient's age, handedness, socioeconomic status, and similar variables are clues to his or her overall premorbid cognitive functioning, these parameters do not offer the precision required (e.g., actual test performance scores) to estimate such functioning accurately.

It would be useful to have precise and quantifiable premorbid cognitive indices for several methodological reasons. For example, if a researcher were interested in the breakdown of semantic memory in a neurological patient, there would be an obvious advantage in having a premorbid test score available that could provide a baseline estimate, no matter how crude, of semantic memory functioning (e.g., scores from a naming, vocabulary, or fluency test). Another reason for obtaining an estimate of premorbid cognitive functioning is to compare the contribution that stored knowledge makes, relative to the location, size, and type of brain lesion in predicting level of performance on a dependent variable (not necessarily the same measure that is available from premorbid testing). A third reason would be to determine the capability of a modular cognitive system to learn new information after injury. Similarly, it would be useful to know whether the severity of emotional and behavioral disorders following brain injury is consistent with the patient's preinjury interpersonal state.

Despite the usefulness of acquiring such premorbid data, investigators are typically left with utilizing nonpsychometric variables (e.g., achieved educational level) along with the family history of the patient's functioning. There are some isolated exceptions to this state of affairs and they will be presented, along with some suggested remedies for when such data are not available. In this chapter we describe what is reliably known about the effects of premorbid psychological functioning upon postmorbid functioning. We first examine the effects of preinjury intelligence and education upon postinjury test performance. Next we will present what is known about the effects of preinjury language ability (in particular, bilingualism) and whether multilingual ability protects against severe language disability postinjury. We then examine whether preinjury personality affects postinjury behavior and mood regulation. Finally, we review the effects of having special skills upon postinjury recovery. We end the chapter with a discussion of the theoretical and methodological implications of our review.

The comparison between premorbid (in humans) and preoperative (in animals) effects on postmorbid behavior is primarily inferential. Both the precision of the lesion and cognitive capacity of varied species are too different to equate. Despite the scarcity of human data, the research that is available suggests the relevance of premorbid data for understanding postmorbid cognitive and behavioral performance.

EFFECTS OF PREINJURY
INTELLIGENCE

In this section we review what is known about the relationship between preinjury intelligence level and outcome. We also will comment upon some attempts to estimate preinjury intelligence, based on patient history and postinjury test performance. The majority of studies examining the effects of preinjury performance upon postinjury recovery of cognitive functions have usually relied upon a single-score estimate of intelligence. Most typically, it has been the soldier injured during combat who has such information available. These patients usually have an extensive military record, including test scores they received during their induction into the military. The qualification test score is a summary percentile score that reflects performance on several subtests (e.g., vocabulary, mental arithmetic, object knowledge, and spatial processing). The classification score may also represent several subtests too, but these subtests tend to demand aptitude that is more related to eventual job assignments. For example, a subtest measuring reading speed might be related to a clerical assignment on a military base. These scores have fortunately been made available to researchers interested in recovery of function. An additional advantage in studying wounded soldiers is that they are representative of the community at-large in age, education, socioeconomic status, and sociocultural habits. This might not be the case for soldiers who suffer accidental head injuries during peacetime.

When civilian patients have been studied, it has proven very difficult to obtain preinjury information about their cognitive abilities. There have been few studies of adults that have obtained either preinjury school test score data or if the patient served in the military, their military test score data. Most typically an index of educational level achieved is used along with occupational, and perhaps, socioeconomic status. Even when these cognitive indices are available, they have been primarily used as matching variables to reduce between-group variance, rather than to explore the recovery issues that are the focus of this chapter.

Weinstein and Teuber (1957a) had the opportunity to examine World War II veterans with penetrating head injuries and a group of matched controls on a military classification test (Army General Classification Test [AGCT]) that they had been administered prior to injury during induction when they were presumably normal and healthy. All the soldiers had been injured 1 to 3 years after induction and were retested approximately 10 years later. Location of brain injury was based on surgical notes and skull X-rays. The controls and brain-injured patients were matched on their preinjury scores and the controls on retesting gained an average of 13 points. Test–retest correlations were high ($r = .92$), indicating an orderly increase in scores among the controls. Among the brain-injured, only the patients with left temporal and temporal-parietal insult showed a decline in test scores from their premorbid performance, whereas all other brain-injured groups enjoyed at least a modest increase in test performance. Even after aphasics were eliminated from the left temporal and temporal-parietal groups, their performance remained the most impaired on the classification tests. In contrast to the specific effects of left temporal and temporal-parietal lesions on performance on this classification test, brain lesions, regardless of site, seemed to impair performance on specific visuospatial tests, such as the Hidden Figures Test.

In a subsequent paper, Weinstein and Teuber (1957b) attempted to analyze more carefully the effects of preinjury education and intelligence upon postinjury test scores, again using the Army General Classification Test score as the dependent variable. They found no relationship between preinjury education level and postinjury intelligence test performance. In fact, they also found that *lower* preinjury test scores tended to result in higher postinjury test scores. There was a positive correlation ($r = +.56$) between *preinjury* educational level and test performance. What was surprising was the lack of "functional protection" offered by advanced preinjury educational attainment or test performance on postinjury recovery.

Teuber (1960) cautioned against generalizing from these findings to postinjury recovery on all cognitive tests, since his research suggested that tests such as the Hidden Figures Test, which requires visuoanalytical processing, appear to be affected by lesions in disparate brain areas. In addition, since Teuber did not report on preinjury scores that represented visuospatial processes, it would be hard to argue with certainty that such tests do not show the same sensitivity to lesion location and size.

More recently, Grafman, Salazar, Weingartner, Vance, and Amin (1986) re-examined the relationship of brain tissue loss volume, lesion location, and pre-injury intelligence upon postinjury recovery on cognitive tasks. They studied veterans who suffered penetrating head wounds while in combat and a matched control group 15 years after their service in Vietnam. Unlike the studies conducted by Teuber and his coworkers, Grafman et al. had access to detailed CT scans on each patient (Fig. 14.1) for accurate localization and were able to examine three times as many subjects. They relied on stepwise multiple regression procedures to compare directly the percentage of variance of cognitive test performance postinjury that could be accounted for by the location of the lesion (verified by CT scan), size of lesion (CT scan summation), or the preinjury level of intellectual functioning (Armed Forces Qualification Test percentile score). In addition, Grafman et al. chose postinjury test scores that either represented a relatively unique cognitive process or were composite scores representing numerous cognitive operations. They found that preinjury intelligence level predicted a significant amount of the variance on postinjury cognitive testing, being a better predictor for tests requiring complementary cognitive processes (e.g., an intelligence test score) than for tests measuring a specific cognitive process (e.g., face recognition). Brain tissue loss volume was found to play a larger role when a global cognitive measure was used, but a smaller role when a specific cognitive process was measured. Finally, lesion location was shown to be a significant predictor of performance only for specific cognitive processes. Nevertheless, preinjury intelligence appeared to assume an even larger role in postinjury cognitive performance than either brain tissue loss volume or a particular structural loss (Figs. 14.2 and 14.3). This finding was weaker for patients with right hemisphere lesions, presumably because test selection was less appropriate. The authors felt that brain tissue volume loss may inhibit recovery of general cognitive processes because the remaining adjacent tissue fails to assume compensatory processing. Discrete structural loss would tend to inhibit recovery of specific cognitive processes but allow the use of compensatory cognitive processes subserved by spared adjacent or distant tissue to help patients perform on a cognitive task that allows for the use of alternate cognitive strategies to solve a problem, answer a question, or recognize previously shown information.

Grafman et al. (1988) more precisely evaluated the effects of premorbid intellectual function on postinjury intelligence test performance by focusing on the Armed Forces Qualification Test (AFQT), a test composed of four subtests assessing vocabulary knowledge, arithmetic word problem solving, object function recognition, and the ability to construct mental representations of geometrical figures (Fig. 14.4). A multiple regression analysis used to predict the veterans' postinjury intelligence test score found that preinjury intelligence was most predictive, size of lesion was next, and lesion location was least important. When predicting postinjury subtest scores from the same intelligence test, lesion location assumed a much greater predictive value. Specifically, left temporal and occipital lesions impaired performance on vocabulary and object function subtests. These findings essentially replicated their earlier study but made an additional statistical point. That is, a regression to the mean effect and high intercorrelation coefficient values will almost always be found with pre- and postinjury scores on the same test (Figs. 14.5 and 14.6). Thus, it is necessary to account for the effect of preinjury test scores prior to considering the effects of any other variable on the pre- to postinjury difference score. It can be shown that the "residualized gain," namely, the remaining error of prediction after pretest scores are regressed on posttest scores, is uncorrelated with pretest scores. Thus, by adjusting for pretest variance first (when a pretest score is available), an investigator can then assess the importance of other variables independent of the pretest score. Finally, the study by Grafman et al. (1988) (as opposed to studies by Teuber's group) found that preinjury education level had a mild association with postinjury AFQT performance, but only in the group of patients whose preinjury score on the AFQT fell below the 50th percentile.

In children, Rutter (Rutter, Chadwick, & Shaffer, 1983) reported that social class or socioeconomic status is of little importance in predicting cognitive outcome following head injury. He noted that while higher social class marginally benefits recovery, it never approaches statistical significance. In general, he dismissed any profound effects of preinjury intellectual achievement on postinjury recovery. Levin and Eisenberg (1979) had access to preinjury Performance IQ data in children. They found that a higher preinjury Performance IQ scale score was not protective and that in fact, the higher the preinjury Performance IQ score, the more likely they were to find a downward deviation in score on postinjury testing. At least for head injuries, Levin, Ewing–Cobbs, and Benton (1984) subscribe to a psychiatric (Tsuang, Boor, & Fleming, 1985), but not intellectual, risk factor importance for the *occurrence* of head injury.

The majority of studies referred to, with the exception of Grafman, Salazar et al. (1986), minimize the effects of premorbid learning aptitude and intelligence on recovery. Despite these negative results, clinical researchers are continuously trying to develop accurate estimators of premorbid intelligence when no test score is readily available. Several investigators (e.g., Hart, Smith, & Swash, 1986; and Larrabee, Largen, & Levin, 1985; O'Carroll & Gilleard, 1986) have attempted to estimate premorbid intellectual functioning in patients with Alzheimer's disease.

These studies have utilized either reading tests or "hold" tests (e.g., vocabulary) from the Wechsler Adult Intelligence Scale to make predictions about

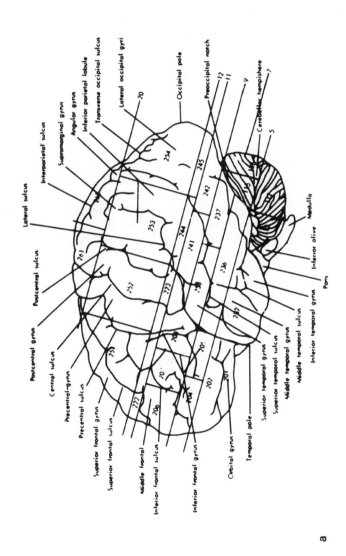

Lateral sulcus

Interparietal sulcus

Supramarginal gyrus

Angular gyrus

Inferior parietal lobule

Transverse occipital sulcus

Lateral occipital gyri

Occipital pole

Preoccipital notch

Cerebellar hemisphere

Postcentral gyrus

Postcentral sulcus

Central sulcus

Precentral gyrus

Precentral sulcus

Superior frontal gyrus

Superior frontal sulcus

Middle frontal

Inferior frontal sulcus

Inferior frontal gyrus

Orbital gyrus

Temporal pole

Superior temporal gyrus

Superior temporal sulcus

Middle temporal gyrus

Middle temporal sulcus

Inferior temporal gyrus

Pons

Medulla

Inferior olive

a

282

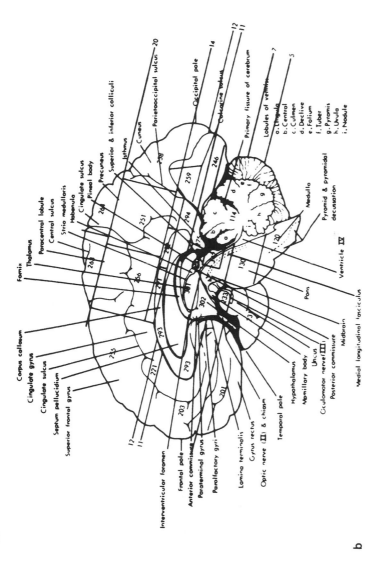

b

Corpus callosum
Cingulate gyrus
Cingulate sulcus
Septum pellucidium
Superior frontal gyrus

Fornix
Thalamus
Paracentral lobule
Central sulcus
Stria medullaris
Habenula
Cingulate sulcus
Pineal body
Precuneus
Superior & inferior colliculi
Isthmus
Cuneus
Parietooccipital sulcus — 20

Occipital pole

Calcarine sulcus — 14

Primary fissure of cerebrum — 12
                                — 11

Lobules of vermis — 7
a. Lingula
b. Central
c. Culmen
d. Declive
e. Folium
f. Tuber
g. Pyramis
h. Uvula
i. Nodule — 5

Medulla

Pyramid & pyramidal
decussation

Ventricle IX

Pons

Midbrain
Posterior commissure
Oculomotor nerve (III)
Unus
Mamillary body
Hypothalamus
Temporal pole
Optic nerve (II) & chiasm
Gyrus rectus
Lamina terminalis
Parolfactory gyri
Paraterminal gyrus
Anterior commissure
Frontal pole
Interventricular foramen

Medial longitudinal fasciculus

FIG. 14.1   CT was done with a GE 8800 scanner in standardized 5-mm cuts at about 25 degrees to Reid's baseline, yielding about 24 slices per patient. Involvement of more than 80 specific brain areas was coded for computer entry by the use of standard templates prepared for each slice, assigning code numbers to each area. Structures or areas only partly involved on CT were considered as completely involved for analysis to include possible areas of abnormal tissue around the lesion seen on CT. To aid in localization, we prepared a photographic, anatomical atlas by slicing a fresh-frozen specimen in *situ* at the same angle on a large cryotome and photographed it at 1-mm intervals, yielding more than 130 brain sections. Image analysis included both a subjective morphological interpretation as well as a quantitative lesion analysis, using a light pen to outline the affected area in each slice. Total lesion volume was then calculated from a summation of these areas on relevant slices. The lateral (a) and medial (b) views shown in this figure give an indication of coding assignments.

283

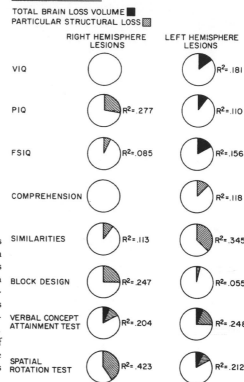

FIG. 14.2. In this figure the circles represent 100% of the variance on a particular test score. The filled-in parts of the circle represent the proportion of variance in test performance accounted for by either total brain loss volume or particular brain structure involvement (e.g., left temporal lobe). The R^2 represents the total amount of variance in performance that could be explained by brain loss volume plus particular brain structure loss.

premorbid functioning. Wilson, Rosenbaum, and Brown (1979) found that demographic factors were reasonable estimates of intellectual functioning pre-morbidly, when compared with intelligence test scores. Karzmark, Heaton, Grant, and Matthews (1984) attempted to replicate Wilson et al.'s (1979) findings and found a somewhat lower predictive accuracy when demographic factors were used. They found greater accuracy in predicting premorbid intel-ligence when just using education level achieved. Goldstein, Gary, and Levin (1986) cautioned that regression equations used to estimate premorbid intellec-tual functioning were adequate for midrange predictions but were likely to distort scores on both tails of the distribution of scores (they used sex, age, race, occupation, and education).

Premorbid intelligence measures are estimates of learned behavior and knowledge. Thus, they have some resemblance to preoperative learned behav-iors in animals. In humans, this type of knowledge is usually acquired over many years, whereas preoperative learning periods in animals may vary. An additional

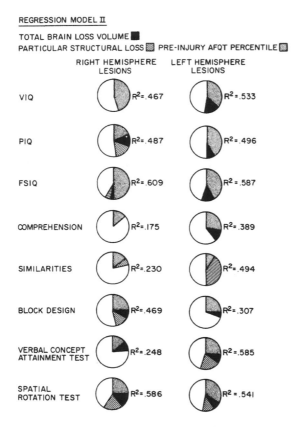

REGRESSION MODEL II

TOTAL BRAIN LOSS VOLUME ■
PARTICULAR STRUCTURAL LOSS ▨   PRE-INJURY AFQT PERCENTILE ▨

	RIGHT HEMISPHERE LESIONS	LEFT HEMISPHERE LESIONS
VIQ	$R^2 = .467$	$R^2 = .533$
PIQ	$R^2 = .487$	$R^2 = .496$
FSIQ	$R^2 = .609$	$R^2 = .587$
COMPREHENSION	$R^2 = .175$	$R^2 = .389$
SIMILARITIES	$R^2 = .230$	$R^2 = .494$
BLOCK DESIGN	$R^2 = .469$	$R^2 = .307$
VERBAL CONCEPT ATTAINMENT TEST	$R^2 = .248$	$R^2 = .585$
SPATIAL ROTATION TEST	$R^2 = .586$	$R^2 = .541$

FIG. 14.3   This multiple regression analysis added the variable of preinjury Armed Forces Qualification Test score. Compared with Fig. 14.2, it can be seen that the preinjury Armed Forces Qualification Test score accounts for more variance in postinjury test performance than either brain loss volume or brain structure loss.

factor that can be controlled for in animals, that is, learning to various criterion levels, would be very difficult to control in humans, although a good sample of human subjects will have an approximately normal distribution of a test score obtained premorbidly so that levels of ability can be a factor.

As reported here, general knowledge levels are well maintained postinjury in humans if assessment takes place beyond the acute recovery period. Thus, we can infer that there is not an overall loss in cognitive functioning. In addition, we noted that lesions to particular brain regions are more important than overall brain tissue loss in predicting postinjury performance on tasks requiring specific cognitive processes suggesting that the brain has a modular organization. This

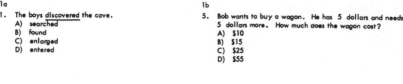

1a
1. The boys discovered the cave.
A) searched
B) found
C) enlarged
D) entered

1b
5. Bob wants to buy a wagon. He has 5 dollars and needs 5 dollars more. How much does the wagon cost?
A) $10
B) $15
C) $25
D) $55

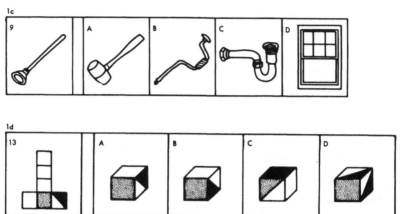

FIG. 14.4 Shows sample items from the vocabulary (1a) arithmetic (1b), objects (1c), and boxes (1d) subtests of the Armed Forces Qualification Test. For the objects and boxes subtests, the stimulus item is on the far left and subject must choose either the correct associate (1c) or the correct figure from the four choices to the right.

suggests that cortical "cognitive modules" may have linked to them specific encoding and retrieval processes that are unaffected by lesions to other cognitive modules. In addition, the effects of subcortical lesions to memory registration systems seems to affect new learning in almost all cognitive modules.

Aphasia in Bilinguals

As a group, polyglot and bilingual aphasics present like monolingual aphasics with respect to general aphasic impairments, when compared retrospectively (Albert & Obler, 1978). There are a few reports that language recovery in polygots is faster than in monolinguals (Holland et al., 1985), but these studies have methodological problems, including not considering recovery relative to the etiology of the reported case (e.g. sarcoidosis cannot be compared with cerebrovascular accidents, nor to tumors). Moreover, treatment factors are usually not mentioned. Unfortunately, there has been no prospective study that directly analyzes the size and topography of the lesion, symptomatology, and

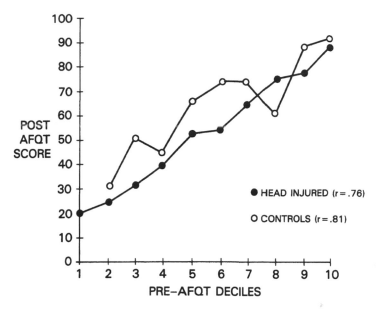

FIG. 14.5 This figure shows the relationship between pre- and postinjury Armed Forces Qualification Test scores for men with penetrating brain wounds and controls.

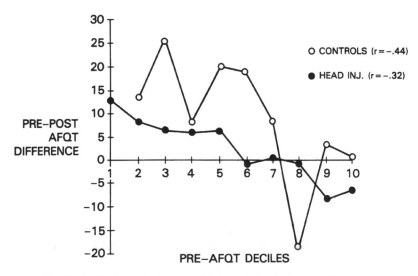

FIG. 14.6 This figure demonstrates the varied relationship between the preinjury Armed Forces Qualification Test (AFQT) and the pre post AFQT difference score for head-injured and controls. Note that subjects with lower preinjury scores tend to show greater improvement than those with higher scores.

recovery rates of monolinguals versus bilinguals, but from the data presented in the literature (and from our own clinical experience with a Catalan-Spanish community) there is generally no difference in the types of aphasias or in the rate of recovery given a similar lesion and etiology.

The typical case of a polyglot aphasia is one in which all languages are impaired to an equal degree (Albert & Obler, 1978; Charlton, 1964; Paradis, 1977). But in some cases, languages are lost in different degrees, sometimes even resulting in completely different syndromes in different languages. There have been several patterns of recovery of language described, beginning with Ribot (1882), who stated that the selective return of the "mother tongue" was merely a particular case of the law of regression, that is, the most recent episodes committed to memory are the first destroyed, the older the episode, the more stable it should be. This was referred to as "Ribot's rule," and also implied that the linguistic habits acquired in early childhood were more resistant to aphasic changes than those acquired subsequently, irrespective of the relevant degree of fluency at the time of the insult. Pitres (1895) showed that the "mother tongue" was not always the one best recovered, rather more often the language recovered was the most familiar or conversant to the patient at the moment of the insult, that is, the language of the milieu (e.g., the language of the country that the patient was living in at the time of the insult). Minkoswki (1927) suggested that emotional factors, through a powerful psychoneurobiological dynamic force, are capable of playing a decisive role during recovery in the struggle to select a particular language to be used. Later on, Minkowski (1963) emphasized that although several factors interacted during recovery none were predictive of outcome.

Paradis (1977, 1986; Paradis, Goldblum, & Abidi, 1982) has extensively described several possible patterns of restitution: (1) synergistic: in which the progress in one language is accompanied by similar progress in another (the most frequent); this type can be subdivided into (a) differential: The impairment in each of the languages is different, but progress in one language is nevertheless accompanied by progress in the other, (b) parallel: There is a similar impairment and recovery of both languages at the same rate and to the same extent relative to their premorbid fluency (the most common), (2) antagonistic: One language regresses; meanwhile the other progresses, (3) successive: One language does not reappear until the other is completely restored, (4) mixed: The patient mixes words or intonation among the different languages, (5) selective: The patient recovers some languages but not others, and (6) alternate antagonism: The patient can speak only one language for a given period of time, with languages alternating for consecutive periods.

In discussing recovery, one must address whether there is a greater participation of the nondominant hemisphere in the representation and/or processing of language in bilinguals. Some authors (such as Gloning & Gloning, 1965; Minkowski, 1963) proposed an increased participation of the right hemisphere.

However, the participation of right hemisphere mechanisms in language recovery is far from clear considering the data collected with several experimental methods, including the Wada Test and cortical stimulation (Rapport & Tan, 1983). Some authors (Stark, Genesee, Lambert, & Seitz, 1977) conclude that bilingualism actually intensifies the development of cerebral dominance; others (e.g., Gordon, 1980) do not see any difference in lateralization. Most researchers agree, however, that all languages are subserved by a common cortical region or are jointly distributed over the classical language areas. The two most favored hypotheses used to explain unrecovered language are that (1) Language is not lost but inhibited, and (2) That there is a locus in the brain that acts as a switch mechanism, which allows the patient to shift from one language to another.

Thus, an increased level of linguistic proficiency can be inferred in patients who were premorbidly fluent in more than one language. The effects of this proficiency on recovery from brain damage can be compared with those people who only speak one language premorbidly. In this case, the "preoperative factor" would be degree of language ability and its effect upon postinjury language functioning.

Unfortunately, it is currently difficult to determine the frequency of occurrence of nonparallel recoveries, since information relating to parallel recoveries is not generally published. Furthermore, it is difficult to compare the various published cases with each other because of the lack of standardization of assessments and a lack of important details from most descriptions. There is an ongoing multicenter study developed by the department of linguistics at McGill University in Montreal, in conjunction with neuropsychologists and neurolinguists from the l'Institute National de la Santé et de la Recherche in Paris, that utilizes a recently created Bilingual Aphasic Test that has been translated into 40 languages, including those spoken by large bilingual populations around the world. This multicenter effort will eventually provide us with several answers to the issue of types of aphasia and patterns of recovery among bilinguals.

Premorbid Personality

In the wake of an acute or a chronic, deteriorative brain disorder, the patient often experiences changes in temperament or personality, sometimes with psychotic-like or schizophreniform features, particularly if the neural damage is pervasive and severe, due to encephalitis, cortical or subcortical dementia, neurotoxic, endocrinological, or metabolic disorders (Lishman, 1983).

The available data, albeit sparse, suggest that psychiatric sequelae of brain damage are variable and unlikely to be produced by a single factor. This view was articulated nicely by Lishman (1983) and others who described primary, secondary, and tertiary (reactive) components which promote neuropsychiatric deficits following brain disorders; sex, age at onset, preinjury personality and cognitive capabilities, severity and locus of injury, the regimen of medication, socioeconomic and employment status, extent and type of cognitive-physical-social defects, the veridicality of the patient's (and family's) perception of changes, environmental and societal reactions and those by the patient and family, status of litigation/compensation, sensorimotor defects, and the emergence of epilepsy. Several recent texts offer excellent overviews of the psychosocial and educational problems associated with the neurobehavioral consequences of traumatic brain damage and the harsh compromises these deficits impose on the patient, family and support individuals (Brooks, 1984; Goldstein & Ruthven, 1983; Jennett & Teasdale, 1981; Levin, Benton, & Grossman, 1982; Lishman, 1983; Prigatano, 1986; Rosenthal, Griffith, Bond, & Miller, 1983).

That distinct personality patterns have not been aligned with specific neurological disorders may be due to the use of diagnostic behavioral indices with psychiatric patients and the absence of a comprehensive neural theory of emotions (Bear, 1983). As a result, there have been numerous, but equivocal attempts to profile premorbid personality traits which might identify individuals at risk for emotional disorders following neurological dysfunction (see Lishman, 1983). Scattered efforts have failed to codify pre- versus postinjury personality changes, and in most instances, test results are not usually available except retrospectively, and then, by inventory or interview with a risk of overstatement (Brooks, 1984; Jennett & Teasdale, 1981).

Moreover, in select cases with premorbid psychometric and personality test results, the patients were usually referred for diagnostic and treatment purposes, casting suspicion about pre-existing maladjustment. Preinjury behavioral observations, regardless of less than ideal methodology or format, are deemed valuable to chart treatment and prognosis, and provide the "best prediction of the degree to which the patient and his family will make a satisfactory post-injury adaptation" (Rosenthal et al., 1983, p. 410).

Rehabilitation specialists dealing with neurological patients usually concur that individuals with prior emotional or characterological instability may be at risk to display an organic mental syndrome, postconcussion or posttraumatic stress disorder, depending on the severity of the injury (Brooks, 1984; Prigatano, 1986). Thus, a premorbidly hostile, carping, and overly anxious individual is likely to manifest irritability, anger, or belligerence; emotional dyscontrol after head injury is more probable by patients who evinced emotional lability before the accident (Panting & Merry, 1972).

Teuber (1960) noted that preinjury attitudes may exert a positive or negative influence on postinjury losses and reactions, but these effects vary in accordance with lesion size and location. Strategically located lesions may interfere with the patient's ability to act on or remember intent and motives; the original resilience commanded by the patient improves his or her reactions to injury. Oddy and Humphrey (1980) reported that 2 years after head injury, patients who remained unemployed were described as "nervous and suspicious" prior to the accident, suggesting that such patients were premorbidly disposed to mood changes postinjury.

A cadre of workers (Brooks & McKinlay, 1983; Jennett & Teasdale, 1981; Prigatano, 1986) have challenged the assumption that premorbid personality precisely predicts psychiatric sequelae after craniocerebral injury. Earlier, Kozol (1946) reported "no correlation between pre-traumatic personality and the liability to development of post-traumatic mental symptoms"; his work was based on an historical-biographical inventory of 60 traits. Whereas neurotic patients offered persistent complaints about fatigue, insomnia, headaches, and dizziness, neurotic symptoms also appeared in patients who were relatively well adjusted before the accident. In some cases, totally new and unexpected behaviors emerged, related in part to the extent and locus of lesion, and the reaction by the patient to the perceived changes. Interestingly, normal individuals ran a close second in reporting postinjury symptoms. In turn, the psychopathic individual showed elevated euphoria, and a lack of concern and seriousness after injury; this impression had to be tempered by evidence of alcohol dependency in this group.

Brooks and McKinley (1983) requested relatives to rate emotional changes in patients retrospectively and at 3, 6, and 12 months after head injury. The changes were adverse and centered on emotional dyscontrol, unhappiness and immature, child-like behavior. The ratings revealed a triad of complaints: irritability, dependency, and insensitivity, traits which were unrelated to their premorbid personality. These authors also found a relation between negative features and "subjective burden." That is, unresolved emotional and behavioral residua were more likely than physical disabilities to encumber and stress the family. Durable posttraumatic emotional defects were highly disruptive to relationships, especially with spouses and children, as opposed to parents.

With closed head injury, guarded expectations are usually affixed to cases with severe and multiple trauma, lengthy coma, and an amnesia which envelopes events after (and to lesser degree, before) the accident. These patients are likely to incur irreparable psychosocial maladjustment regardless of their pretraumatic personality or temperament (Bond, 1986; Brooks, 1984; Levin et al., 1982). Their psychoaffective changes may be plotted along a continuum of anxiety–depression, withdrawal and interpersonal isolation, and disorganized ideational processes (Bond, 1986; Prigitano, 1986). Such changes may also obscure other intrusive determinants identified as distractibility, perplexity, and reduced stamina, which were uncharacteristic in the patient's premorbid history (Lezak, 1978).

In many instances and in spite of obvious impairment in memory and socialization, many patients fail to recognize and acknowledge their problems (Tyerman & Humphrey, 1984). In clinical practice, there is an inclination to interpret "denial of illness" (anasognosia) by neurological patients within the realm of psychological defenses, for example, repression, suppression, or displacement (Prigatano, 1986). Accordingly, the patient more likely to have right-brain injury and left-hemibody neglect minimizes the disability. During early recovery, this patient may fault therapists or programs for his or her unresponsive hemiparesis and failures. Weinstein (Weinstein & Cole, 1963; Weinstein & Kahn, 1955) examined the premorbid style of hemiparetic patients exhibiting denial and reported that denial was not a consequence of right parietal damage only, and may reflect an imperception. This trait was more likely to occur in individuals who even before injury or disease tended to discount personal shortcomings. However, the disturbances in emotional orientation and surveillance by patients with right-brain lesions (Bear, 1983) cannot be explained solely on the basis of pretraumatic personality style.

In sum, brain disorders or lesions undeniably alter emotions and behavior, though these defects may initially be eclipsed by life–death issues, physical disabilities, and intellectual impairment. With the passage of time and reluctant acceptance of the cognitive deficits, the personal-social defects of the patient soon threatens the integrity and the emotional and financial resources of the family, the marriage, and employment stability. In this context, the available data posit a link between the premorbid personality and postinjury psychiatric sequelae and changes in emotionality. Recent studies, however, suggest that the locus and extent of injury plays a far more important role than has heretofore been assumed, especially if frontotemporal structures are implicated in the injury or disease process (Grafman, Vance, Weingartner, Salazar, & Amin, 1986).

The Talented Individual

In studying premorbid effects upon recovery from brain damage, one must also examine the effects, if any, of the development of particular skills to exceptionally high levels. The rarity of such individuals, let alone those who have suffered some form of cerebral insult, limits the number of available documented cases. Moreover, many cases have been shrouded in secrecy, probably out of fear of damaging the individual's or organization's public image (e.g., the cases of boxer Muhammad Ali and baseball pitcher J. R. Richards).

There are nevertheless a few exceptional individuals from the literary, musical, and graphic arts who have been extensively studied by Alajouanine (1948), Zaimov (Zaimov, Kitov, Kolev, Regnault, & Perot, 1969), Botez and Wertheim (1959), Wertheim and Botez (1961), Jung, and more recently by Gardner (1975, 1982) and Kornyey (1977). These investigators describe the patterns of lost and preserved linguistic, intellectual, and artistic skills, as well as, changes in aesthetic taste, style, and personality associated with brain injury. The effects of brain damage among literary and graphic artists appear far more consistent then among professional musicians. These apparent differences between groups is thought to be related to the survival value of the underlying cognitive functions which predominantly serve the literary and graphic arts. Our ability to communicate to each other and to orient ourselves visually within the environment are far more important for survival than our ability to perceive or produce music. As such, specific brain regions appear to be genetically committed to serving linguistic and visuospatial functions while musical abilities may be laid down in cortex according to that individual's type of training, if any, and level of expertise.

We begin this survey of the relative resilience of talented individuals to brain damage by looking at a few documented cases of major painters who suffered left-hemisphere lesions. Alajouanine described the case of a major French painter known for his "originality of matter, technical qualities of realization, and intense individualism of each of his works" (p. 235, 1948). At the age of 52 the artist was struck with aphasia of Wernicke's type, sparing phonetic discrimination. He was severely anomic and made numerous paraphasic errors when speaking. Reading and writing were equally disturbed. His comprehension was adequate as he was capable of understanding the general meaning of a conversation. He showed no signs of hemiplegia but had a slight hemianopic defect. The only difference in his paintings before and after the onset of aphasia noted by Alajouanine was that they had "perhaps gained a more intense and acute expression." Zaimov et al. (1969) describe the case of a painter who, prior to an acquired brain injury, was known for his narrative style. His paintings usually depicted pastoral scenes of people and places from his native Bulgaria. In 1951, at the age of 47, he suffered an apoplectic ictus which resulted in paralysis of the right arm and a persistent severe aphasia. His expressive vocabulary was limited to 70 to 80 words and his ability to comprehend spoken language varied from day to day and was limited primarily to concrete words and short sentences. He was unable to resume reading or writing although he could copy written text. Memory and intelligence had, reportedly, remained intact. He first attempted to paint again 3 months after his seizure. The authors describe it as an intensely emotional moment when, during a visit from his mother, he asked to be seated on a chair and began painting with his *left hand,* which he had never done before. The likeness to her was striking. From that point on he continued to paint with his left hand. Despite his continued productivity, he underwent a dramatic change in style going from more narrative to more abstract, ethereal depictions of his subjects. His postinjury paintings lacked perspective and were filled with fantastic elements and condensed images. The control that he had exercised in his preinjury paintings was no longer apparent, as he took liberties with relative size and logical progression.

More recently, Marsh and Philwin (1987) describe the case of 72-year-old man who had a left posterior parietal tumor. He displayed both an expressive and receptive aphasia, was unable to write his name or to draw or copy line drawings of objects on command. A few months prior to his death the patient redid a painting which he had completed and not seen for 4 years. A comparison of the paintings shows extensive right-side neglect, constructional distortions, and heightened emotionality. The authors attribute the greater deficits seen in their patient, as opposed to those previously described with left-hemisphere lesions, to the nature of the lesion. Neglect is more often associated with fast-growing tumors (Heilman, 1979). Moreover, the length of time between the onset of lesion and the resumption of artistic activities seems to be important in the detection of neglect (Engerth & Urban, 1933).

Gardner (1975) described one of Jung's cases (Louis Corinth), an innovative German artist active during the early part of this century. Corinth had established a strong reputation for his expressive portraits and his unsentimental landscapes when, in 1911, he suffered a right-hemisphere stroke which left him with some right-sided weakness. He also suffered from a severe depression following the accident. After several months of recovery, Corinth resumed his work, but the new paintings were now distinctly different. The outlines were more deliberate, features were exaggerated to the point where portraits looked almost like caricatures of the model. Edges and contours became blurred or were missing from the right side of the painting. These changes were interpreted by the art critics of the day as reflecting Corinth's new vision of life stemming from his own experiences. The paintings are, however, strikingly similar to the drawings rendered by right-hemisphere-lesioned patients when *level of ability* is taken into account. The tendency to obscure or omit parts of the left side of space, to omit or misplace details, and generally simplify, are all characteristic of the graphic reproductions of patients with posterior right-hemisphere lesions. The altered emotional nuances, heightened subjectivity and idiosyncrasy seen in Corinth's later paintings are aspects not normally apparent in the relatively primitive drawings of most patients but are qualities which may be expressed in other behaviors.

At first glance, the evidence reviewed here suggests that the graphic artist's artistic abilities seem to be quite resilient to brain damage. The painters who had left-hemisphere damage coupled with hemiplegia were able to create works comparable with those prior to the onset of aphasia by learning to use the other hand, despite only minor recovery of language functions. Although the damaged right-hemisphere case showed signs of left-side neglect, the right side of the paintings showed remarkable preservation of shape and form lacking from the drawings of average right-hemisphere-lesioned persons. However, a closer look into the changes displayed in the paintings before and after the onset of illness suggests patterns of deficits which are similar to those seen in the general population.

The changes in style observed among left-hemisphere-damaged artists can be interpreted as resulting from impaired access to semantic knowledge. Martin (1987) described the case of an Alzheimer's disease (AD) patient who suffered from severe word-finding problems and impaired semantic knowledge but could nonetheless slavishly copy line drawings. Even though he demonstrated relatively intact visuospatial abilities on a route-finding task his errors were primarily related to rule breaking rather than an inability to find his way. The rule breaking seen in his patient may be related to the observed loss of artistic control regarding perspective and relative size. Painters who prior to their brain injury had depicted their subjects with a high level of realism, now tended toward the more abstract. What was thought to be greater artistic license taken by the artist may have, in fact, been more a symptom of the underlying cerebral pathology. Another of Martin's AD patients, who displayed artistic aptitudes, had relatively intact word-finding abilities but suffered from visuospatial and constructive impairments. The accuracy of this patient's copies of various material varied with the level of meaningfulness and the degree of detail. Meaningful material with details such as shadowing were well reproduced while abstract line drawings were poorly reproduced. Martin described this patient as relying on intact semantic representations to copy the material; in instances where semantic categorization was difficult, the patient was unable simply to follow the lines within the drawing. Perhaps Corinth was also relying on intact semantic knowledge to continue his painting.

We now turn to the effects of brain damage on the careers of renowned literary artists. We were unable to document any cases of writers having suffered right-hemisphere lesions. The lack of such studies is probably due to the absence of language deficits that would cause literary problems. It would, nevertheless, be interesting to note changes, if any, in the writer's style or preferred subject matter.

There are, however, cases of famous writers suffering left-hemisphere disease. Charles Baudelaire's talent was abruptly and permanently lost when he was struck down by a right-sided hemiplegia and severe aphasia. According to his friends, the poet could only utter the curse: *cre nom* (Alajouanine, 1948). Unfortunately, there is no record of any attempt by Baudelaire to continue writing with the unaffected hand. Alajouanine (1948, 1973) provides a more recent and in-depth account of the course of a similar affliction to Valery Larbaud, an award-winning French poet and essayist who spoke several languages fluently. At age 57, Larbaud abruptly suffered neurological illness. He initially showed severe right hemiplegia and aphasia; his speech was limited to a macabre *leitmoti* sentence: *Bonsoir les choses d'ici-bas*, which he uttered involuntarily and often inappropriately. Comprehension, however, was good and improved gradually. Reading, memory, reasoning, judgment, spatial orientation, and artistic appreciation all seemed unaffected. His speech and writing improved but he retained agrammatisms which effectively prevented any literary creations. Although he was eventually able to enjoy and critique the works of others by showing signs of approval or disapproval, the remaining aphasic symptoms had robbed him of the cognitive tools necessary for continued artistic expression, despite his premorbid training.

In their classic work on language, Jakobson and Hale (1956) analyzed the writing style of the famous Russian novelist Gleb Ivanovic Uspenskij, who reportedly suffered from a speech disorder during the latter part of his life. They consider his lengthy descriptions of scenes and characters, ladened with synecdochic details, to be symptomatic of, what they called, a similarity disorder. (Briefly, a similarity disorder is exemplified by a person's inability or unwillingness to acknowledge the equivalence of certain terms, i.e., to use two symbols to designate the same thing.) The reader was easily lost in a sea of details, thereby failing to grasp the whole.[1] Jakobson and Halle cannot rule out the influence the literary predilections of the time may have had on Uspenskij. Yet his writings clearly demonstrate an exaggerated metonymic style. Gardner (1975) theorized that the various writing styles used by some of the great authors are mimicked by aphasics but lack the richness of meaning and emotion underlying the great works. For example, the terse recitations of a Broca's aphasic can resemble Hemingway's short-sentenced style. The ramblings of a Wernicke's aphasic can resemble Faulkner's flowing, syntactically complex style. As in the case of great painters who continued to paint after brain injury, perhaps certain literary works distinguished by their peculiar or exaggerated style may have resulted, in part, from brain injury which did not sufficiently impair language functions as to render the authors without the means for continued expression.

The available data pertaining to brain-injured musicians are far less consistent. Lesions to either side of the brain may induce similar or different symptoms. These results may partly be due to changes in the relative salience of various features of music as the musician becomes more proficient. The untrained listener is thought to focus on the "gestalt" of the melody while the musically sophisticated listener focuses more on the relations between sets of musical elements. The former approach is associated with right-hemisphere functioning while the latter is more often associated with the left hemisphere. Hence, the type and level of musical training someone receives may affect the relative salience of certain features of music. The talented musician, by virtue of his or her different approach to music, may therefore also differ in resilience to brain disease.

Luria and his colleagues (Luria, Tsvetkova, & Futer, 1965) described the case of V. G. Shebalin, an accomplished Russian composer. Shebalin suffered vascular lesions to the temporal-parietal and temporal regions, leaving him with a severe auditory aphasia. Reading and writing were largely preserved, although

---

[1]A. Kamegulov cited in Jakobson and Halle (1956), p. 80. "From underneath an ancient straw cap with a black spot on its shield, there peeked two braids resembling the tusks of a wild boar; a chin grown fat and pendulous definitely spread over the greasy collars of the calico dicky and in thick layer lay on the coarse collar of the canvas coat, firmly buttoned on the neck. From below this coat to the eyes of the observer there protruded massive hands with a ring, which had eaten into the fat finger, a cane with a copper top, a significant bulge of the stomach and the presence of very broad pants, almost of muslin quality, in the broad ends of which hid the toes of the boots."

he tired easily and was unable write long words or a series of phrases. He was nevertheless able to continue teaching and composed some of his best works.

In contrast, the outstanding French composer Ravel was unable to compose any new pieces after being struck down by a moderate aphasia. There was no recorded paralysis or hemianopia but certain ideomotor apraxias were present. Alajouanine (1948) attributed the cause of the aphasic breakdown to some form of cerebral atrophy because of the presence of bilateral ventricular enlargement.

Botez and Wertheim (1959) reported a case of expressive amusia resulting from a tumor situated in the posterior third of the first two convolutions of the right frontal lobe. This right-handed patient also exhibited transitory expressive aphasia with dysprosody. Unlike the previous cases, the amusia occurred in the absence of severe aphasia. Although the patient had no formal training, he made his living playing the accordion and singing. The observed deficits were mostly limited to the musical expression. An important exception to his intact receptive musical abilities occurred when the patient was asked to sing and accompany himself on the accordion. He sang with correct intonation but his accordion playing was chaotic. Remarkably, the patient was not the least affected by the "atonalism" of the instrument and kept on singing. Although his receptive musical abilities were largely spared, these subtle deficits may have been the result of his lack of training. His singing was probably subserved more by intact left-hemisphere structures while his inability to play the melody on the accordion simultaneously, or be aware of the discordance between his singing and playing, may have been due to impaired right-hemisphere functioning.

This brief overview of the preserved abilities of distinguished artists after brain injury leads to two general conclusions. First, in most cases where the capacity to express their talents remain, artists are able to resume their activities albeit in an altered way. Secondly, when premorbid level of ability is taken into account, the patterns of changes after the onset of illness suggests that the underlying brain organization of exceptional individuals and the general population is essentially the same. Lastly, the apparent preserved functioning in particularly visual and musical artists may be due to the use of strategies which were acquired during their lengthy and intensive training. For instance, Gombrich (1961) describes many of the painter's strategies which were developed through the ages to render more realistic three-dimensional representations onto a two-dimensional medium. Although Corinth and Martin's patient C had obvious visuospatial deficits, they may have relied on a set of rules or strategies acquired through training and experience in order to accomplish their work. Conversely, Zaimov's patient Z. B. and Martin's patient W either chose not to or were unable to follow specific rules. In Z. B.'s case, the critics interpreted the lack of control in his later paintings to be an increase in artistic licence taken to convey stronger emotions.

These results support the thesis that many independent cognitive modules may contribute to the final artistic creation and that the impairment of certain cognitive processes may alter the patient's performance without robbing him or her completely of his or her artistic abilities. Individuals of average ability may not have enlisted as many cognitive processes and are therefore more susceptible to the ill effects of brain injury on that specific function.

GENERAL DISCUSSION

Our review indicated that there have been few group studies that have directly tested the question of whether premorbid abilities and interpersonal functioning play a significant role in postbrain-injury recovery and outcome. The studies that have shed the most light in this area are those that utilized military veterans and took advantage of the accessibility of preinjury cognitive data in the form of a classification-intelligence test. These studies suggest that despite statistical effects such as "regression to the mean" or "covariate relationships between measures administered twice or more to the same individuals," the protective power of preinjury ability level (as reflected in performance on intelligence tests that measure various knowledge domains and skills) for eventual postinjury outcome is apparent. That is, while obtaining a higher score (i.e., a better performance) in a cognitive domain or skill will not prevent a diminished score postinjury (nor would a poorer score prevent improvement or a practice effect on postinjury testing), the data suggest that patients will generally remain at the same ability level despite size and location of lesion. This deceptively simple finding indicates that when an injury or disease is not all-consuming (as might be the case in a dementing or encephalitic disorder), compensatory cognitive and behavioral processes will subsidize performance on tests postinjury. If we assume that affected cognitive processes in different individuals would be equally impaired following nervous system insult or disease, then the overall ability of patients as measured by a standard test of intellectual ability should remain stable after brain damage. Thus, when assessing group results on a general test of cognitive ability (which requires the contribution of numerous cognitive processes), the protectiveness of premorbid state (whether a person is bright or dull) is observed. An argument could be made that this premorbid ability as reflected by classification-intelligence test performance, at least partly based on exposure to, and training on, specific cognitive skills resembles those paradigms that train animals to learn certain behaviors prior to lesioning and subsequent to the lesion find that the most "expert" of the lesioned animals recovers faster (e.g., Smith, 1959).

Unfortunately, the picture becomes more clouded at the level of the individual patient. This problem has been illustrated by the presentation of skilled artists and musicians who suffered brain damage. Their postinjury deficits reinforce the concept that *specific* cognitive processes are modular and that such processes can be so impaired by brain disease or trauma that the artist never reattains his previous form (although he may resume painting or composing with skill, the representations or compositions differ in style and substance making use of unimpaired cognitive processes). In the group studies we reviewed, this phenomenon was seen when subtests of a classification-intelligence test were used for data analysis. These subtests frequently required specialized cognitive processes (e.g., imaginal generation of visual representations) which were very susceptible to impairment by local/focal lesions and not "protected" by premorbid ability level. This suggests that all functions or abilities rely on a hierarchy of cognitive processes that can be dissociated as a result of brain damage. Functional ability will appear more impaired as the cognitive processes or representations most important for the expression of a functional ability are damaged.

Expertise in languages does not protect against postinjury aphasic deficits although the pattern of recovery may be affected. Bilinguals and monolinguals reportedly share similar recovery rates and also share in the persistence of specific cognitive deficits. However, new language learning following brain injury has not been reported and further studies are needed to control for the methodological problems raised in our review of bilingual language recovery after brain damage.

The issues surrounding premorbid personality and postinjury behavioral changes are clearly too complex to resolve at this time. What is known about pre-existing psychiatric disorder is that it makes an individual more likely to experience a traumatic brain injury (e.g., more likely to be intoxicated and reckless when driving). Studies comparing patients with and without a premorbid documented psychiatric history could be a first step in addressing the role of premorbid personality and mood in recovery of function following brain damage.

On a more positive note, this review has identified several factors that contribute to an understanding of premorbid effects upon postbrain-injury recovery. Premorbid level of cognitive ability remains the most powerful factor in predicting postinjury level of recovery. This is particularly true when the level of recovery is assessed by a general measure of intelligence. More specific cognitive processes, despite the evidence of great proficiency pre-injury, may be permanently impaired post injury the specific process impaired dependent on the location of the lesion. In addition, preinjury psychiatric disorders predispose a patient to experience mood and behavioral changes postinjury. Specific cognitive processes and representations in spatially distinct brain regions suggest the concept of a self-contained information-processing module which would include stimulus/knowledge representations and associated encoding and retrieval mechanisms. These modules would encode information in parallel and redundant fashion. Thus, even though brain damage might affect a specific information-processing module, other modules that participate in stimulus analysis could assume a compensatory role. In the case of partial damage to a module, we would assume that representations within the module are distributed so that postinjury access to at least the most "consolidated" modular representations would be possible.

Finally, our review suggests that, in addition to the concept of modular cognitive representations and processing, a general learning capacity and ability is distributed throughout the brain. This capacity for learning is biologically conservative even in the event of brain injury. Therefore, the advantage in functioning postinjury, which probably also occurs preinjury, goes to the patient who had a relatively greater learning "capacity." Of course, in the face of severe brain damage or a progressive dementia, the predictive factor of learning ability or capacity diminishes in power.

In order to disentangle more completely the effect of preinjury ability upon postinjury performance, we advocate both task analysis and human information-processing approaches. Task analysis to define better the cognitive processes required for performance on neuropsychological tasks used to test patients; the human information-processing approach, because it best specifies and models the kinds and levels of cognitive processes that are required to perform a task. The degree of cognitive specificity identified and in turn the success in localizing the cognitive process to a set of brain structures or regions, will ultimately determine how precisely we can measure and predict the effects of preinjury ability upon postinjury outcome and recovery.

ACKNOWLEDGMENTS

The authors express their gratitude to Mrs. Ruth O'Reilly and Ms. Barbara King for their administrative expertise and their assistance in preparing the manuscript. We thank the National Institute of Neurological Disorders and Stroke, and Medical Neurology Branch for providing the facilities which allowed us to prepare the manuscript.

The opinions and assertions contained herein are the private views of the authors, and are not to be construed as official or necessarily reflecting the views of the National Institutes of Health, the United States Public Health Service, the Department of Health and Human Services, the Uniformed Services University of the Health Sciences, or the Department of Defense.

REFERENCES

Alajouanine, T. (1948). Aphasia and artistic realization. *Brain, 71,* 229–241.
Alajouanine, T. (1973). *Valery Larbaud sous divers visages.* Paris: Gallimard.
Albert, M. L., & Obler, L. K. (1978). *The bilingual brain.* New York: Academic Press.
Bear, D. (1983). Hemispheric specialization and the neurology of emotion. *Archives of Neurology,* 34, 195–384.
Bond, M. R. (1986). Neurobehavioral sequelae of closed head injury. In I. Grant & K. M. Adams (Eds.), *Neuropsychological assessment of neuropsychiatric disorders.* Oxford, England: Oxford University Press.
Botez, M. I., & Wertheim, N. (1959). Expressive aphasia and amusia following right frontal lesion in a right-handed man. *Brain, 82,* 186–203.

Brooks, D. N., & McKinlay, W. W. (1983). Personality and behavioral change after head injury—a relative's view. *Journal of Neurology and Neurosurgical Psychiatry, 46,* 336–344.

Brooks, D. N. (Ed.). (1984). *Closed head injury: Psychological, social and family consequences.* Oxford, England: Oxford University Press.

Charlton, M. (1964). Aphasia in bilingual and polyglot patients: A neurological and psychological study. *Journal of Speech and Hearing Disorders, 29,* 307–311.

Engerth, G., & Urban, H. (1933). Zur kenntnis der gestorten kunstlerischen leistung bei sensorischer aphasie. *Zeitschrift für Die Gesamte Neurologie und Psychiatrie, 145,* 753–787.

Gardner, H. (1975). *The shattered mind: The person after brain damage.* New York: Knopf.

Gardner, H. (1982). *Art, mind and brain: A cognitive approach to creativity.* New York: Basic Books.

Gloning, I., & Gloning, K. (1965). *Aphasien bei poliglotten. Beitrag zur Dynamik des Sprachabbaus sowie zur Lokalisationsfrage dieser Strungen.* Wiener Zeitschrift fur Nervenheilkunde, 22, 362–397.

Goldstein, F. C., Gary, H. E., Jr., & Levin, H. S. (1986). Assessment of the accuracy of regression equations proposed for estimating premorbid intellectual functioning on the Wecheler Adult Intelligence Scale. *Journal of Clinical and Experimental Neuropsychology, 8,* 405–412.

Goldstein, G., & Ruthven, L. (1983). *Rehabilitation of the brain-damaged adult.* New York: Plenum Press.

Gombrich, E. H. J. (1961). *Art and illusion: A study in the psychology of pictorial representation.* New York: Pantheon Books.

Gordon, H. (1980). Cerebral organization in bilinguals: Lateralization. *Brain and Language, 9,* 255–268.

Grafman, J., Jonas, B. S., Salazar, A. M., Weingartner, H., Ludlow, C., Smutok, M. A., & Vance, S. C. (1988). Intellectual function following penetrating head injury in Vietnam veterans. *Brain, 111,* 169–184.

Grafman, J., Salazar, A., Weingartner, H., Vance, S., & Amin, D. (1986). The relationship of brain-tissue loss volume and lesion location to cognitive deficit. *Journal of Neuroscience, 6,* 301–307.

Grafman, J., Vance, S. C., Weingartner, H., Salazar, A. M., & Amin, D. A. (1986). The effects of lateralized frontal lesions on mood regulation. *Brain, 109,* 1127–1148.

Hart, S., Smith, C. M., & Swash, L. M. (1986). Assessing intellectual deterioration. *British Journal of Clinical Psychology, 25,* 119–124.

Heilman, K. M. (1979). Neglect and related disorders in clinical neuropsychology. In K. M. Heilman & E. Valenstein (Eds.), *Clinical neuropsychology.* New York: Oxford University Press.

Holland, L. A., Miller, J., Reinmuth, O. M., Bartlett, C., Fromm, D., Pashek, G., Stein, D., & Swindell, C. (1985). Rapid recovery from aphasia: a detailed language analysis. *Brain and Language, 24,* 156–173.

Jakobson, R., & Halle, M. (1956). *Fundamentals of language.* Gravenhage, Netherlands: Mouton.

Jennett, B., & Teasdale, G. (1981). *Management of head injuries.* Philadelphia: Davis.

Karzmark, P., Heaton, R., Grant, I., & Matthews, C. G. (1984). Use of demographic variables to predict overall level of performance on the Halstead–Reitan Battery. *Journal of Consulting and Clinical Psychology, 52,* 663–665.

Kornyey, E. (1977). Aphasie et creation artistique. *L'Encephale, 111,* 71–85.

Kozol, U. L. (1946). Pretraumatic personality and psychiatric sequelae of head injury. II. Correlation of multiple, specific factors in the pretraumatic personality and psychiatric reaction to head injury, based on analysis of 101 cases. *Archives of Neurology and Psychiatry, 56,* 245–275.

Larrabee, G. J., Largen, J. W., & Levin, H. S. (1985). Sensitivity of age-decline resistant ("hold") WAIS subtests to Alzheimer's disease. *Journal of Clinical and Experimental Neuropsychology, 7,* 497–504.

Levin, H. S., & Eisenberg, H. M. (1979). Neuropsychological impairment after closed head injury in children and adolescents. *Journal of Pediatric Psychology, 4,* 389–402.

Levin, H., Ewing–Cobbs, L., & Benton, A. L. (1984). Age and recovery from brain damage: A review of clinical studies. In S. W. Scheff (Ed.), *Aging and recovery of function in the central nervous system.* New York: Plenum Press.

Levin, M. S., Benton, A. L., & Grossman, R. G. (1982). *Neurobehavioral consequences of closed head injury*. Oxford, England: Oxford University Press.

Lezak, M. (1978). Living with the characterologically altered brain injured patient. *Journal of Clinical Psychiatry, 39*, 592–598.

Lishman, W. A. (1983). *Organic psychiatry*. Oxford, England: Blackwell Scientific Publications.

Luria, A. R., Tsvetkova, L. S., & Futer, D. S. (1965). Aphasia in a composer. *Journal of the Neurological Sciences, 2*, 288–292.

Marsh, G. G., & Philwin, B. (1987). Unilateral neglect and constructional apraxia in a right-handed artist with a left posterior lesion. *Cortex, 23*, 149–155.

Martin, A. (1987). Representation of semantic and spatial knowledge in Alzheimer's patients: Implications for models of preserved learning in amnesia. *Journal of Clinical and Experimental Neuropsychology, 9*, 191–224.

Minkowski, M. (1927). Klinischer Beitrag zur Aphasie bei Polyglotten speziell im Hinblik aufs Schweizerdeutsche. *Schweizer Archiv für Neurologie und Psychiatrie, 21*, 43–72.

Minkowski, M. (1963). On aphasia in polygoys. In L. Halpern (Ed.), *Problems of dynamic neurology* (pp. 119–161). Jerusalem: Hebrew University.

O'Carroll, R. E., & Gilleard, C. J. (1986). Estimation of pre-morbid intellectual in dementia. *British Journal of Clinical Psychology, 25*, 157–158.

Oddy, M., & Humphrey, M. (1980). Social recovery during the year following severe head injury. *Journal of Neurology, Neurosurgery and Psychiatry, 43*, 798–802.

Panting, A., & Merry, P. (1972). The long-term rehabilitation of severe head injuries with particular reference to the need for social and medical support for the patient's family. *Rehabilitation, 38*, 33–37.

Paradis, M. (1977). Bilingualism and aphasia. In H. A. Whitaker & H. Whitaker (Eds.), *Studies in neurolinguistics* (vol. 13, pp. 65–121). New York: Academic Press.

Paradis, M. (1986). Neurolinguistic Perspectives on Bilingualism. In *The assessment of bilingual aphasia*, (pp. 1–17). Hillsdale, NJ: Lawrence Erlbaum Associates.

Paradis, M., Goldblum, M. C., & Abidi, R. (1982). Alternate antagonism with paradoxical translation behavior in two bilingual aphasic patients. *Brain and Language, 15*, 55, 69.

Pitres, A. (1895). Etude sur l'aphasie chez les polyglottes. *Revue de Medicine, 15*, 873–899.

Prigatano, G. (1986). *Neuropsychological rehabilitation after brain injury*, Baltimore: Johns Hopkins Press.

Rapport, R. L., & Tan, C. T. (1983). Language function and dysfunction among chinese and English speaking polyglots: Cortical stimulation, wada testing, and clinical studies. *Brain and Language, 18*, 342–366.

Ribot, T. (1882). *Diseases of memory: An essay in the positive psychology*. London: Kegan Paul. Originally published in 1881 as Les maladies de la memoire (Paris: G. Baillere).

Rosenthal, M., Griffith, E. R., Bond, M. R., & Miller, J. D. (Eds.). (1983). *Rehabilitation of the head injured adult*. Philadelphia: Davis Co.

Rutter, M., Chadwick, O., & Shaffer, D. (1983). Head injury. In M. Rutter (Ed.), *Developmental neuropsychiatry*. New York: Guilford Press.

Smith, C. J. (1959). Mass action and early environment. *Journal of Comparative and Physiological Psychology, 52*, 154–156.

Stark, R., Genesee, F., Lambert, W., & Seitz, M. (1977). Multiple language experience and cerebral dominance. In S. Segalowitz & F. Bruber (Eds.), *Language Development and Neurological Theory*. Orlando, FL: Academic Press.

Teuber, H. L. (1960). The premorbid personality and reaction to brain damage. *Journal of Orthopsychiatry, 30*, 322–329.

Tsuang, M. T., Boor, M., & Fleming, J. A. (1985). Psychiatric aspects of traffic accidents. *American Journal of Psychiatry, 142*, 538–546.

Tyerman, A., & Humphrey, M. (1984). Changes in self-concept following severe head injury. *International Journal of Rehabilitation Research 11–23*.

Weinstein, E. A., & Cole, M. (1963). Concepts of anosognosia. In L. Halpern (Ed.), *Problems in dynamic neurology.* Jerusalem: Hebrew University Medical School.

Weinstein, E. A., & Kahn, R. L. (1955). *Denial of illness: Symbolic and physiological aspects.* Springfield, IL: Thomas.

Weinstein, S., & Teuber, H.-L. (1957a). Effects of penetrating head injury on intelligence test scores. *Science, 125,* 1036–1037.

Weinstein, S., & Teuber, H.-L. (1957b). The role of pre-injury education and intelligence level in intellectual loss after brain injury. *Journal of Comparative and Physiological Psychology, 50,* 535–539.

Wertheim, N., & Botez, M. I. (1961). Receptive amusia: A clinical analysis. *Brain, 84,* 19–30.

Wilson, R. S., Rosenbaum, G., & Brown, G. (1979). The problem of pre-morbid intelligence in neuropsychological assessment. *Journal of Clinical Neuropsychology, 1,* 49–53.

Zaimov, K., Kitov, D., Kolev, N., Regnault, M., & Perot, F. (1969). Aphasie chez un peintre. *L'Encephale, 58,* 377–416.

Commentary 1

Preoperative Events and Brain Damage: A Commentary

Bryan Kolb
Department of Psychology
University of Lethbridge, Canada

The task I was assigned was "to comment on the chapters and to integrate them." This has not proven to be an easy task! The challenge for me, and indeed for any reader, is to extract a message from each chapter and somehow to integrate this collage of facts and experiments into a meaningful gestalt. As in any gestalt, the details are not especially important and while some of the details may influence the gestalt (and there are details of individual chapters that I might take issue with), it is the overall story that is important. Thus, it is here that I shall focus. I must add, however, that many of the chapters are excellent reviews. Good examples are Singh's and Grijalva et al.'s reviews of the effects of VMH and LH lesions, respectively, Ward's review of the effects of visual cortex lesions in bushbabies, and Overmier's review of the effects of forebrain lesions in teleosts. Grafman et al. probably had the most difficult task, that of looking at the effects of premorbid factors upon outcome of brain damage in humans. The variance in effects of similar brain damage in different people is a major puzzle and can often shake the confidence of the most unashamed localizationists. Indeed, it is in this chapter, and to some extent in Donovick and Burright's chapter that we get a feeling for the problems of variance, an important issue that I will return to later.

I have divided my commentary into several components. In the first, I shall review briefly the nature of the effects summarized in the chapters. I shall then consider the question of why such effects might or might not occur.

A PRECIS OF THE BOOK

While all of the chapters deal with preoperative events, the definition of what a preoperative event might be is broad and in different chapters the concept is used differently. Table 1 summarizes many of the preoperative events discussed and places them into three categories. The first category, nonspecific experience, refers to general conditions such as housing in enriched environments or in social groups, and level of education, as well as general factors, such as intelligence as measured by IQ. All of these factors are nonspecific because they influence many behaviors. For example, Albert and his colleagues emphasize the role of social housing on predatory aggression, but the effects are clearly much broader than this. They include effects on other aspects of social interaction and probably on general problem solving as well as food preferences and other behaviors.

The second category is that of specific effects of experiences such as the preoperatively solving of various problems such as visual discriminations or the acquisition of "knowledge" about specific stimuli, such as salt or other foods. The effects of these experiences would seem to be fairly specific to the particular behaviors being measured. For example, preoperative exposure to salt appears to influence changes in salt preference after gustatory thalamus lesions. I note that some of the effects appear to be specific to particular behaviors, but they are

TABLE 1
The Types of Preoperative Events that Affect
Lesion Outcome

Nonspecific Experience
  Social factors
  Environmental enrichment
  General intelligence
  Education
  Personality
Specific Experience
  Preoperatively learned habits
  Exposure to specific stimuli (e.g., tastes or foods)
  Restricted feeding or drinking
  Restricted sensory experience immediately pre-lesion
Neural Manipulations
  Previous brain damage
  Alterations in transmitter, modulator, or hormone levels
  Alterations in blood sugar level
  Castration

---

often not specific to particular brain treatments. Thus, preoperative dieting reduces feeding deficits and weight loss not only from lateral hypothalamic lesions, but also from orbital frontal lesions.

Finally, there are preoperative manipulations of the brain itself. For example, prior brain damage often alters the effects of later damage, as in the "serial lesion effect" discussed in many of the chapters. Curiously, there appears to be considerable variance in the consequences of preoperative neural manipulations. For example, whereas many authors reliably find serial lesion effects from forebrain lesions in rats, Overmier finds no such effects in teleosts and indeed, many authors, such as myself, have difficulty in reliably demonstrating these effects in rats when a broad test battery is used.

A review of Table 2, which is a simple summary of some of the major points about preoperative effects (at least to this reader), leads me to the conclusion that although preoperative effects can often be demonstrated, and are associated with lesions in many different regions, the fact of positive preoperative effects of experience is not ubiquitous. Even though absence of evidence of preoperative effects is hardly evidence of absence of the effects, it is clear that the effects are variable, a result that suggests that there must be modulating factors that somehow predispose the organism's response to the preoperative events. This strikes me as a central issue for it is in the variance in the effects of preoperative treatments that we may find the key to understanding, and to predicting, the action of preoperative events, and indeed, to understanding the mechanisms underlying the preoperative events.

Why Do Preoperative Events Affect Subsequent Behavior?

An initial step in understanding a phenomenon is to describe it. Once described, the next step is to dissect the phenomenon, in order to explore its basis. This dissection can be done in many ways. One approach is to manipulate variables and to examine the behavioral outcome. This is legitimate and it is the intent of many chapters in this book. There is danger here, however, as we must remember that explanations need to go beyond behavior at some point. Thus, to appeal to a mechanism of "learning" as an explanation may be useful but our explanation cannot stop there. It is not helpful to make statements such as "the brain compensates for . . . loss using mnemonic mechanisms in the initial regulation" or that the brain compensates using "conditioning mechanisms." What mechanisms are we talking about? How do these work? Why do they only work some times and for some behaviors?

It strikes me that there are at least three things to consider here. I shall call these things "the unstable environment," "the response to lesions," and "the mechanism of action."

TABLE 2
Summary of the Chapters

First Author	Conclusions Regarding Preoperative Experience
Albert	Social contact alters normal as well as lesion-potentiated predatory aggression.
Braun	No evidence for preop effects on the outcome of lesions in primary sensory regions.
Donovick	Preop castration and social factors have opposite effects on emotional change following septal lesions
Grafman	Preinjury abilities in humans are best predictors of postinjury ability level, although the precise ability measured is important. General intelligence has greatest effect.
Grijalva	Preop experiences have both central and peripheral effects. Behavioral effects may be related to the peripheral, rather just the central effects.
Lepore	Preop overtraining may lead to positive or negative transfer following callosal transections.
Kemble	Age and environment interact in effects of amygdala lesions. These effects are also task-dependent.
Krieckhaus	Highly specific preop effects of MTT lesions on avoidance learning.
Olton	Task-specific preop effects on septal/hippocampal lesions; show both positive and negative transfer.
Overmier	No unambiguous effect of preop training on outcome of forebrain lesions in teleosts depending on test conditions.
Schallert	Preop experiences, such as feeding or drinking regime, affect not only recovery but also postop drug effects.
Schulkin	Even brief preop exposure to specific sensory events (e.g., salt) may protect animals from lesion-induced behavioral changes. These preop events are highly specific to test conditions.
Singh	VMH syndrome modified by social experience and specific training. Peripheral changes (e.g., vagotomy) also affect lesion outcome.
Ward	Preop overtraining on specific problems has specific postop effect after lateral occipital lesions.

The Unstable Environment. It is implicit in the theme of this book that the environment has significant effects on both brain and behavior and that these effects somehow interact with the effects of lesions. There is little reason to doubt this is a general phenomenon, but there is a problem. It cannot be assumed that the effect of preoperative events is static. This is demonstrated beautifully in an experiment by Sutherland and Arnold (1987). Rats were preoperatively trained in the Morris water task (see Olton & Markowska's chapter

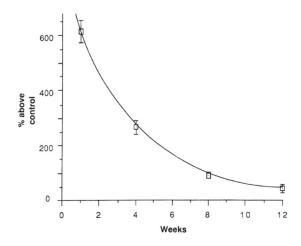

FIG. 1. Summary of the effects of hippocampal lesions performed at different intervals after training in the Morris water task. The effect of the lesion decreases markedly from 1 week after training to 12 weeks after training. All animals received the same postoperative recovery period (from Sutherland & Arnold, 1987).

for details of this task) before receiving injections of neurotoxins into the hippocampus, which produced a large hippocampal lesion. It has been shown previously in several labs that this procedure leads to a significant chronic deficit in spatial navigation (e.g. Morris, Garrud, Rawlins, Rawlins, & O'Keefe, 1981; Sutherland, Kolb, & Whishaw 1982). In Sutherland and Arnold's experiment, however, the animals did not all receive their lesions immediately; they received lesions from 1 to 12 weeks after training. The result was unambiguous: Preoperative training produced a greater beneficial effect with longer intervals between training and brain damage. In other words, animals that were trained, given lesions, and then retrained had larger impairments than animals that were trained and held for 3 months prior to surgery (Fig. 1). This result is important because it shows that the effect of the same environmental treatment varies over time. Consider the complications in humans who are constantly in an unstable environment in which they are learning and experiencing. It is hardly any wonder that there is such variability in the effects of similar brain damage to different people.

The Response to Lesions. If one is considering the effects of preoperative effects on postlesion behavior it is crucial to consider what lesions do to the brain. The effect of brain damage can be considered on two different levels: effects on behavior and effects on the brain. Behavioral effects of brain lesions can be sorted into three quite different classes: (1) loss of function, (2) release of function, and (3) disorganization of function. Nearly all of the chapters dealt largely with loss of function and its return under different preoperative treatments (but see Lepore). What about the latter two effects? Are there parallel data here, too?

Damage produces many effects in the brain, each of which is likely to respond differently to preoperative events. These include: (1) cell death, (2) gliosis, (3) edema, (4) calcification, (5) loss of synapses, (6) reactive synaptogenesis, (7) sprouting of axon collaterals and terminals, (8) sprouting of dendritic or axonal arbors, (9) changes in transmitter synthesis, release, reuptake, and so on, (10) changes in receptor sensitivity or receptor numbers, (11) changes in blood flow and metabolism, and (12) the production of trophic factors. In addition, of course, there are changes in physiological properties or characteristics of cells or aggregates of cells, as well as changes in the interactions of different areas of the brain. Which of these is affected by preoperative events? We have no idea but our explanations of preoperative effects depend on our having at least some vague notion of what the effects might be. Indeed, as Grijalva, Lindholm, and Roland show nicely, the effects need not even be central but could be peripheral, a possibility that has scarcely been considered to date.

The Mechanism of Action. The question of "why" preoperative effects influence the outcome of brain damage leads us directly to the question of what preoperative effects do to behavior and to the brain. Many of the chapters addressed the former question and proposed psychological explanations especially with respect to conditioning phenomena. What is needed now, however, is to focus our attention on what the physiological or morphological mechanisms might be. We know from more than 20 years of study that experience changes many morphological features of the brain, particularly the cortex. For example, different experiences produce specific and reliable changes in dendritic arborization and synapse formation with experiences (e.g., Greenough, 1984). Since parallel changes occur following brain damage, it is reasonable to suppose that preoperative events influence lesion outcome via such mechanisms. Further, it is likely that the brain is conservative, so that when behavioral plasticity occurs, whether it be in learning problems, experiencing events, or recovery from brain damage, the neural mechanisms underlying the plasticity will be similar. A significant challenge will be to determine what the neural changes are, to determine why and what way they change after experiences, and how they influence recovery from brain damage. As we begin to study these questions further behavioral questions will emerge and further behavioral work will be needed.

In conclusion, it seems reasonable to suggest that the brains of different individuals must be different in some nontrivial way, and thus the variance in the effect of treatments such as lesions or drugs may be accounted for, in part, by pretreatment variance in the brains themselves. The fact of pretreatment effects on lesion outcome is well documented in this volume but so too is the fact that pretreatment effects are not always beneficial, sometimes are without effect, and that they vary over time. We still must address the question of "why," however, and although one approach to this question is behavioral, the answer must go beyond a psychological level to a morphological or physiological explanation if we are to lay claim to understanding the question of how preoperative events influence the outcome from brain injury.

REFERENCES

Greenough, W. T. (1984). Possible structural substrates of plastic neural phenomena. In G. Lynch, J. J. McGaugh, & N. M. Wienberger (Eds.), *Neurobiology of learning and memory*. New York: Guilford Press.

Morris, R. G. M., Garrud, P., Rawlins, P., Rawlins, J. N. P., & O'Keefe, J. (1982). Place navigation impaired in rats with hippocampal lesions. *Nature, 297*, 681–683.

Sutherland, R. J., & Arnold, K. (1987). Anterograde and retrograde effects on place memory after limbic diencephalic damage. *Society for Neuroscience Abstracts, 13*, 1066.

Sutherland, R. J., Kolb, B., & Whishaw, I. Q. (1982). Spatial mapping: definitive disruption by hippocampal or medial frontal cortex damage in the rat. *Neuroscience Letters, 31*, 271–276.

Commentary 2

Commentary on the Protective Effects of Preoperative Experience

Eliot Stellar
Department of Anatomy and Institute of Neurological Sciences
University of Pennsylvania

This book is based on the very interesting idea that preoperative experience may protect brain-damaged animals against deficits that would normally occur after brain lesions and that the same may be true for brain-injured humans. In some ways, it is the opposite side of the coin from recovery of function after brain injury, since the preoperative experience eliminates, reduces, or gets around the deficits before they occur rather than after they occur. In this light, much is to be gained by analyzing the various kinds of preoperative protective effects along the same lines as we classically have analyzed postoperative recovery effects.

At one extreme, there may be various kinds of anatomical and neurochemical synaptic changes that broaden and deepen the brain mechanism underlying the behavior, in one case before injury, and in the other, after. At the other extreme, is the animal's ability to learn to solve a problem presented by brain injury, either by developing a coping strategy before injury (devised by the experimenter) or after injury (demanded by the need to adapt to the deficit). In the latter case, the solution to the problem may involve a different pathway in the brain than that subserving the original function, such that one kind of test reveals the deficit and another kind of test reveals brisk, normal function.

An example from a thesis by Evan Snyder, in the laboratories of W. W. Chambers and C. N. Liu (personal communication) at the University of Pennsylvania Medical School will illustrate the point. He cut one pyramidal tract of rhesus monkeys at the level of the rostral medulla, above the decussation (Fig. 1), and the animals developed a number of marked motor deficits on the opposite side. Among these deficits was the failure to give a placing response of the hind leg when the animals were held with legs suspended and the hairs of the

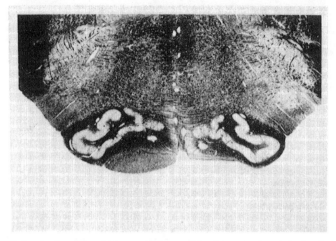

FIG. 1.   Lesion of the right pryamidal tract of the rhesus monkey at the level of
the inferior olive in the rostral medulla, above the level of the decussation.

dorsum of the hind foot were touched by the edge of a table. These monkeys,
however, had been trained preoperatively, while sitting in a chair, with the
sight of their legs occluded, to place their hind legs on a board when the hairs on
the dorsum of the foot were touched, as an instrumental response to obtain food.
Following the pyramidal tract lesion, this instrumental response remained intact
as long as the animals were tested in the food-getting instrumental situation. But
the placing response to touch of the same hairs in the reflex-testing situation
continued to be absent, even though the monkeys were tested repeatedly over a
period of 2 years postoperatively. To the eye of the observer, the two responses
appeared identical, yet one survived pyramidal lesion (the instrumental placing
response) and the other did not (the reflex placing response).

This volume is filled with many fascinating experiments to test the hypothesis that preoperative experience protects against the effects of brain lesions. In
most instances, evidence is brought forward to show that some aspect of preoperative experience, in some way, attenuates the effects of brain injury. In a
few cases, no preoperative experience effect was found: after telencephalic lesions in teleost fish, after very extensive hippocampal lesions. In some interhemispheric transfer of training paradigms, initial overtraining seemed to
inhibit transfer to the second side after corpus callosum section rather than
facilitate transfer.

In the main, however, positive results are reported. In some instances the
animal learned something preoperatively that stood it in good stead when faced
by the postoperative deficit. For example, lesions of the thalamic taste pathway,
that prevent salt-depleted, naïve rats from drinking selectively from a tube with

salt solution rather than a water tube, did not have this effect on rats that had been trained preoperatively to drink salt from a tube in a very distinctive location in the home cage. Even though they had lost their ability to taste, they went right to the familiar salt tube when salt-needy, quite unlike naïve taste-blind rats.

In other cases, the preoperative experience was not something the animal learned, but rather a treatment effect that obviated the postoperative symptom. For example, following bilateral lateral hypothalamic lesions, rats refuse to eat until they reduce their body weight to some low level; then after a few days to a few weeks, depending on the size of the lesion, they begin to eat, but they maintain a subnormal body weight postoperatively. If rats are starved down to this low body weight preoperatively, then they never go through the period of starvation, but rather begin to eat immediately after lateral hypothalamic lesions. It is as though a body weight set point is lowered by the lesion and all the preoperative experience has to do is reach that lower set point by starvation.

In still other cases, there is evidence to suggest that the preoperative training protected against the brain lesion by changes in the neural mechanism involved. In one ingenious study reported here by Grijalva, it was found that preoperative treatment with intraperitoneal alpha-methyl-para-tyrosine (AMT) reduced levels of dopamine (DA) and norepinephrine (NE) in the nigrostriatal pathway, producing a supersensitivity in the lateral hypothalamic system that attenuated the effects of lateral hypothalamic lesions. Interestingly enough, the same supersensitivity can be produced postoperatively to attenuate lateral hypothalamic symptoms.

Except for such inferences about anatomical and neurochemical changes in the neurons involved in the brain mechanisms controlling behavior, there is little direct information to say how preoperative experience produces its protective effects. We are not yet at that state of the art. But the chapters here have begun the process of localizing the brain mechanisms involved: to the striate cortex, the hippocampus, the amygdala, the nigrostriatal pathway, for example. And there is evidence, in studies from Merzenich's laboratory (Clark, Allard, Jenkins, & Merzenich, 1988) of how rapidly changes in synaptic connections can take place in a structure as complex as the primate cortex, as a function of specific tactile experience or altered peripheral input. The next step is to identify the strongest instances of the protective effects of preoperative experience and to explore the synaptic changes involved (cf. Greenough, 1975). Such a line of investigation should be productive of ideas of how postoperative recovery might come about, what changes take place at the synaptic level, and how treatments might be devised to facilitate those synaptic changes and thus facilitate recovery from brain injury. Since one of the chapters in this volume makes it clear that brain-injured people are also protected by their preoperative capacities and experience, it is not unreasonable to hope that the work reported here would eventually contribute to practical as well as theoretical endpoints.

REFERENCES

Clark, S. A., Allard, T., Jenkins, W. M., & Merzenich, M. M. (1988). Receptive fields in the body-surface map in adult cortex defined by temporally correlated inputs. *Nature, 332,* 444–445.

Greenough, W. T. (1975). Experimental modification of the developing brain. *American Scientist, 63,* 37–46.

Commentary 3

A Commentary as a Suggestion

Jay Schulkin
Department of Anatomy and Institute of Neurological Sciences
University of Pennsylvania

Two brain regions may be critically involved in many of the protective effects. The first is the amygdala, the second is the extrapryamidal motor region of the basal ganglia. Consider the amygdala first.

The amygdala is known to play a role in regulatory behaviors (e.g., Fonberg, 1974; Schulkin, Marini, & Epstein, in press; chap. 7 in this volume). The major taste-visceral pathway to the forebrain terminates in the central nucleus of the amygdala (Norgren, 1984). In fact, the amygdala has been viewed not only as playing a role in basic motivated regulatory behavior, but also as playing a role in the recognition of positive rewards in learning and memory (Mishkin & Appenzeller, 1987). The experience of hunger and thirst, the recognition of gustatory sources and other sensory information relevant to behavior, memory for the location of rewards and their anticipation, and the beneficial effects of enriched experience (e.g., first seven chapters) all seem to be part of normal amygdala function. Therefore, I suggest that the protective effects on regulatory behavior may be due to amygdala function. The fact that there appear to be little or no preoperative protection following amygdala damage supports this hypothesis (Fonberg, 1974; chaps. 2, 5, and 7).

The extrapyramidal regions of the basal ganglia have been thought to mediate simple motor habits (Mishkin & Appenzeller, 1987) or memories (Squire, 1987). Simple preoperatively learned discriminations and motor habits are spared postoperatively (chaps. 8, 11, and 13; Squire, Cohen, & Zouzounis, 1984). The fact that the protective effects on discrimination learning and learned motor patterns are limited and confined to what was learned preoperatively, (e.g., Held, Gordon, & Gentile, 1985), suggests that the extrapyramidal system may be importantly involved in the protective effects on maze learning, motor coordination, and overtrained discriminations that are habitually performed. The limitations of these protective effects to what was learned preoperatively, and the fact that the experience does not generalize to new postoperative tasks, lend credence to the view that this brain region may be involved in protecting preoperatively learned habits and discriminations.

Importantly, there are parallel examples in humans. The evidence in humans also suggests that simple motor habits or memories are often left intact following brain trauma (Squire et al., 1984). This is a preoperative effect. Moreover, preoperative intelligence is a factor with regard to the effects of the brain damage on behavior (chap. 14). The same holds for rats with cortical damage (Lansdell, 1959). Other evidence in humans suggests that the preoperative psychological state of the person affects postoperative recovery following brain damage (e.g., Johnston & Carpenter, 1980; chap. 6). Similar observations have been put forward for experimental animal subjects (Balagura, Harrell, & deCastro, 1978). However, despite extensive preoperative practice and overtraining of language use, there appears to be little or no protective effects on language use with damage to specific regions of the human brain (Geschwind, 1974; chap. 14). Similarly for experimental animal subjects, the greater the dependence of a function on a brain region the less liklihood of any protection if the area is damaged (chaps. 8 and 9).

Finally, while the major focus of this book was Behavioral Neuroscience, documenting protective effects on behavior as a result of preoperative experiences, it is equally important that future research continue to study the effects of experience on brain function, morphology, and physiology (e.g., Greenough, 1975; Rosenzweig, 1984). After all, I do believe that the preoperative experiences that this book is testimony to produce critical brain changes (morphological, synaptic organization, neural connectivity, etc.) that provide for the physical basis of the protection.

REFERENCES

Balagura, S., Harrell, L. E., & DeCastro, J. M. (1978). Organismic states and their effect on recovery from neurosurgery: A new perspective with implications for a general theory. *Brain Behavior Evolution, 15,* 19–40.

Fonberg, E. (1974). Amygdala functions within the alimentary system. *Acta Neurobiology Experimentalis, 34,* 435–466.

Geschwind, N. (1974). Late changes in the nervous system: An overview. In Stein, D. J., Rosen, J. F., & Butters, N. (Eds.), *Plasticity and recovery of function in the central nervous system.* New York: Academic Press.

Greenough, W. T. (1975). Experiential modification of the developing brain. *American Scientist,* *63,* 37–46.

Held, J. M., Gordon, J., & Gentile, A. M. (1985). Environmental influences on locomotor recovery following cortical lesions in rats. *Behavioral Neuroscience, 99,* 678–690.

Johnston, M., & Carpenter, L. (1980). Relationship between preoperative anxiety and post-operative state. *Psychological Medicine, 10,* 361–367.

Lansdell, H. C. (1959). Effect of brain damage on intelligence in rats. *Journal of Comparative Physiological Psychology,* 461–464.

Mishkin, M. (1954). Visual discrimination performance following partial ablations of the temporal lobe, 11. Ventral surface vs. hippocampus. *Journal of Comparative and Physiological Psychology, 47,* 187–193.

Mishkin, M., & Appenzeller, P. (1987). The anatomy of memory. *Scientific American,* May, 80–89.

Norgren, R. (1984). Central neural mechanisms of taste. *Handbook of Physiology Sec. 1, The Nervous System. Vol. 3, Sensory Processes.* American Physiological Society, Washington, DC: pp. 1087–1128.

Rosenzweig, M. R. (1984). Experience, memory and the brain. *American Psychologist, 39,* 365–376.

Schulkin, J., Marini, J., & Epstein, A. N. (1989). A role for the medial region of the amygdala in mineralocorticoid induced salt hunger. *Behavioral Neuroscience 103,* 178–185.

Squire, L. R., Cohen, N., & Zouzounis, J. A. (1984). Preserved memory in retrograde amnesia: Sparing of a recently acquired skill. *Neuropsychologia, 22,* 145–152.

Squire, L. R. (1987). *Memory and brain.* New York: Oxford Press.

Author Index

321

Subject Index

A

Abdominal vagotomy, and hyperphagia and
  obesity, in VMH syndrome, 73–74
Ablation(s)
  neocortical
    and memory-related disorders, 233–250,
      see also Amnestic sensory agnosia
    and recovery from lateral hypothalamic
      damage, 47–48
    telencephalon, in teleost fish, 191–208, see
      also Telencephalon ablated teleost fish
    visual capacity following, see Striate/-
      extrastriate lesion deficit analysis
Accumbens, medial, predatory behavior and,
  140, 143
Active avoidance test, VMH lesions and, 75–
  77
Adipsia, in lateral hypothalamic syndrome,
  36, see also Lateral hypothalamic
  syndrome
Affective behavior, see also Personality
  and amygdaloid damage, 104
  in VMH syndrome, 66, 74–77, see also
    Ventromedial hypothalamic syndrome
Age-experience interactions, 98–99
Age-related sparing, amygdaloid damage and,
  96–98
Aggressive behavior, see also Predatory
  behavior

amygdaloid damage and, 104–105
Agnosia, 233–250, see also Amnestic sensory
  agnosia
Aldosterone, and salt hunger, 29–30
Alimentary experiences, see also Ingestive
  behavior
  preoperative, effects on regulatory neuro-
    behavioral system of, 21–31, see also
    Salt hunger
Alpha-methyl-para-tyrosine, and recovery from
  lateral hypothalamic damage, 44
Alzheimer's disease, premorbid effects in, 294–
  295
Amnesia, anterograde, 175
Amnestic sensory agnosia, 233–250
  experiences between sequential lesions and,
    247–248
  historical observations of, 233–238
    latent preoperative memory retrieval and,
      236–238
    theoretical considerations of, 235–236
    ubiquity in, 234–235
  preoperative overtraining effects on, 238–
    244
    gustatory neocortex and, 243–244
    intrinsic neocortex and, 244
    massive visual neocortex ablations and,
      239–241
    partial visual neocortex ablations and,
      241–242